Echocardiography: Techniques and Interpretation

Echocardiography: Techniques and Interpretation

SONIA CHANG
Allied Health Professional,
Riverside Hospital, Toledo, Ohio;
Consultant in Echocardiography

with the assistance of:

JOHN K. CHANG
Director, Echocardiography Laboratory,
Riverside Hospital, Toledo, Ohio

2nd Edition

LEA & FEBIGER *Philadelphia* *1981*

Lea & Febiger
600 Washington Square
Philadelphia, PA   19106
U.S.A.

Library of Congress Cataloging in Publication Data

Chang, Sonia.
  Echocardiography, techniques and interpretation.

  Rev. ed. of: M-mode echocardiographic techniques
and pattern recognition.
  Bibliography: p.
  Includes index.
  1. Ultrasonic cardiography. I. Chang, John K.
(John Kai) II. Title. [DNLM: 1. Echocardiography.
WG 141.5,E2 C456m]
RC683.5.U5C48   1981   616.1′207543   81-2200
ISBN 0-8121-0784-5   AACR2

PRINTED IN THE UNITED STATES OF AMERICA

Print No.   4   3   2   1

To our children,
Gina
Lilah
Michael

Foreword

It is with great pleasure that I write the foreword of this book. It gives me the chance to recognize publicly the talent of Sonia and John Chang.

Sonia Chang was one of the obstetricians who assisted in the delivery of echocardiography. She worked with the master of echocardiography, Harvey Feigenbaum, at the University of Indiana. I first learned of her meticulous work through mutual friends, but later observed the records she produced. I became convinced that she was a superb technician who was making a great contribution to a fledgling new discipline.

I then discovered her ability to teach. She taught hundreds of physicians the importance of "getting the picture right." She also taught many cardiology fellows and technicians. There are few great teachers and Sonia is one of them.

Because of her technical ability and her ability to teach, I urged her to join the Department of Medicine at Emory University School of Medicine at a time we were beginning to develop echocardiography. She did so and remained with us from August 1975 to August 1976. Emory University School of Medicine has always been an exciting place to work. It is old enough to be stable and young enough to be flexible. This is why I was able to move Sonia from the status of Research Associate to Assistant Professor of Medicine. The Department of Medicine at Emory has about 130 full-time faculty members. Ninety-five percent of these are physicians. Five percent of them have their doctorates in other fields such as biochemistry. A few are recognized because of their unique ability to do things that others cannot do. Sonia was warmly received in the latter category. This enabled her to influence a larger audience than she could otherwise reach.

After her arrival at Emory, I discovered the depth of her intellect. She knew cardiac anatomy and physiology. She was eager to learn more about the problems of patients so that she could be more helpful in the electrocardiographic laboratory. Her husband, John, began to learn echocardiography at Emory and he became an expert in the environment we provided.

Sonia and John moved to the Medical College of Ohio in 1976. We at Emory are indebted to her for assisting us in developing echocardiography in our area.

My spies tell me that they sold their Atlanta home, but I have always been lucky; maybe she will return. In the meantime, we will profit from her written word.

J. Willis Hurst, M.D.
Chairman of the Department of Medicine
Emory University School of Medicine

Professor of Medicine (Cardiology)
Physician and Chief
Emory University Hospital and Clinic

Physician and Chief
Grady Memorial Hospital
Atlanta, Georgia

Preface

Echocardiography has grown up. In 1960, it was of some academic interest and of marginal clinical use. Now, 20 years later, it is an important diagnostic procedure in the management of heart disease. It has moved from the laboratory into the classroom to explain the physiology of normal and abnormal cardiac anatomy. An explosion of medical literature has explored echocardiography as a tool to evaluate acquired and congenital cardiovascular disease, to measure the effects of pharmacologic applications, and to assess the quality of myocardial function in health and disease.

The embryo of Echocardiography: Techniques and Interpretation began in 1968 as a collection of echocardiographic patterns of motion acquired through instruction of techniques and interpretation to visiting cardiologists and physicians in cardiology fellowship programs. Popular demand for copies of this collection precipitated its publication as M-Mode Echocardiographic Techniques and Pattern Recognition in 1976.

This completely revised and enlarged edition of Echocardiography: Techniques and Interpretation incorporates the newer techniques of two-dimensional echocardiography correlated with M-mode techniques for practical clinical cardiovascular evaluation. The text directs the reader toward important clinical findings, correct recording techniques, pitfalls, and interpretation of the echographic patterns of motion—all supported by invasive procedures: catheterization, operations, and necropsy. Illustrations and line drawings are fully labeled and are accompanied by legends requiring little reference to the text for explanation. Photographs of surgical or necropsy specimens complement echocardiographic and catheterization findings. Pediatric echocardiography is interwoven throughout the book. Following each chapter, an exhaustive bibliography provides easy access to the world's English-language literature, categorized by specific diseases or common echocardiographic observations.

Each chapter mirrors personal interests and laboratory experience with regional populations of patients. One-on-one technical and interpretative instruction now encompasses echocardiography laboratories nationally and internationally, providing new insights and knowledge concerning examination techniques, clinical application, and equipment expertise. The third edition has already begun.

Without the patients, this book would not exist. A thorough M-mode and two-dimensional echocardiogram takes a long time. While we sit beside the patients examining the mechanics of their hearts, we listen to them talk. They worry, about themselves, their families, and their futures. They want to feel better and to be productive citizens. It is for these patients that we again offer Echocardiography: Techniques and Interpretation to the medical community.

Toledo, Ohio   Sonia Chang

Acknowledgments

Two men contributed most to my career. Interest, involvement, and an insatiable desire to contribute to the field of echocardiography was stimulated by Harvey Feigenbaum, M.D., Professor of Medicine, Indiana University Medical Center, Indianapolis, Indiana.

J. Willis Hurst, M.D., Professor and Chairman of the Department of Medicine of Emory University School of Medicine and Editor-in-Chief of The Heart, Arteries and Veins, was most influential in my quantum career leap from technologist to Assistant Professor of Emory University's medical faculty, providing an academic vehicle to express my work most effectively. Infrequent, but valued, communications with Dr. Hurst helped to nourish the incentive to complete this extensive revision of Echocardiography: Techniques and Interpretation. The zeal to finish wavered many times as other areas of my life demanded "equal time."

I wish to thank Erie Chapman, III, President of Riverside Hospital, and Harold Crary, Director of Professional Services, Riverside Hospital, Toledo, Ohio, for their support of diagnostic and investigative efforts. Through the generosity, enthusiasm, and encouragement of Riverside Hospital's administration and medical staff, my husband, John Chang, and I have been able to establish a modern, high-quality diagnostic echocardiographic laboratory in this progressive and innovative community hospital.

I am indebted to the physicians of Riverside Hospital, Toledo, Ohio; Medical College of Ohio, Toledo, Ohio; and Emory University Hospital and Clinic, Atlanta, Georgia. Their patients were a rich source for these few echocardiograms representing a spectrum of cardiovascular anatomy, physiology, and dysfunction.

An echocardiogram should be beautiful as well as diagnostic. It was our good fortune to find illustrators who shared our passion to "get the picture right." For the past four years, talented photographic and artistic work flowed from the cameras, developing trays, and drawing boards of Carol Perkins, Jerry Lubinski, Tony Flawinski, Josephine Cole, and

Edward Joseph of the Audiovisual Department, Medical College of Ohio, Toledo, Ohio.

M-Mode Echocardiographic Techniques and Pattern Recognition was translated into Italian and Spanish in 1978. These beautiful and competent translations were the work of Tommaso Morlino, M.D., Edizione Italiana a cura del, and Professor Mario Vincenzi, Piccin Editore, Padova, Italy; and Mario A. Marino, M.D., Editorial Medica, Panamericana, Buenos Aires, Argentina.

Guidance, constructive criticism, and extended deadlines were gratefully accepted from R. Kenneth Bussy, Executive Editor, and the staff of Lea & Febiger in Philadelphia, Pennsylvania.

Finally, my appreciation is extended to Mary Clifford, M.D., for new beginnings, and to members of the medical community throughout the world who find Echocardiography: Techniques and Interpretation to be a useful source book in their laboratories, classrooms, and libraries.

Contents

1

Basics

A diagnostic echocardiogram must accurately reflect a patient's cardiac anatomy and ability to pump blood. To record and to interpret the echocardiogram correctly, the physician and the nonphysician echocardiographer must be knowledgeable about some of the physical principles of ultrasound and their interaction with soft tissue and fluids.

The techniques necessary to produce an echocardiogram of diagnostic quality are the core of this monograph. The basic techniques for M-mode and two-dimensional echocardiographic examination are adaptable to most commercially available echographic equipment.

PRINCIPLES

Source of Ultrasound

An echocardiographic examination begins by placing a transducer along the patient's parasternal border. The choice of an appropriate transducer depends upon the size of the patient and the intrathoracic depth of the cardiac structures under investigation.

A transducer's sound source or *active element* is usually a circular lead zirconate titanate crystal ranging from 6 to 13 mm in diameter. Following a two-microsecond application of alternating electric current from the echograph, the active element expands and contracts, initiating mechanical vibrations. These mechanical vibrations are transmitted as periodic oscillations or sine waves through a coupling gel into the body tissue. These oscillations will be referred to as *sound waves*.

Echoes are reflected sound waves returning to the transducer during a quiet period when no sound waves are being transmitted. Echoes impinging upon the active element cause it to change shape again. An electric current is processed through a receiver and signal amplifier for display on an oscilloscope. Crystalline deformation, secondary to electrical current or mechanical vibrations, is known as the *piezoelectric effect*. The piezoelectric effect is convenient because it allows the same active element to function as a receiver as well as a sound source. The shape, size, and thickness of the active element determines how rapidly it can change shape. The more rapidly the active element can change shape, the higher its frequency.

Cycles, Wavelengths, and Pulses

Following application of electrical voltage from the echograph, a four-cycle pulse of ultrasound (Fig. 1–1) is transmitted into the elastic tissue of the chest. The sound waves are transmitted through the tissue in a series of molecular disturbances called *compressions and rarefactions* (Fig. 1–2). The distance between the beginning of one molecular compression to the beginning of the next molecular compression is one *pressure cycle* or one *wavelength.*

The *frequency* of an active element is equal to the number of pressure cycles directed past a fixed observation point in a known amount of time. For example, if the transducer could send one cycle (1 molecular compression + 1 molecular rarefaction) past a fixed observation point in one second, this transducer would have a frequency of one cycle per second or one *hertz (Hz).* Echocardiography uses transducers capable of sending millions of cycles per second or *megahertz (MHz).* Ultrasound is inaudible, since it is far above the audible range of 20,000 cycles/sec.

At normal body temperature, a sound wave travels through soft tissue at approximately 1540 m/sec. This velocity is constant, regardless of the number of sound waves being

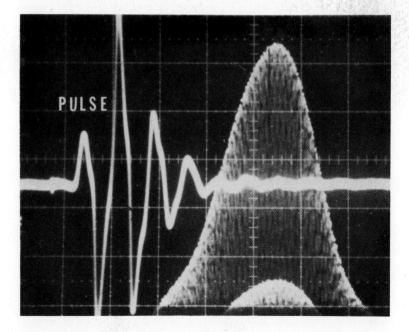

Fig. 1–1. In this photograph of a reflected pulse, the pulse is superimposed over a 2.25 MHz transducer's frequency spectrum showing the transducer's maximum sensitivity at varying distances from the sound source. (Photograph courtesy of KB-Aerotech, Krautkramer-Branson, Inc., Lewistown, Pennsylvania.)

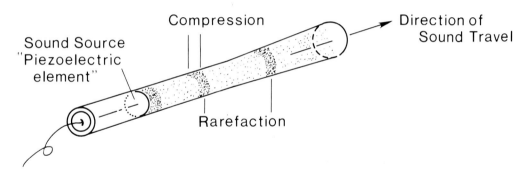

Fig. 1–2. This diagram shows molecular *compression* (increased molecular density) and *rarefaction* (decreased molecular density) as an ultrasonic pulse is transferred through soft tissue at the rate of 1540 m/sec. The distance between the onset of one compression to the beginning of the next compression is equal to one wavelength or cycle. In terms of frequency, one cycle per second is equal to one hertz.

transmitted. The length of a cycle (wavelength) can be estimated from the following formula if the frequency of the transducer is known:

$$\text{Wavelength (mm)} = \frac{\text{velocity of sound through soft tissue}}{\text{frequency of transducer}} = \frac{1.5}{f}$$

Table 1–1 shows the estimated wavelength of six transducers used for echocardiographic examination.

A *pulse* is composed of two to five cycles, but most of the newer transducers emit pulses having four cycles. From Table 1–1, notice that a high-frequency transducer has a shorter pulse length than have transducers with lower frequencies. With short pulses, one is more likely to record separate echoes from structures positioned closely together *(resolution)*. However, short cycles cannot travel far before their energy dissi-

Table 1–1.
Estimated Cycle Length and Pulse Length of Six Echocardiographic Transducers

Transducer frequency (MHz)	Cycle length (mm)	Pulse length (mm)
1.6	0.937	3.74
1.9	0.789	3.16
2.25	0.666	2.66
3.5	0.428	1.71
5.0	0.300	1.20
7.0	0.214	0.85

MHz, megahertz; pulse length = four cycles

pates into the tissue as heat or becomes scattered by particulate matter within the cardiac muscle. This energy loss is called *attenuation*. Thus, high-frequency transducers, emitting short cycles, are suitable for examination of neonates and infants whose cardiac structures are less than eight centimeters from the transducers. They are inadequate for examination of adolescent or adult patients whose cardiac tissue is more distant from the active element.

REMEMBER

*High-frequency transducers = more cycles/sec =
shorter cycles = less penetration*

*Low-frequency transducers = fewer cycles/sec =
longer cycles = more penetration*

Echograph System

The transducer is attached to the echograph, which contains a timer and a transmitter to supply intermittent external energy to the piezoelectric crystal. Electrical currents are generated and processed through a receiver and amplifier for display as moving patterns on monitoring oscilloscopes (cathode ray tubes). Interfacing this system with a recorder provides a means to capture these motion patterns on light-sensitive paper for analysis.

The intrathoracic depth of cardiac tissue, with respect to the transducer, is electronically calculated and displayed as depth markers on the recording paper (Fig. 1–3). The distance between two markers is equal to one centimeter of tissue depth, regardless of the markers' physical distance from each other on the oscilloscope or paper.

Beam Width

Following each electrical excitation of the active element, a column of ultrasound is transmitted into the body's tissue. Up to now, the discussion was limited to a single sound wave. The diameter of this column or *sound beam* is equal to the diameter of the active element. The sound beam remains collimated for several centimeters. The length of this collimation or *near field* depends upon the active element's wavelength and diameter (Table 1–2). The depth of most echocardiographic tissue examinations exceeds the length of the near field (Fig. 1–4). Fortunately, nonfocused transducers can be used to examine tissue nearly twice the depth of the near field before resolution and *acoustic sensitivity* deteriorate. Under test conditions, acoustic sensitivity is loosely defined as a transducer's ability to detect a 6-mm steel rod in a water bath at definite distances from the active element. Many

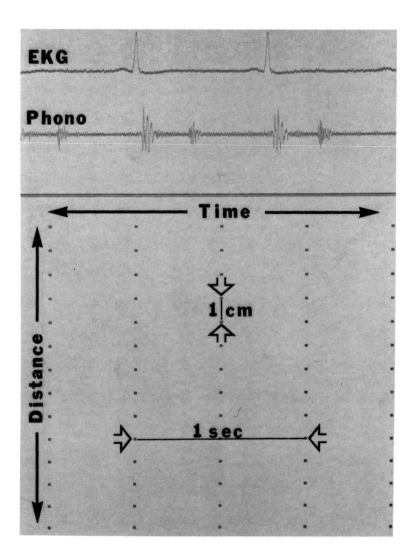

Fig. 1–3. Electronically calculated tissue depth markers. The distance between two markers is equal to 1 cm tissue depth. The duration of echographic events and paper recording speed could be measured from 0.5-second time intervals.

Table 1–2.
Estimated Length of Near Field for Five Nonfocused Transducers

Transducer frequency (MHz)	Diameter of active element (mm)	Wavelength (mm)	Length of near field (mm)
1.9	19	0.789	114
2.25	6	0.666	14
2.25	13	0.666	63
3.5	6	0.428	21
5.0	6	0.300	30

$$\text{Length of near field} = \frac{D^2}{(4)\,(\text{wavelength})}$$

D = diameter of piezoelectric crystal

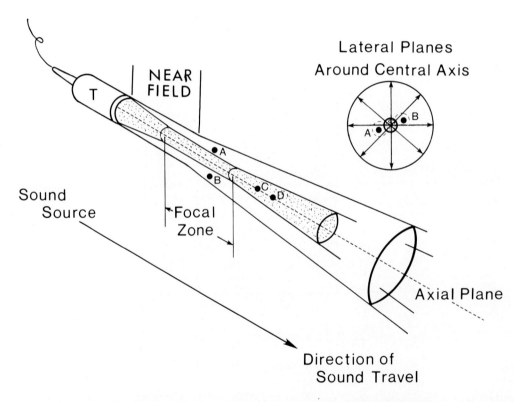

Fig. 1–4. Diagram showing the beam widths diverging beyond the *near field*. The divergent area is called the *far field*. Targets C and D are positioned serially within the sound beam's central axis. These targets return separate echoes to the transducer if the pulse length does not exceed the distance between targets. Targets A and B are positioned peripherally in relation to the sound beam's central axis. A wide beam width (unshaded) senses two targets, but their relative positions cannot be determined by an observer. The beam width can be decreased or focused by the application of curved lenses placed in front of piezoelectric crystal to bend emitted sound waves inward (shaded beam). The focused beam width must be less than the distance between targets A and B to obtain information about them individually.

factors affect a transducer's sensitivity, including the echographic system to which it is attached. The interested reader is referred to the bibliography following this chapter.

Beam pattern diagrams and amplitude curves of four transducers are shown in Figures 1–5 to 1–8. An amplitude curve shows the transducer's acoustic sensitivity at various distances from the active element, measured in decibels. A decibel is a mathematic unit to express the intensity of one sound as compared to another. Manufacturers of transducers use the following equation to express sound intensity:

$$dB = 20 \log (A_1/A_2)$$

dB = decibel
A = reflected sound intensity

As seen in Figures 1–5 to 1–8, a transducer's maximum sensitivity coincides with the sound beam's minimum diameter. Tissue examinations in these areas provide the best definition of a reflector's location and thickness.

Axial Resolution

Part of the diagnostic quality of an echocardiogram depends upon how well the echographic system can *resolve* (identify separately) two structures that are close together but are

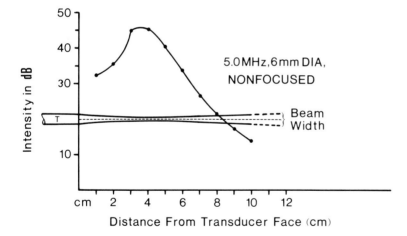

Fig. 1–5. Beam pattern diagram for a nonfocused 5.0 MHz transducer, showing the minimum beam width 4 cm from the transducer. Each point on the superimposed amplitude curve represents the maximum acoustic sensitivity of that portion of the beam. The curve as a whole depicts the sensitivity distribution across the sound beam at known distances from the transducer, as measured in decibels (dB). dB = 20 log (A₁/A₂) (Courtesy of John Nanasi, KB-Aerotech, Krautkramer-Branson, Inc., Lewistown, Pennsylvania.)

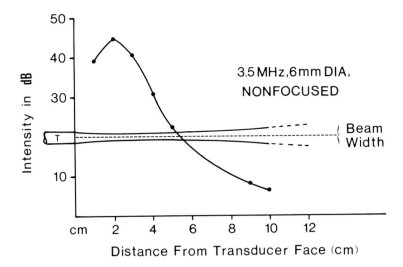

Fig. 1–6. Beam pattern diagram for a nonfocused 3.5 MHz transducer, showing the minimum beam width 2 to 3 cm from the transducer and maximum acoustic sensitivity 2 cm from the transducer. At 5 cm, acoustic sensitivity is equal to or exceeds half the maximum acoustic sensitivity. Thereafter, sensitivity deteriorates rapidly. (Courtesy of John Nanasi, KB-Aerotech, Krautkramer-Branson, Inc., Lewistown, Pennsylvania.)

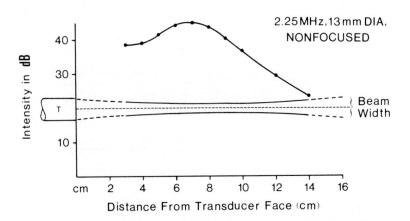

Fig. 1–7. Beam pattern diagram for a nonfocused 2.25 MHz general-purpose transducer, showing the minimum beam width 7 to 10 cm from the transducer. The maximum acoustic sensitivity occurs 7 cm from the transducer. All points on the amplitude curve equal or exceed half the maximum amplitude to a depth of 14 cm. (Courtesy of John Nanasi, KB-Aerotech, Krautkramer-Branson, Inc., Lewistown, Pennsylvania.)

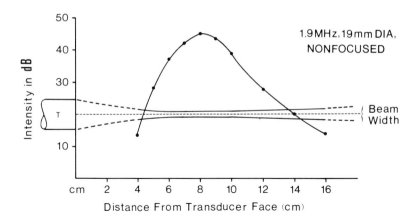

Fig. 1–8. Beam pattern diagram for a nonfocused 1.9 MHz transducer, showing the minimum beam width 6 to 10 cm from the transducer. The maximum acoustic amplitude is 8 cm from the transducer. All points on the amplitude curve equal or exceed half the maximum amplitude to depth of 16 cm. Resolution of echoes is poor in the area near the transducer and at depths exceeding 16 cm. (Courtesy of John Nanasi, KB-Aerotech, Krautkramer-Branson, Inc., Lewistown, Pennsylvania.)

positioned at different depths along the central axis, with respect to the sound beam's direction of travel (Fig. 1–4, targets C and D). Layers of tissue will reflect separate echoes *if* the length of the pulse does not exceed the distance between the targets. At the present time, commercially available echographs have an axial resolution of between 1.0 and 1.5 mm.

Lateral Resolution

We often refer to "ice-pick" views in which we envision sound waves being transmitted along a narrow pathway to the tissue of interest. This is an erroneous concept. A sound beam has circumferential size with a diameter equal to or greater than the diameter of the active element. It is able to reflect sound waves from tissue located peripherally around the beam's central axis (Fig. 1–4, targets A and B). When the echoes are displayed on the oscilloscope or paper, the echocardiographer does not know how the reflecting tissues were positioned with respect to each other or to the transducer. They could be side by side or offset.

The lateral resolution of most echographs is many times worse than their axial resolution. Lateral resolution can be improved by using focused transducers. By placing a curved lens between the active element and its protective epoxy faceplate, the sound beam can be narrowed within and beyond the near field, thereby decreasing the quantity of beam divergence in the far field. More ultrasonic energy is concentrated over a smaller tissue area. To identify off-axis targets individually, the beam width must be narrow enough to pass between two entities without intercepting either one. Each target may then be identified separately by directing the sound beam toward its location. The disadvantage of a focused transducer is its loss of sensitivity at both ends of the sound beam. Our preference is for a family of high- and low-frequency nonfocused transducers, reserving high-frequency focused transducers for the examination of premature infants.

Absorption

A sound wave has a perilous journey once it leaves the transducer; it loses energy at the rate of 1 dB/Cm/MHz as the sound travels through tissue of different densities. Some of the energy is dissipated (absorbed) as heat into the tissue by mechanisms not fully understood.

Deflection and Refraction

As long as the sound wave travels through tissue of a homogeneous density, little refraction (bending) or *deflection* (altered direction of travel) takes place. Sound waves travel through homogeneous blood at approximately 1500 m/sec. When the sound waves intercept tissue of a different density, such as a ventricular wall, there is an acoustic mismatch between blood and tissue that creates a boundary or *interface*

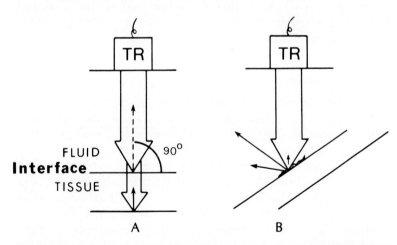

Fig. 1–9. *A,* The angle of incidence equals 90° when a sound wave's direction of travel intercepts a reflector's maximum plane of motion. Some sound waves are reflected back to the transducer (TR), while others enter a new medium across the fluid-tissue boundary or *interface.* Energy loss occurs in the form of heat dissipation into tissue *(absorption). B,* Curved and irregular or roughened cardiac structures change the sound wave's direction of travel away from the original line of incidence *(deflection).*

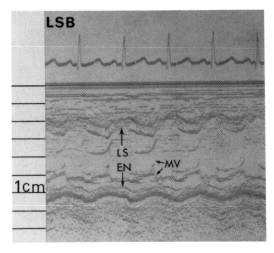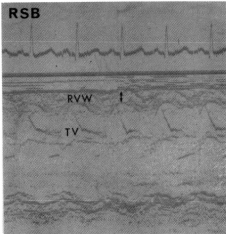

Fig. 1–10. *A*(LSB), The transducer was positioned along the left parasternum, directing the sound beam inferiorly and laterally to obtain septal and posterior left ventricular wall motion. Insignificant reflections from the area of the right ventricular wall suggest that the line of incidence was too oblique and caused too many echoes to be deflected from the area, or that the right ventricular wall was absent. *B* (RSB), The transducer was repositioned along the right parasternum, directing the sound beam medially toward the tricuspid valve (TV). The sound waves were perpendicular to the right ventricular wall (RVW), reflecting more sound waves back to the transducer. This pediatric patient had a pressure gradient across the pulmonary valve of 20 mm Hg. LS, left septum-blood interface; EN, posterior left ventricular endocardium-blood interface; MV, mitral valve motion.

(Fig. 1–9). Some sound waves are reflected back toward the transducer, whereas others continue through the interface into the new tissue medium and lose some of their energy through absorption and scattering. A few low-intensity echoes are returned to the transducer from particulate matter within the muscle itself. These echoes assist in the identification of cardiac muscle.

Sound waves travel more rapidly through nonfluid tissue, averaging 1540 m/sec. Although there may be slight bending or refraction of the sound waves as they cross an interface, the quantity of refraction is probably insignificant in echocardiography.

Few reflecting surfaces in the heart are smooth. They are either curved, irregularly shaped, or roughened. Sound waves striking oblique or roughened surfaces are deflected away from their direction of travel (Fig. 1–9). If too many sound waves are deflected, some areas of the cardiac anatomy appear to be absent (Fig. 1–10).

Angles of Incidence

Much of the time allotted to an echocardiographic examination is consumed by the necessity to align the sound wave's

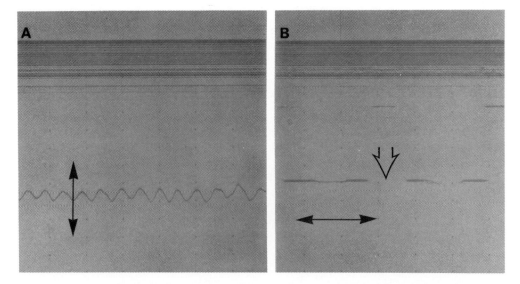

Fig. 1–11. *A,* Stationary transducer is positioned in coupling gel on the surface of the hand. The hand was moved up and down perpendicular to the sound beam (arrow). This paper recording shows the intact inscription of motion with the maximum amplitude of hand displacement. *B,* The hand changed to a sliding movement across face of the transducer (arrow). Since the distance of the hand surface did not change with respect to the transducer, no displacement movement was registered. When the hand did not intercept the sound beam, no reflections were received; this caused fragmentation of the tracing (open arrow).

direction of travel perpendicular to the maximum plane of movement by various cardiac structures. The angle of this alignment is called the *angle of incidence.*

This angle is equal to 90° if the sound wave's direction of travel is exactly perpendicular to the tissue's maximum plane of movement. When the angle of incidence is less than 90°, sound waves are deflected away from the tissue of interest, and reflections will not be received by the transducer. Moving structures appear to have less excursion—or no excursion, if the structure's plane of movement is parallel to the sound beam's direction of travel (Fig. 1–11). The validity of every echographic measurement depends upon the achieving of maximum structural motion. Anything less produces erroneous information concerning the quality of cardiac perfusion, contraction and compliance, chamber dimensions, and valvular velocities and excursions.

Coupling Gel

Because ultrasonic waves pass through air so slowly (about 330 m/sec), the echocardiographer must exclude air between the transducer and the patient's skin with the generous use of a coupling medium. Of the products that can be used, one should consider those most favorably that contain little dissolved air, do not stain clothing, are hypoallergenic, and will not melt at an elevated body temperature.

Reverberations

The trained echocardiographer habitually expands an echocardiographic tracing to exclude ultrasonic reverberations most frequently seen behind the left ventricle in an area anatomically occupied by the lung (Fig. 1–12). Reverberations result when reflected sound waves rebound from the transducer's faceplate and are retransmitted into the tissue. These sound waves are reflected a second time from the original interface or from another interface and are received on the second return trip to the transducer.

Reverberations cause most interpretation difficulties when one is considering the presence of pericardial thickening. I

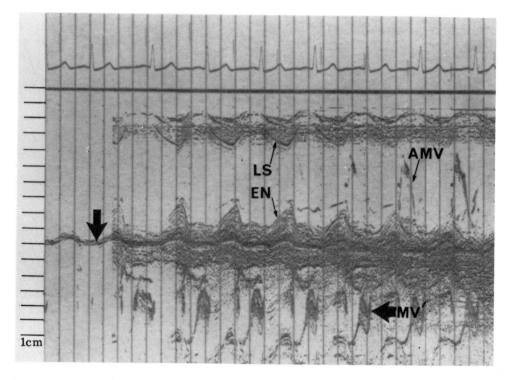

Fig. 1–12. Reverberations of mitral leaflet (MV') appearing in area anatomically occupied by lung. The leaflet appeared to be unusually echoreflective, consistent with tissue thickening. The patient had infective endocarditis three years prior to this echogram. These excessive reflections may have been caused by rough leaflet surfaces secondary to healed vegetations. (Unmarked bold arrow), Primary pericardial-lung interface. Echoes immediately behind the primary pericardium do not represent pericardial thickening. LS, left septal-blood interface; EN, posterior left ventricular endocardial-blood interface; AMV, anterior mitral leaflet motion. (From Feigenbaum, H.: Echocardiography. 3rd Ed. Philadelphia, Lea & Febiger, 1981.)

have found good surgical correlation of thickened pericardium with its echographic evidence by observing a simple rule: the primary pericardial echo must be positioned *behind* weaker, synchronously moving echoes (Fig. 1–12). Low-intensity echoes positioned behind the primary pericardial echo are ignored, as are echoes moving in areas that should be occupied by the lung.

INSTRUMENTATION

At the beginning of each echocardiographic examination, controls are preset on the instrument panel (Fig. 1–13). An arbitrary *depth* of 15 cm is selected for adults and of 8 to 10 cm for pediatric examinations. The depth may then be expanded or compressed, depending upon the patient's heart size, thoracic diameter, and the contrast quality of the echogram on the recording paper. The contrast deteriorates with too much depth expansion.

One should use moderate settings for *echo amplification (gain), damping, and reject.* For an adult examination, *depth compensation* begins 3 cm from the transducer and ends at 5

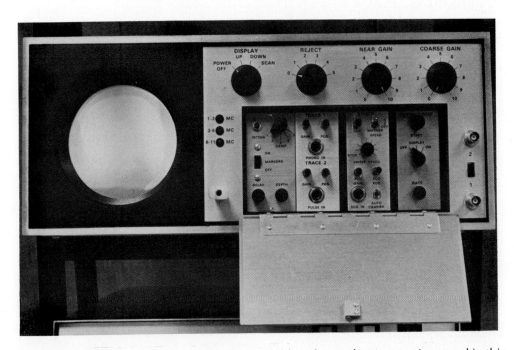

Fig. 1–13. Front panel of a commercially available echograph. Most tracings used in this monograph were *begun* at the following settings: Reject, 2; near gain, 4; coarse gain, 7; damping, 3; depth compensation began arbitrarily at 3.0 cm and ended at a depth of 5.0 cm. The minimum rate of compensation was equal to 1.0 cm and was used for neonatal examination. The rate of compensation could be increased as desired for examination of adults by turning control clockwise. (Courtesy of Smith-Kline Instruments, Inc., Sunnyvale, California.)

or 6 cm. The *rate of compensation* is set fully counterclockwise. Throughout the examination, damping is periodically increased to isolate the pericardial-lung interface. Near
gain and coarse gain are manipulated as necessary throughout
the entire examination to visualize all desired interfaces.

Reject

Reject eliminates low-intensity echoes from the echographic system (Fig. 1–14). A minimum of reject should be
applied to maintain maximum system sensitivity.

Depth Compensation

Low-intensity sound waves are reflected from tissue located
distantly from the transducer. For example, echoes reflected
from the vicinity of the posterior left ventricular wall lose
considerable energy because of absorption and deflection. By
the time these echoes return to the transducer, they have
much less amplitude than do those echoes reflected from
structures positioned closer to the transducer. Depth compensation amplifies the intensity of these distant reflections and
suppresses the intensity of echoes near the transducer.

Superimposition of a depth compensation curve on an
echocardiogram is shown schematically in Figure 1–15. The
beginning of depth compensation must be adjusted for each
patient. If it begins too near the transducer, controls for
increasing or decreasing amplification in this area become
ineffective. If it begins behind the left septal-blood interface

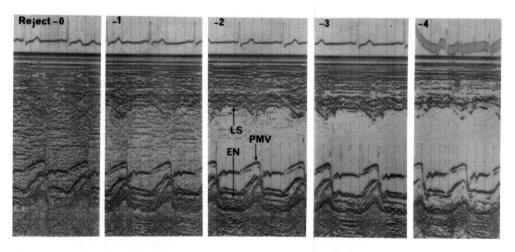

Fig. 1–14. Reject is used to eliminate low-intensity echoes from the echographic system.
0 and 1, Too little reject allows too many low-intensity echoes to obscure useful motion.
2 and 3, An appropriate reject level showing good separation between tissue and
blood-filled areas. 4, Too much reject decreased sensitivity and eliminated useful
information. LS, left septal-blood interface; EN, posterior left ventricular endocardial-
blood interface; PMV, posterior mitral leaflet motion.

or behind the mitral valve-blood interface, these structures
might not be seen at all without high, near-field amplification.
I prefer to begin depth compensation arbitrarily in front of the
presumed right septal-blood interface (Fig. 1–15, A to B).
When the septum is located, the near gain is turned off. The
beginning of depth compensation is moved into the right
septal-blood interface. The near gain is then increased mini-
mally to amplify echoes from the chest and the right ventricular wall.

In some cases, the left septal-blood interface is unclear in
patients with aortic insufficiency or anteroseptal infarction.
Then the rate of compensation is increased over a distance of 5
or 6 cm. If the right septal-blood interface is unclear, it would
be wise to move the beginning of depth compensation nearer
to the right ventricular wall and to increase the rate of
compensation to extend past the left septal-blood interface

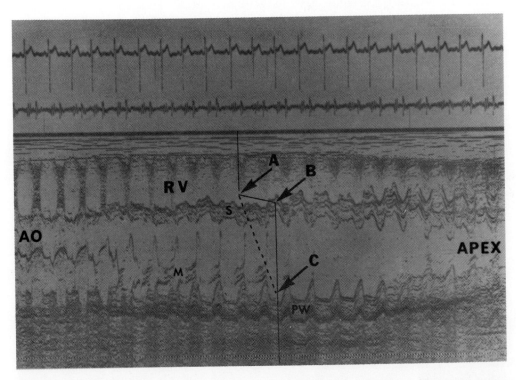

Fig. 1–15. A scan from the aorta toward the left ventricular apex. A to B, Depth
compensation began in the right ventricular cavity and ended in the vicinity of the right
septal-blood interface. A to C, The clockwise rotation of rate control increased the distance
over which depth compensation was effective. The beginning of compensation may need
to be moved closer to the right ventricular wall to avoid loss of septal echoes. An increased
rate of compensation is desirable in patients with asymmetrical septal hypertrophy, aortic
insufficiency, and septal myocardial infarction. AO, aorta; RV, right ventricle; S, interventricular septum; M, mitral valve motion; PW, posterior left ventricular wall.

(Fig. 1–15, A to C). This procedure prevents the accidental loss of important reflections from the septum.

Gain

Gain controls the amplification of received echoes. Gain has no effect upon the intensity of sound wave transmission nor does it select those echoes that are most useful for evaluation. It will not improve the quality of the echocardiogram if the transducer is incorrectly positioned with respect to the tissue of interest.

1. *Near gain.* When depth compensation is applied, near gain amplifies echoes between the transducer and the end of depth compensation (Fig. 1–15, B or C).

2. *Coarse gain.* With or without depth compensation, coarse gain or overall gain amplifies all echoes equally. Too much amplification diminishes *resolution,* the ability to visualize two reflectors in close proximity to each other. Too little amplification causes fragmentation of a structure's movement pattern, even though the transducer may be perpendicular to the tissue's maximum plane of movement (Fig. 1–16).

Depth and a Rule of Fourths

Depth must be adjusted for each patient. This control is used to display selected depths of tissue relative to the sound

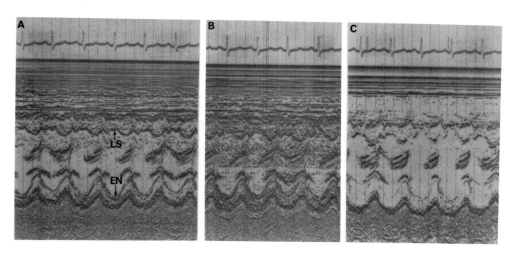

Fig. 1–16. Coarse gain amplifies sound waves received through piezoelectric crystal. *A,* The appearance of a left ventricular study when the amplification is correctly adjusted. The myocardial-blood interfaces are clearly defined with completely inscribed patterns of movement. The weaker reflections provide a texturing of the myocardium that helps to identify the cardiac muscle. *B,* Too much amplification reduces the resolution of closely related echoes. *C,* Too little amplification causes fragmentation of movement patterns, but does not affect the amplitude of the tissue motion. Coarse gain has no influence over the angle of incidence between the sound beam and the plane of tissue movement. LS, left septal-blood interface; EN, endocardial-blood interface.

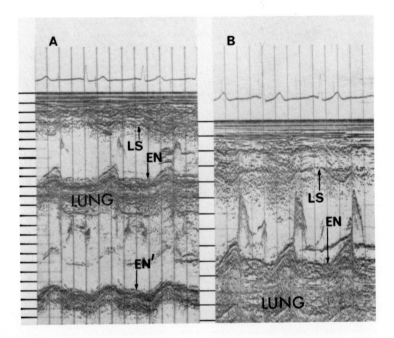

Fig. 1–17. A 44-year-old female patient with *Streptococcus viridans* two years prior to this echocardiogram, lupus erythematosus, and moderately severe mitral insufficiency. Depth control governs the quantity of tissue that is displayed on the oscilloscope or paper recording. *A,* Depth was too compressed, showing reverberations from the posterior wall in the area anatomically occupied by lung. *B,* Depth was expanded to eliminate visualization of reverberations and to observe "rule of fourths;" that is, the available paper width was divided so that the electrocardiogram could occupy the upper one-fourth of paper, the echocardiogram occupied the middle half of the paper, and the lower fourth was allotted to extracardiac anatomic and pathologic study behind the heart. LS, left septal-blood interface; EN, endocardium-blood interface. Unusual echo-reflective quality inscribed below the anterior mitral leaflet motion is consistent with roughened leaflet surfaces.

source. A parasternal examination of the adult heart requires visualization of 12- to 17-cm tissue depth. Subcostal examination requires a minimum of 15 cm and often requires a depth exceeding 20 cm. Less tissue depth is required when examining patients with small thoracic diameters. Depth expansion eliminates visualization of reverberations on the paper record or on the oscilloscope (Fig. 1–17).

It is my practice to follow a *rule of fourths*. The width of the recording paper is roughly divided into four segments. The upper fourth is for ancillary recordings—electrocardiogram and phonocardiogram. The middle half is occupied by the echocardiogram, and the lower fourth is reserved for extracardiac anatomic and pathologic abnormalities.

Damping

Damping, or pulse power, regulates the quantity of voltage delivered to the piezoelectric crystal. Little damping increases the intensity of the sound waves and allows deeper penetration into the tissue, but only at the expense of deteriorating resolution (Fig. 1–18). Too much damping reduces sound wave penetration. Resolution is good, but the ability to obtain echoes from distant tissue is diminished (Fig. 1–18). Moderate damping is sufficient for most transducers whose

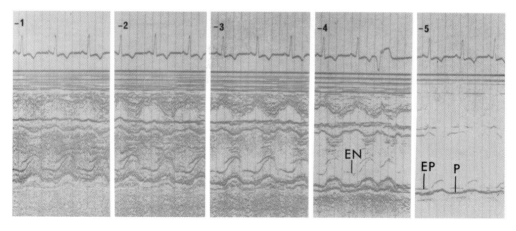

Fig. 1–18. A 68-year-old female patient with angina pectoris. Damping or attenuation has several functions. It controls the quantity of the voltage delivered to the piezoelectric crystal to initiate the pulse. After pulse initiation, damping absorbs leftover ultrasonic energy. 1 and 2, Minimum damping is used to drive the sound waves deeper into the tissue, but at the expense of resolution. 3, Moderate damping is sufficient for most echocardiographic studies. 4, Excessive damping results in decreased sensitivity in the area of the left ventricular endocardial-blood interface (EN). Increased amplification improves this tracing. 5, Maximum damping is most useful for intermittent isolation of the epicardial-pericardial-lung interfaces for identification of pericardial effusion and occult pericardial disease. LS, left septal-blood interface; P, primary pericardial-lung interface; EP, epicardial-pericardial fluid interface.

frequency is appropriate for the examination. Less damping will not change the active element's frequency, but it will serve to drive the available sound waves more deeply into the soft tissue.

REMEMBER

Too little damping = excessive ultrasonic energy = increased penetration = decreased resolution
Too much damping = insufficient ultrasonic energy = decreased penetration = decreased sensitivity

ANGLES AND SCANS

The mitral valve is a suitable reference point at which to begin an echographic examination, since it is located close to the center of the heart. Movement from surrounding cardiac structures is obtained by redirecting the transducer from the mitral valve toward other areas of the heart (Fig. 1–19). The pulmonary valve lies superiorly to the mitral valve in a plane

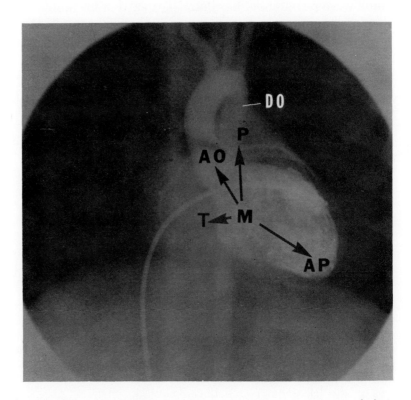

Fig. 1–19. Interrelationship of intracardiac structures and their directional scan planes from the mitral valve (M). AO, aorta; P, pulmonary artery; T, tricuspid valve area; AP, left ventricular apex; DO, descending aorta.

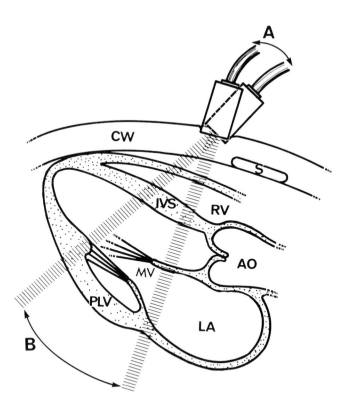

Fig. 1–20. Relationship between sound beam, septum, mitral valve, and posterior left ventricular wall during a scan (directional change of sound beam's position). The scan interrogated unequal quantities of septal and posterior wall tissue. Novice echocardiographers angle the transducer too much and bypass areas of tissue interest. CW, chest wall; IVS, interventricular septum; RV, right ventricle; MV, mitral valve; AO, aorta; PLV, posterior left ventricular wall; LA, left atrium.

with the left ear. The aortic valve lies in a sector between the throat and the right shoulder. The tricuspid valve is positioned directly medial and slightly inferior to the mitral valve, and the left ventricular apex lies in an inferior and lateral plane below the mitral valve.

The term *scan* is used frequently throughout this monograph. A scan results when one changes the angle of the transducer in a deliberate attempt to interrelate one area of the heart with another (Fig. 1–20). If the recorder is activated, a paper copy is made of the movement of intracardiac structures transected by the sound beam during the scan (Fig. 1–15).

BIBLIOGRAPHY

Anon.: Lateral resolution. Lewistown, Pa., KB-Aerotech, Krautkramer-Branson, Inc., *1*(4), 1979.

Anon.: Properties of sound waves. *In* An Introduction to Echocardiography — Physics. Edited by G. Leech, G. Sutton, and P. Wells, London, Medi-Cine, 1978.

Anon.: Sensitivity I. Lewistown, Pa., KB-Aerotech, Krautkramer-Branson, Inc., *1*(4), 1979.

Arditti, A., et al.: Single channel dual echocardiography. Am. J. Cardiol., *46*:277, 1980.

Baker, B.: Physical and technical principles in diagnostic ultrasound. *In* Diagnostic Ultrasound. Edited by D. King. St. Louis, C.V. Mosby, 1974.

Bansal, R., et al.: Feasibility of detailed two-dimensional echocardiographic examinations in adults. Prospective study of 200 patients. Mayo Clin. Proc., *55*:291, 1980.

Baum, G., et al.: Fundamentals of Medical Ultrasonography. New York, G.P. Putnam's Sons, 1975.

Benassi, A., et al.: A buffered video interface for cardiac imaging. J. Nucl. Med. Allied Sci., *23*:129, 1979.

Bernstein, A.: Analog storage of M-mode echocardiograph signals using video tape. IEEE Trans. Biomed. Eng., *27*:448, 1980.

Bernstein, A.: Microcomputer editing of M-mode echocardiograms for semiautomatic analysis. IEEE Trans. Biomed. Eng., *27*:472, 1980.

Brown, R.: Overview of diagnostic ultrasound. Semin. Roentgenol., *10*:255, 1975.

Carlsen, E.: Ultrasound physics for the physician: a brief review. J. Clin. Ultrasound, *3*:69, 1975.

Davidovits, P.: Physics in Biology and Medicine. Englewood Cliffs, N.J., Prentice-Hall, 1975.

Edler, I.: The use of ultrasound as a diagnostic aid and its effects on biological tissues. Continuous recording of the movements of various heart structures using an ultrasound echo-method. Acta Med. Scand. [Suppl.], *170*:7, 1961.

Feigenbaum, H.: Echocardiography, 2nd Ed. Philadelphia, Lea & Febiger, 1976.

Feigenbaum, H.: Principles of echocardiography. Am. J. Med., *62*:805, 1977.

Fleischer, A., et al.: Introduction to Diagnostic Sonography. New York, John Wiley & Sons, 1980.

Fry, W.: Mechanism of acoustic absorption in tissue. J. Acoust. Soc. Am., *24*:412, 1952.

Fry, W., et al.: Ultrasound transmission in tissue visualization. *In* Diagnostic Ultrasound. Edited by C. Grossman, J. Holmes, C. Joyner, and E. Purnell. New York, Plenum Press, 1966.

Geiser, E., et al.: A framework for three-dimensional time-varying reconstruction of the human left ventricle: sources of error and estimation of their magnitude. Comput. Biomed. Res., *13*:225, 1980.

Goldman, D., et al.: Tabular data of the velocity and absorption of high-frequency sound in mammalian tissues. J. Acoust. Soc. Am., *28*:35, 1956; Errata: J. Acoust. Soc. Am., *29*:655, 1957.

Griffith, J., et al.: Switch gain: a technique for simplifying ultrasonic measurement of cardiac wall thickness. IEEE Trans. Bio. Med. Eng., *22*:337, 1975.

Henry, W., et al.: Report of the American Society of Echocardiography Committee on nomenclature and standards in two-dimensional echocardiography. Circulation, *62*:212, 1980.

Hertz, C.: Ultrasonic engineering in heart diagnosis. Am. J. Cardiol., *19*:6, 1967.

Hertz, C.: The interaction of physicians, physicists and industry in the development of echocardiography. Ultrasound Med. Biol., *1*:3, 1973.

Hostetler, M., et al.: A microprocessor-controlled echocardiographic tracking system. IEEE Trans. Biomed. Eng., *27*:249, 1980.

Kadaba, M., et al.: Attenuation and backscattering of ultrasound in freshly excised animal tissues. IEEE Trans. Biomed. Eng., *27*:76, 1980.

Kelly, E.: Ultrasonic Energy — Biological Investigations and Medical Applications. Urbana, Ill., University of Illinois Press, 1965.

Kessler, L.: Ultrasonic attenuation in mammalian tissue. J. Acoust. Soc. Am., *53*:1759, 1973.

Kingsley, B., et al.: Another look at echocardiography: concepts in biomedical engineering. Am. J. Cardiol., 19:108, 1967.

Kisslo, J.: Two-dimensional echocardiography. Radiol. Clin. North Am., 18:105, 1980.

Kleid, J., et al.: Echocardiography: Interpretation and Diagnosis. New York, Appleton-Century-Crofts, 1978.

Kossoff, G.: Principles of two-dimensional echocardiography and real-time imaging. Med. J. Aust., 1:7, 1977.

Kremkau, F.: Physical principles of ultrasound. Semin. Roentgenol., 10:259, 1975.

Ludwig, G.: The velocity of sound through tissue and the acoustic impedance of tissues. J. Acoust. Soc. Am., 22:862, 1950.

McMaster, R.: Nondestructive Testing Handbook. New York, Ronald Press, 1959.

Meltzer, R., et al.: The source of ultrasound contrast effect. J. Clin. Ultrasound, 8:121, 1980.

Meltzer, R., et al.: Why do the lungs clear ultrasonic contrast? Ultrasound Med. Biol., 6:263, 1980.

Meyer, R.: Pediatric Echocardiography. Philadelphia, Lea & Febiger, 1977.

Mimbs, J., et al.: The dependence of ultrasonic attenuation and back scatter on collagen content in dog and rabbit hearts. Circ. Res., 47:49, 1980.

Mortimer, A., et al.: A relationship between ultrasonic intensity and changes in myocardial mechanics. Can. J. Physiol. Pharmacol., 58:67, 1980.

Ramana, Y., et al.: Shear velocity of muscle tissues. J. Biomech. Eng., 2:211, 1980.

Reid, J.: A review of some basic limitations in ultrasonic diagnosis. In Diagnostic Ultrasound. Edited by C. Grossman, J. Holmes, C. Joyner, and E. Purnell, Proceedings of the First International Conference. Univ. of Pittsburgh, 1965. New York, Plenum Press, 1966.

Roelandt, J.: Practical Echocardiology. Forest Grove, Oreg., Research Studies Press, 1977.

Vas, R., et al.: Analysis of cardiac kinetics: use of a new photo-optic technique. Am. J. Physiol., 238:98, 1980.

Venrooij, G.: Measurement of ultrasound velocity in human tissues. Ultrasonics, 9:240, 1971.

Wells, P.N.T.: Absorption and dispersion of ultrasound in biological tissue. Ultrasound Med. Biol., 1:369, 1975.

Wells, P.N.T.: Biomedical Ultrasonics. London, Academic Press, 1977.

Yeh, E.: Reverberations in echocardiograms. J. Clin. Ultrasound, 5:84, 1977.

2
The Normal Heart

NORMAL MITRAL VALVE

The mitral valve is located between the left atrial and left ventricular chambers. A large, apron-shaped anterior leaflet is suspended from the fibrous tissue of the aortic root, in close proximity to the left and posterior noncoronary aortic leaflets. The rectangular posterior mitral leaflet is attached to the atrioventricular annulus. The filmy leaflets are thickened near their free edges, owing to the insertion of many chordae tendineae.[1]

In their closed position, the rough edges of the mitral leaflets are pressed tightly together, effectively preventing the re-entry of blood into the left atrium during systole. When open, the leaflets assume a conical shape that funnels left atrial blood inferiorly along the posterior aspect of the left ventricle toward the apex. This is the inflow tract. The direction of blood flow is then reversed and is directed superiorly along the anterior aspect of the left ventricle toward the aorta. This is the left ventricular outflow tract. The anterior mitral leaflet serves a secondary function as the posterior boundary of the left ventricular outflow tract.

Recording Technique

Since the mitral valve is centrally located in relation to all other cardiac structures, a routine echocardiographic examination is begun by searching for mitral valve motion. The anatomic area of the mitral valve can be located by hand palpation of the right ventricular outflow tract along the left parasternum. The transducer should be placed perpendicularly over this pulsation and angled slightly medially and cephalad (Figs. 2–1 and 2–2). If the mitral valve's motion is fragmented, then one should move the transducer systematically over the precordium, shifting to higher or lower intercostal spaces. Mitral valve motion may be monitored from the second, fifth, and sixth intercostal spaces. If mitral valve motion is unavailable at the left parasternum, it may be successfully recorded from the subcostal (subxiphoid) examination site.

Normal motion of the anterior mitral leaflet is "M-shaped," opening soon after the second heart sound and closing simultaneously with the onset of the first heart sound (Figs. 2–3 and

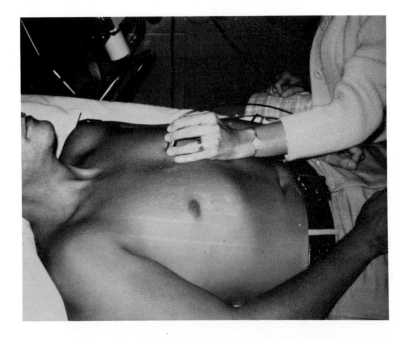

Fig. 2–1. Interrelationship of patient, echocardiographer, and equipment. It is a matter of preference whether an examination is conducted from the right or the left side of the patient.

2–4). When the heart rate exceeds 110 beats per minute, the pattern is more similar to an upside-down "V." Opposing posterior mitral leaflet motion is found by the slightest inferior and lateral angulation of the transducer. Too much angulation causes the sound beam to bypass this leaflet, and its movement is not seen.

Mitral valve motion should be recorded from the free edges of the anterior mitral leaflet to its basilar attachment near the aortic annulus. One should begin this "scan" by directing the transducer inferiorly and laterally into the left ventricle until mitral motion is nearly gone (Fig. 2–5, section 1). While recording continuously, the transducer is then angled superiorly and medially towards the aorta (Fig. 2–5, sections 2 to 4). One may scan from the aorta to the left ventricle if it is easier to do so.

Reflected echo intensity is greatest when the sound beam is most perpendicular to the leaflet's plane of movement. At the same time, the transducer will probably be perpendicular to the chest wall, but this will not always be true. Variation of body habitus from one patient to another requires some flexibility in examination technique. Those who interpret an echocardiogram must be aware of the various methods one

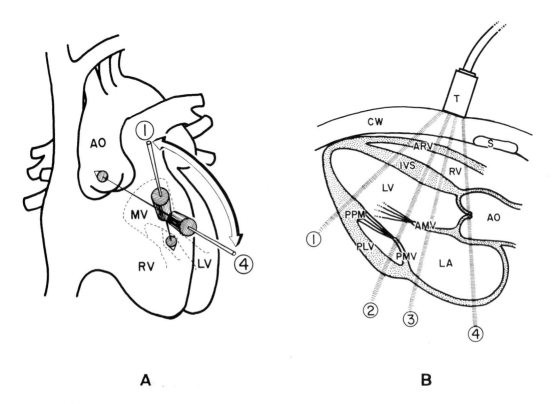

A   **B**

Fig. 2–2.   *A,* Angulation of the transducer from the mitral valve (MV) to the aorta (AO). *B,* Structures transected as the transducer is angled from the mitral valve to the aorta. RV, right ventricle; LV, left ventricle; CW, chest wall; T, transducer; ARV, anterior right ventricular wall; PPM, posterior papillary muscle; PLV, posterior left ventricular wall; AMV, anterior mitral valve; PMV, posterior mitral valve; LA, left atrium; S, sternum; IVS, interventricular septum. (From Feigenbaum, H.: Clinical applications of echocardiography. Prog. Cardiovasc. Dis., *14*: 531, 1972.)

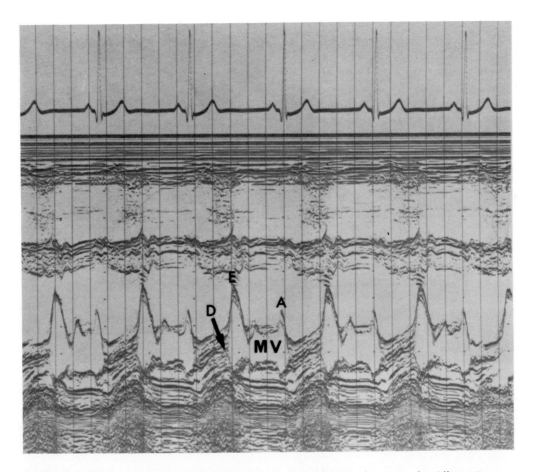

Fig. 2–3. MV, normal mitral valve motion; D, onset of rapid ventricular filling; E, most open position of anterior mitral leaflet; A, leaflet's opening response to left atrial contraction.

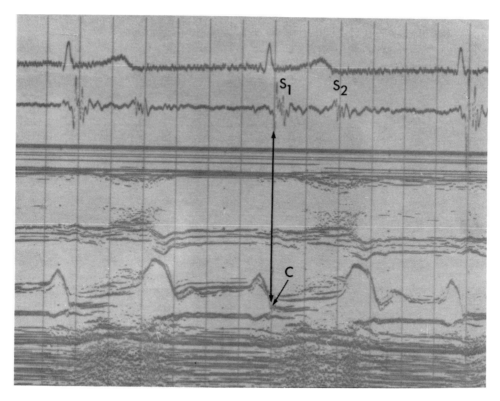

Fig. 2–4. Onset of the first heart sound (S_1) correlating closely with end-diastolic closure of the mitral leaflets. A simultaneous phonocardiogram is useful to identify the termination of mitral leaflet closure when echographic mitral valve closure cannot be obtained. S_2, second heart sound, coincident with aortic valve closure; C, end-diastolic coaptation of mitral leaflets.

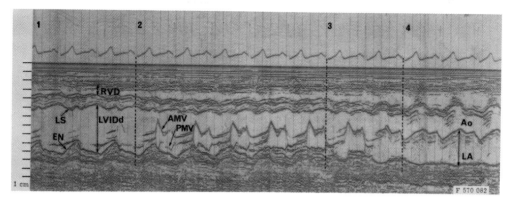

Fig. 2–5. A routine scan from the left ventricle to the aorta (sections 1 through 4). LS, left septum; EN, endocardial surface of posterior left ventricular wall; RVD, right ventricular dimension; $LVID_d$, left ventricular diastolic internal dimension; AMV, anterior mitral valve; PMV, posterior mitral valve; A, aorta; LA, left atrium.

may use to obtain an echocardiogram. Some of these methods deviate from routine "standards" and are discussed throughout this text as the appropriate occasion arises.

Measurements from Mitral Valve Echogram

Measurements of mitral valve motion are customarily taken from that area where the anterior and posterior leaflets exhibit maximum excursion or separation from each other. This area is just before the approach to the atrioventricular junction as one scans from the left ventricle to the aorta. If the transducer should be angled more superiorly, posterior leaflet motion would be lost. Left atrial wall motion would be seen posterior to the anterior mitral valve (Fig. 2–5, sections 3 and 4). A slight inferior angulation of the transducer recovers posterior mitral leaflet motion.

Opening and early diastolic closing velocities of the mitral valve vary considerably secondary to the relationship of the mitral leaflet with the interrogating sound beam. It is important to understand that the position of the patient alters the velocity of valvular motion, and one should be cautious when seeking to extrapolate indices of left ventricular function from mitral valve movement.

Early Diastolic Opening Velocity. Within 50 to 70 msec of the onset of diastole, anterior and posterior mitral leaflets

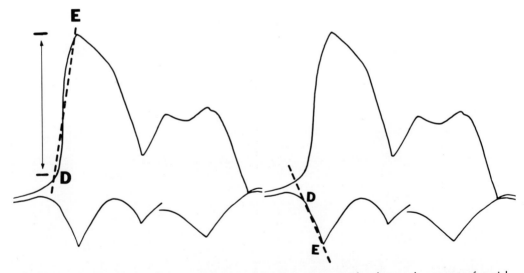

Fig. 2–6. A, D-E is the opening velocity of the anterior mitral valve at the onset of rapid ventricular filling. The opening velocity is expressed as mm/sec. The measurement of the opening velocity is facilitated if the mitral echogram is recorded at 50 to 100 mm/sec with 100 to 200 msec time line intervals. The perpendicular line from D to E shows an opening excursion or amplitude of the anterior mitral leaflet. B, D-E is the opening movement of the posterior mitral leaflet. The maximum opening excursion of the mitral leaflets is infrequently recorded from the subcostal examination site because the sound beam is not perpendicular to the valve's opening movement.

Table 2–1.
Effect of the Position of the Patient upon the Opening Velocity of Normal Anterior and Posterior Mitral Leaflets

Patient	Age (yr)	ANTERIOR VALVE			POSTERIOR VALVE		
		Supine (mm/sec)	LL (mm/sec)	Subxiphoid (mm/sec)	Supine (mm/sec)	LL (mm/sec)	Subxiphoid (mm/sec)
A	41	250	305	165	120	105	45
B	54	345	285	160	70	—	45
C	41	365	405	—	90	130	155
D	42	155	210	275	60	100	150
E	56	385	275	360	65	140	100
F	46	330	290	270	85	145	95
G	50	235	155	400	85	105	140
H	46	315	280	265	75	140	75
I	41	275	315	545	95	95	128

Abbreviations: mm/sec, velocity in millimeters per second; LL, left lateral decubitus, torso elevated 20 to 30 degrees.

separate with a velocity exceeding 150 mm/sec, allowing blood to flow from the left atrium into the left ventricle. The opening velocity of the anterior leaflet is variable within the same patient and from one patient to another and is influenced by the patient's position, respiration, and the relationship of the transducer with the opening leaflet.

Measurement of the opening velocity of the anterior and posterior mitral leaflets is shown in Figure 2–6. Some normal individuals were examined to show the different opening velocities as the valve was examined from several sites (Table 2–1). These measurements were obtained from complexes exhibiting maximum excursion and completeness of movement throughout diastole and systole. The transducer was either perpendicular to the chest wall or angled slightly superiorly and medially. None of these measurements were derived from tracings requiring inferior angulation to record leaflet motion.

Opening Excursion of Anterior Mitral Leaflet. The most pliable portion of the anterior mitral leaflet lies between its midsection and free edges. During diastole, the valve opens widely into the body of the left ventricle (Fig. 2–5). The anterior mitral leaflet opening excursion ranges from 16 to 30 mm and is influenced by respiration, Valsalva maneuvers, and the position of the patient (Table 2–2). When wide open, the anterior mitral leaflet approaches the left side of the septum within 0 to 8 mm if the inner circumference of the left ventricle is not enlarged (Fig. 2–7). This measurement is one variable used to evaluate left ventricular function.

Early Diastolic Closure of Anterior Mitral Leaflet. Early diastolic mitral valve closure begins just after the maximum

Table 2–2.
Effect of the Position of the Patient upon the Opening Amplitude of Anterior and Posterior Mitral Leaflets

Patient	ANTERIOR VALVE (mm)			POSTERIOR VALVE (mm)		
	Supine	LL	Subxiphoid	Supine	LL	Subxiphoid
A	20	20	20	9	8	—
B	23	22	21	3	5	—
C	21	20	23	10	9	—
D	21	20	18	5	—	8
E	14	16	21	—	9	9
F	19	19	23	9	10	10
G	25	22	29	9	10	10
H	21	25	24	9	10	7
I	21	23	25	9	10	8
J	20	19	23	10	10	8

Abbreviations: LL, left lateral decubitus (partial).

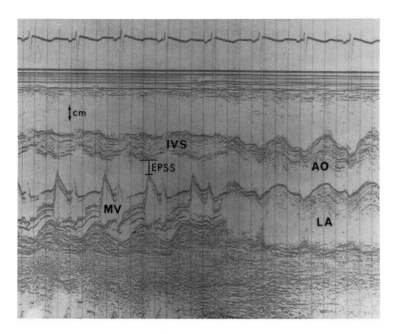

Fig. 2–7. A scan from the mitral valve to the aorta, showing the relation of the open mitral valve to the left side of the septum. The normal distance between the mitral E-point and the septum (EPSS) does not often exceed 8 mm, compatible with ejection fractions exceeding 55%. This measurement is not applicable in patients with mitral stenosis, aortic insufficiency, or left anterior descending artery disease. MV, diastolic mitral valve motion; IVS, interventricular septum: AO, aorta; LA, left atrium.

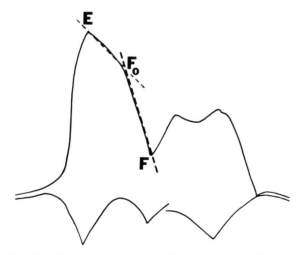

Fig. 2–8. The E-F_0 slope is the deceleration phase of early diastolic mitral valve closure. F_0-F slope is the acceleration phase of early diastolic closure. F_0 is infrequently seen in mitral valve tracings with slow recording speeds. The use of digitizing tables and computer analysis probably reflects a more accurate rate of diastolic closure. Manual measurement usually ignores the F_0 component and assumes the E-F slope to be an average of deceleration-acceleration phases.

Table 2–3.
Effect of the Position of the Patient upon Diastolic Mitral Valve Closure

Patient	$E-F$ (mm/sec)			$E-F_o$ (mm/sec)			F_o-F (mm/sec)		
	Supine	LL	Subxiphoid	Supine	LL	Subxiphoid	Supine	LL	Subxiphoid
A	130	110	155	50	40	50	295	210	230
B	105	70	80	45	45	—	150	110	—
C	110	85	75	100	85	30	300	155	155
D	110	110	50	45	60	25	205	180	80
E	125	155	215	40	55	—	230	345	—
F	105	105	65	85	95	—	315	219	—
G	140	160	95	65	85	—	240	210	—
H	75	75	105	36	38	48	160	250	140
I	90	55	60	55	40	50	150	100	205
J	140	145	155	35	45	60	170	215	140

Abbreviations: E–F, diastolic closure of mitral valve prior to atrial contraction; E–F$_o$, deceleration phase of mitral valve early diastolic closure; F$_o$–F, acceleration phase of diastolic leaflet closure; LL, left lateral decubitus (partial).

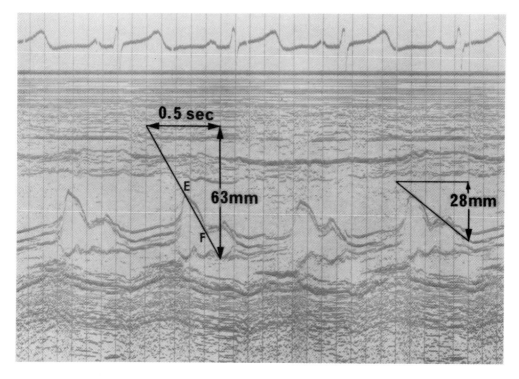

Fig. 2–9. Measurement of the early diastolic closing velocity of the anterior mitral leaflet. The E-F closing velocity was 63 mm in 0.5 sec or 126 mm in 1 sec. The E-F$_0$ closing velocity was 28 mm in 0.5 sec or 56 mm in 1 sec.

leaflet opening (E-point) and terminates at the F-point (Figs. 2–8 and 2–9). Early E to F diastolic closure velocity is affected by the position of the patient and of the transducer (Table 2–3). It is also affected by a poorly compliant ventricle, low cardiac output, mitral valve obstruction, right heart failure, and pulmonary hypertension.

At paper recording speeds exceeding 50 mm/sec, the normal mitral valve often exhibits a deceleration–acceleration closure pattern. The deceleration phase (E to F$_0$) is slow and is related to the rate of left ventricular filling. The acceleration phase (F$_0$ to F) is rapid. The measurements of closing velocity from these different phases are not interchangeable. Common practice is to measure the mitral valve closing velocity from the E-point to the F-point.

Late Diastolic Mitral Valve Opening (Atrial Contraction). If the heart rate is slow, a secondary late diastolic opening of the mitral valve is preceded by an electrically quiet interval. At this time, there is an equalization of pressure between the left atrium and the left ventricle. Blood flows into the left ventricle without any contractile forces by the left atrium. This interval is known as the *conduit* phase. The mitral leaflets

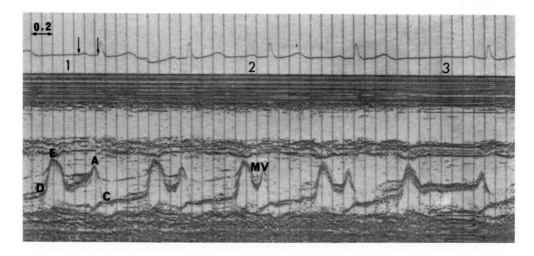

Fig. 2–10. Sinus arrhythmia. Atrial contraction was preceded by conduit phases of varying length (complexes 1, 2, 3). D, initial onset of rapid left ventricular filling; E, maximum opening of anterior mitral leaflet; A, leaflet opening secondary to atrial contraction; C, mitral leaflet closure at the end of diastole; MV, diastolic mitral valve motion. Arrows denote the P-R interval on the electrocardiogram.

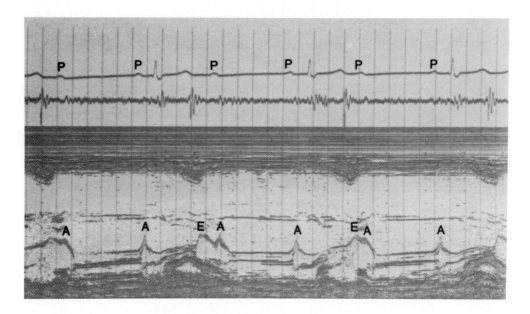

Fig. 2–11. A 73-year-old female patient with atrioventricular dissociation and hypertension. A, irregular atrial contraction; E, maximum open position of anterior mitral leaflet during early diastole; P, electrical depolarization of atrium.

fluctuate slightly as blood continues to flow through them from the pulmonary veins and the left atrium (Fig. 2–10, complexes 1 and 3). With increasing heart rates, the conduit phase is abbreviated or absent. Atrial contraction and mitral valve opening immediately follow early diastolic valve closure (Fig. 2–10, complex 2). With atrial fibrillation, the conduit phase is prolonged to the end of diastole. The mitral valve opens in response to atrial contraction, whether it occurs regularly during sinus rhythm or irregularly as with atrioventricular dissociation (Fig. 2–11).

Ambiguous Mitral Valve Closure

Figure 2–12 A demonstrates mitral valve motion that seems to close before the onset of ventricular systole. This type of closure occurs with acute aortic insufficiency or a slow heart rate, neither of which were present in this patient with cardiomyopathy. The transducer was angled slightly anteriorly to reveal closure of the anterior and posterior mitral leaflets following left ventricular depolarization (Fig. 2–12 B). The premature mitral valve closure in the patient in Figure 2–12 A was an artifact introduced by an incorrect relationship between the sound beam and the mitral leaflet's plane of movement. If there is doubt about the mitral valve's closure point, one should record a simultaneous phonocardiogram to

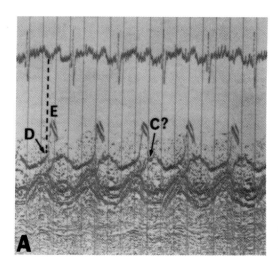
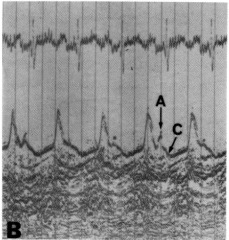

Fig. 2–12. *A,* The mitral valve appeared to close prematurely, a clinically incompatible finding in a patient with cardiomyopathy and heart rate of 85 beats per min. *B,* The transducer was tilted slightly superior from same examination site to show mitral valve's response to atrial contraction and valve closure following ventricular depolarization. The recording speed was 20 mm/sec and 0.2 sec time line intervals. D, onset of rapid left ventricular filling; E, maximum excursion of anterior mitral leaflet; A, leaflet's opening response secondary to atrial contraction; C, end-diastolic closure of anterior and posterior mitral leaflets.

time echocardiographic mitral valve closure with the onset of the first heart sound. These events should occur simultaneously (Fig. 2–4).

Normal Mitral Valve with Arrhythmia

Patterns of mitral valve motion vary from one diastolic cycle to the next, depending upon the length of the diastolic period. Figure 2–10 shows five mitral complexes in a normal individual who had sinus arrhythmia. The diastolic intervals of complexes 1, 2, and 3 were all different, thus changing the pattern of valvular motion. This pattern was not indicative of mitral valve dysfunction. It did reflect the variability of time elapsed during the conduit phase of diastole and the valve's response to passive blood flow.

Premature ventricular contractions shorten the duration of diastolic mitral valve opening and shorten left ventricular filling time (Figs. 2–13 and 2–14). In Figure 2–14, the source of the arrhythmia was a malfunctioning pacemaker. The patient's own rhythm and premature ventricular contractions were interjected when the pacemaker failed to function. During premature ventricular contraction, the mitral valve could not open because left ventricular pressure exceeded left atrial pressure. The anterior mitral leaflet's opening velocity was reduced during the unpaced beats, showing amputated or

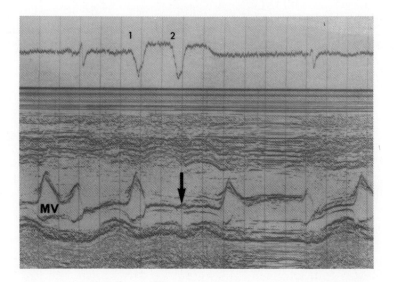

Fig. 2–13. A 34-year-old male patient with cardiomyopathy. There was shortened left ventricular filling time with premature ventricular contractions. The arrow indicates the failure of the mitral valve to open during a second premature ventricular contraction. MV, mitral valve motion during diastole.

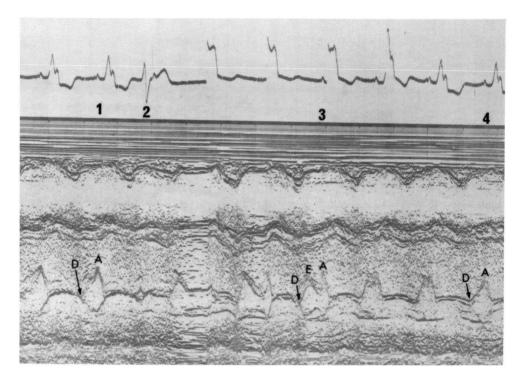

Fig. 2–14. A 72-year-old male patient with coronary artery disease and a malfunctioning pacemaker. The normal mitral valve shows the effects of premature ventricular contraction (complex 2), regular paced beat (complex 3), and return to the patient's own rhythm (complex 4). The markedly diminished velocity of the mitral valve opening in complexes 1 and 4 is associated with elevated left ventricular diastolic pressure. D, onset of rapid left ventricular filling; E, maximal excursion of anterior mitral leaflet; A, leaflet's response to left atrial contraction.

absent E-points. This type of pattern has been seen in patients with significantly elevated left ventricular diastolic pressure.[2] Since this patient did not undergo cardiac catheterization, correlative pressures were not obtained. However, no other hemodynamic or anatomic entity has been found to cause an otherwise normal mitral valve to exhibit such poor leaflet opening at the onset of diastole.

In the presence of atrial fibrillation, the mitral valve shows some coarse fluctuation that should not be mistaken for aortic regurgitation. One complex of motion seen in Figure 2–15 is particularly interesting in that the leaflets did not exhibit motion following early diastolic closure. Then, in the last fourth of a long and apparently nonconductive phase, the leaflets again fluctuated, even though blood flow through the mitral valve had to be minimal. This patient had intermittent atrial fibrillation and flutter on a routine electrocardiogram.

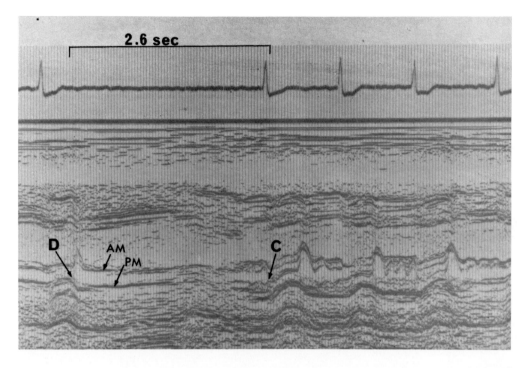

Fig. 2–15. A 68-year-old female patient with pancreatic carcinoma. On hospital admission, the electrocardiogram showed supraventricular tachycardia. The rhythm changed to atrial fibrillation-flutter 24 hours later. The first mitral valve complex shows immobile leaflets throughout most of diastole with resumption of leaflet fluctuation in latter fourth of diastole. D, onset of rapid left ventricular filling; AM, anterior mitral leaflet motion; PM, posterior mitral leaflet motion; C, end diastolic valve closure.

Conceivably, the patient's mitral valve was quiescent during atrial fibrillation and showed movement during atrial flutter.

NORMAL LEFT ATRIUM

The left atrium serves two functions: (1) as a reservoir for oxygenated blood returning from the lungs and (2) as a pump to aid the movement of blood from the left atrium into the left ventricle during late diastole. Unlike the heavily trabeculated endocardium of the left ventricle, the endocardial surface of the left atrial chamber is smooth. Left atrial wall thickness is approximately 3 mm, thicker than the right atrial wall. Hence a strong signal is returned from the posterior atrial wall when the ultrasonic beam is perpendicular to this structure (Fig. 2–16).

Systolic movement of the left atrial wall is unlike left ventricular wall motion (Fig. 2–17). Coincident with mitral valve closure, the posterior left atrial wall moves away from the transducer, remaining in this position throughout systole. At the onset of diastole, the mitral valve opens and blood

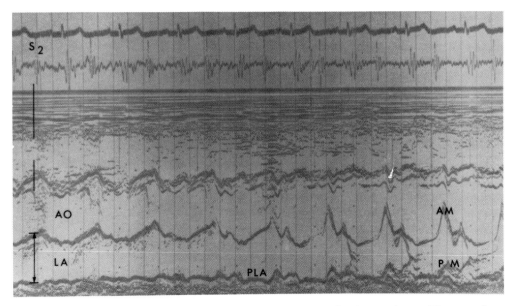

Fig. 2–16. A 17-year-old male patient with a silent mitral valve prolapse. The scan from the aorta toward the left ventricle demonstrated a smooth transition from passive to mobile segments of the left atrial wall. The posterior aortic root demonstrated continuity with the anterior mitral leaflet. AO, aorta; LA, left atrium; PLA, posterior left atrial wall motion; AM, anterior mitral leaflet motion; PM, posterior mitral leaflet motion; S_2, second heart sound.

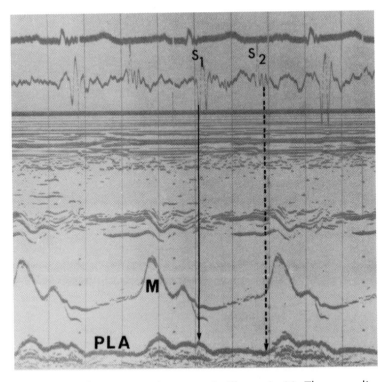

Fig. 2–17. The same patient seen in Figure 2–16. The recording speed was increased to clarify the posterior left atrial wall movement during diastole and systole. PLA, posterior left atrial wall motion; M, mitral valve motion; S_1, first heart sound; S_2, second heart sound.

rushes into the left ventricle. This evacuation of blood from the left atrium is accompanied by a rapid movement of the atrial wall toward the transducer. With early diastolic mitral valve closure, the left atrial wall again moves away from the transducer. During mid-diastole, the left atrium acts as a conduit for blood flowing from the pulmonary veins into the left atrium and through the semiclosed mitral leaflets.

Additional blood is forcefully ejected from the left atrium during atrial contraction and contributes up to one fifth of the total volume received by the left ventricle during diastole. Patients with atrial fibrillation lose this valuable "booster" for late diastolic ventricular filling.

Recording Technique

Left Parasternum. After locating mitral valve motion along the left parasternum, one should angle the transducer superiorly and medially in a sector between the right neck and the right shoulder. The septum attenuates and gradually becomes the anterior aortic wall (Fig. 2–18). The mobility of the anterior mitral leaflet steadily lessens as one approaches the fibrous mitral-aortic junction. Motion patterns of the posterior left ventricle change as the sound beam passes from the left ventricle to the atrioventricular junction to the left atrium. Posterior left atrial wall movement becomes nearly passive if the scan is continued even more superiorly into the aorta.

Identification of posterior left atrial wall motion must be established during the examination. With adjustment of the

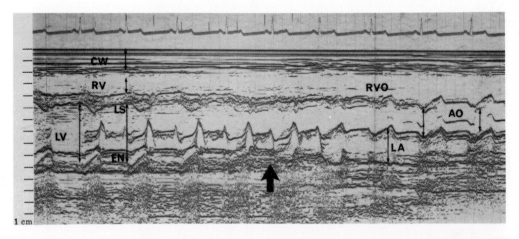

Fig. 2–18. A normal 18-year-old male. The scan from the left ventricle to the aorta demonstrated the transition from the septum to the anterior aortic wall, from the anterior mitral leaflet to the posterior aortic wall, and from the left ventricular wall to the posterior left atrial wall. CW, chest wall; RV, right ventricle; LV, left ventricle; LS, left side of the septum; EN, endocardial surface of posterior left ventricular wall; RVO, right ventricular outflow tract; AO, aorta; LA, left atrium; bold arrow, atrioventricular junction.

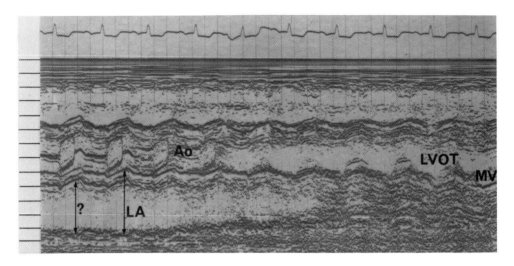

Fig. 2–19. Scan from the aorta toward the mitral valve. The left atrial dimension was measured from the top of the posterior aortic wall echo (showing continuity with mitral valve) to the top of the posterior left atrial wall echo. The origin of the echo without mitral valve continuity is unknown. Ao, Aorta; LA, left atrium; LVOT, left ventricular outflow tract; MV, mitral leaflet motion.

transducer's angle in relation to the atrial wall, multiple scans should show continuity between the left atrial wall and the atrioventricular junction (Fig. 2–18). Reduction of signal amplification (coarse gain) eliminates many low-intensity echoes and should clarify the atrial wall-blood interface.

Figure 2–19 is a scan from the aorta toward the mitral valve. There are two high-intensity echoes inscribed in the vicinity of the posterior aortic root. For consistency, I prefer to measure the left atrial dimension from the top of the echo that has the most continuity with the anterior mitral leaflet.

Suprasternal Examination. Suprasternal examination of the left atrium was described by Goldberg (1971)[3a] and was further validated by Allen (1977),[4] using saline contrast injection techniques. This type of examination is best performed on a sleeping child or a cooperative older child. A thimble- or hammer-shaped transducer (0.25 inch, 3.5 MHz, or 5.0 MHz) can be positioned in the suprasternal notch (Fig. 2–20). One has more room to maneuver if a small rolled towel is placed behind the child's shoulders. The head may be tilted about 45° to the left. Turning the head to the right displaces the ascending aorta rightward. By directing the sound beam inferiorly, caudally, and slightly left laterally, the transverse aorta, right pulmonary artery, and left atrium are transected by the ultrasound (Fig. 2–21 B). Since the left atrium is roughly symmetrical in all directions,[3] measurements from the left sternal border (Z axis) and suprasternally (Y' axis) are compa-

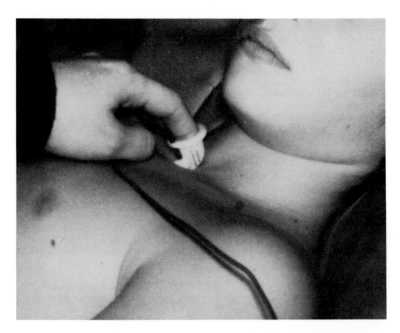

Fig. 2–20. Transducer placement during M-mode suprasternal examination of the ascending aorta, right pulmonary artery, and left atrium. The thumb of the echocardiographer has been retracted to show the relationship between the suprasternal notch and the transducer. Otherwise, the thumb is used for transducer stabilization as needed.

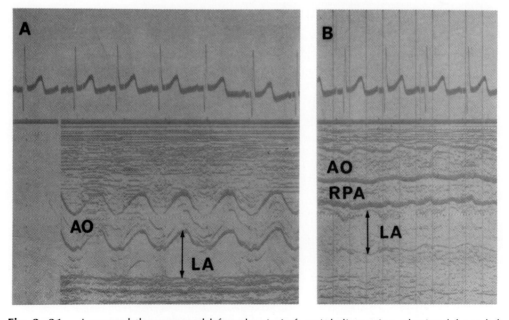

Fig. 2–21. A normal three-year-old female. *A,* Left atrial dimension obtained from left sternal border (Z axis); *B,* Left atrial dimension obtained from suprasternal examination site (Y′ axis). Ao, Aorta; LA, left atrium; RPA, right pulmonary artery.

rable[4] (Fig. 2–21 A and B). Increased left atrial dimension in one plane is usually accompanied by a reduced dimension in another examination plane. This unilateral compression or "pancaking" of the left atrium has been observed in patients with pectus excavatum, pulmonary artery dilatation, and patent ductus arteriosus with respiratory distress syndrome.

Measurement of Left Atrial Dimension

A left atrial dimension is measured at the end of systole, when the aortic and mitral valves are closed. Left atrial blood volume is greatest at this time. The end of systole may be identified on the echocardiographic tracing by (1) aortic valve closure, (2) end of electrocardiographic ventricular repolarization, or (3) onset of the second heart sound identified on a simultaneously recorded phonocardiogram. The left atrial dimension is obtained by drawing a perpendicular line from the top of the posterior aortic root echo to the top of the passive left atrial wall echo (see Fig. 2–16).

Left atrial dimensions are influenced slightly by the patient's position during examination (Tables 2–4 and 2–5). The

Table 2–4.
Effect of the Postion of the Patient upon the Left Atrial Dimension in 21 Adult Females Without Clinical Evidence of Cardiovascular Disease

Patient	Age (yr)	BSA (m²)	Supine (cm)	LL (cm)	Difference (mm)
A	50	1.72	2.1	3.0	9
B	57	1.70	2.5	3.0	5
C	41	1.64	3.1	3.3	2
D	46	1.53	2.4	2.9	5
E	45	1.58	3.0	3.0	0
F	51	1.67	2.8	2.8	0
G	56	1.71	3.8	3.7	−1
H	60	1.70	2.7	2.9	2
I	57	1.52	2.5	3.0	5
J	65	1.57	3.0	3.2	2
K	42	1.84	2.8	3.0	2
L	55	1.67	3.2	3.5	3
M	50	1.80	2.9	2.9	0
N	56	1.64	2.9	2.9	0
O	55	1.74	3.0	3.1	1
P	61	1.64	2.2	3.6	14
Q	58	1.63	2.5	2.9	4
R	43	1.67	2.9	2.9	0
S	53	1.66	3.1	3.7	6
T	65	1.64	2.9	3.3	4
U	52	1.62	3.2	2.9	−3

Abbreviations: BSA, body surface area (per square meter); LL, left lateral decubitus position, torso elevated 20 to 30 degrees; difference, change in cavity dimension.

atrial diameter tends to be smaller when the patient is supine and increases as the patient is turned toward a partial left lateral decubitus position. If a tracing suitable for measurement cannot be achieved in one position, alternative positions should be tried. I found little difference between measurements of left atrial dimension in 30 morbidly obese patients as compared with patients of normal weight (Table 2–6).

NORMAL AORTIC ROOT

The aortic root is positioned in front of the left atrium. This relationship allows structural motion of the aorta to be recorded simultaneously with some portion of the left atrium (see Fig. 2–2 *B*). The relation of the aortic root to the mitral valve is superior and medial, the anterior mitral leaflet having continuity with the left aortic cusp and the posterior or noncoronary aortic cusp.[5] The walls of the aortic root are composed of smooth, elastic muscle, an excellent reflector of

Table 2–5.
Effect of the Position of the Patient upon the Left Atrial Dimension in 24 Adult Males Without Clinical Evidence of Cardiovascular Disease

Patient	Age (yr)	BSA (m²)	Supine (cm)	LL (cm)	Difference (mm)
A	45	2.08	3.0	2.9	−1
B	40	2.31	3.5	3.8	3
C	62	1.89	3.3	3.7	4
D	62	2.12	3.4	3.7	3
E	46	1.90	3.0	3.2	2
F	42	2.00	2.9	3.0	1
G	57	1.66	3.3	3.5	2
H	41	2.05	4.0	4.0	0
I	47	2.16	3.9	4.1	2
J	50	1.80	3.3	3.3	0
K	48	2.02	3.0	3.3	3
L	41	1.99	3.0	3.0	0
M	46	1.97	3.1	3.6	5
N	41	1.91	2.6	3.3	7
O	46	2.04	2.9	3.5	6
P	58	2.03	2.8	3.0	2
Q	41	2.02	2.9	3.2	3
R	41	1.67	3.6	3.8	2
S	55	1.96	4.0	4.0	0
T	45	2.02	3.3	3.5	2
U	56	1.71	2.3	2.5	2
V	43	2.18	4.1	4.3	2
W	63	1.98	3.3	3.8	5
X	43	2.14	4.1	3.8	−3

Abbreviations: BSA, body surface area (per square meter); LL, left lateral decubitus position, torso elevated 20 to 30 degrees; difference, change in cavity dimension.

Table 2–6.

Dimension of the Left Atrium in 30 Morbidly Obese Patients Without Cardiovascular Disease Prior to Ileobypass Operations

Patient	Age (yr)	Height (cm)	Weight (kg)	BSA (m²)	LAD (cm)	LAD/M² (cm)
A	46	157	77.3	1.78	2.3	1.29
B	44	155	93.2	1.92	3.5	1.82
C	54	157	96.3	1.97	4.0	2.03
D	42	157	104.0	2.02	3.0	1.48
E	32	160	103.2	2.04	3.1	1.52
F	32	157	110.9	2.08	3.4	1.63
G	42	155	113.6	2.08	3.1	1.49
H	43	163	108.2	2.12	3.4	1.60
I	30	160	110.9	2.12	3.3	1.56
J	21	160	112.7	2.12	3.0	1.42
K	25	157	116.8	2.14	3.5	1.64
L	31	155	120.9	2.14	3.5	1.64
M	32	164	115.7	2.18	3.7	1.69
N	23	163	121.3	2.23	4.0	1.79
O	38	166	119.0	2.24	3.0	1.34
P	38	163	127.5	2.25	3.5	1.56
Q	34	173	116.8	2.28	4.2	1.84
R	29	171	117.7	2.28	3.6	1.57
S	35	173	120.4	2.32	2.7	1.16
T	26	169	127.7	2.32	3.8	1.64
U	21	170	131.4	2.32	2.8	1.21
V	36	165	133.2	2.34	2.7	1.15
W	22	165	137.5	2.36	3.8	1.61
X	28	173	132.7	2.39	3.0	1.26
Y	42	165	135.9	2.42	3.6	1.49
Z	27	165	154.1	2.45	3.5	1.43
AA	30	178	138.2	2.50	2.7	1.08
BB	30	180	143.6	2.55	3.9	1.53
CC	22	175	172.7	2.72	3.8	1.39
DD	34	175	190.9	2.84	4.1	1.44
RANGE	21–54			1.78–2.84	2.3–4.2	1.08–2.03
MEAN	33			2.25	3.4	1.51
SD					±0.48	±0.22

Abbreviations: BSA, body surface area (per square meter); LAD, left atrial dimension; LAD/m², left atrial dimension corrected for body surface area; SD, 1 standard deviation from mean.

ultrasound. In fact, the intensity of the reflections from the aortic walls serve to differentiate wall tissue from the thinner aortic leaflets whose reflections are comparatively weaker.

Recording Technique

Whenever possible, mitral leaflet motion is recorded first. Then the transducer is slowly angled cephalad until characteristic mitral motion is lost (Fig. 2–22). Some portion of the muscular ventricular septum is still evident. With continued cephalad transducer angulation, the sound beam transects the membranous septal tissue and the right anterior aortic cusp. This is the junction between the most distal aspect of the left ventricular outflow tract and the fibrous aortic root. If one wishes to "size" the aortic annulus prior to the prosthetic aortic valve replacement, measurements should be taken in this area (Fig. 2–23). To complete the scan through the aortic root, the transducer must then be angled slightly medially while continuing cephalad angulation. The aortic root widens into two, thin, synchronously-moving echoes, as the beam traverses the sinuses of Valsalva and the aortic leaflets (see Fig. 2–18). Echoes from the aortic root and the leaflets are often obscured by too much amplification (Fig. 2–24). Because the aortic leaflets and aortic root are much closer to the transducer, reflections from these structures do not need as much amplification as do reflections from the posterior ventricular wall. Therefore, during a scan from the ventricle to the aorta, amplification should be decreased as the aorta is approached.

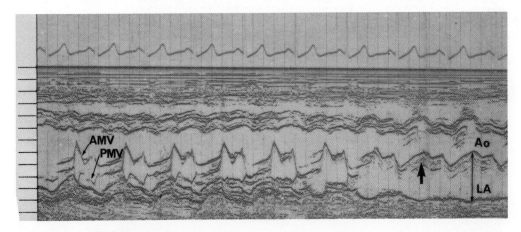

Fig. 2–22. A normal 18-year-old male. The scan from the mitral valve to the aortic root demonstrated tissue transitions from the muscular septum to the anterior aortic root and from the anterior mitral leaflet to the posterior aortic wall. AMV, anterior mitral valve motion; PMV, posterior mitral valve motion; Ao, Aorta; LA, left atrium; bold arrow, multiple echoes often seen in the vicinity of the posterior aortic root below the level of the posterior sinus of Valsalva.

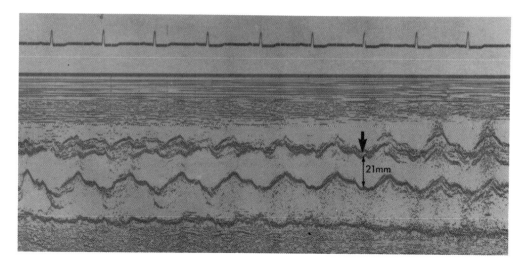

Fig. 2-23. A 21-year-old female patient with aortic insufficiency referred for an echocardiogram to evaluate the dimension of her aortic annulus prior to aortic valve replacement. The dimension measured 21 mm on the echocardiogram and 24 mm on the supravalvular aortogram. The patient's aortic valve was replaced with the smallest-diameter Bjork-Shiley tilting disc prosthesis. Bold arrow, junction between the membranous septum and the aortic root.

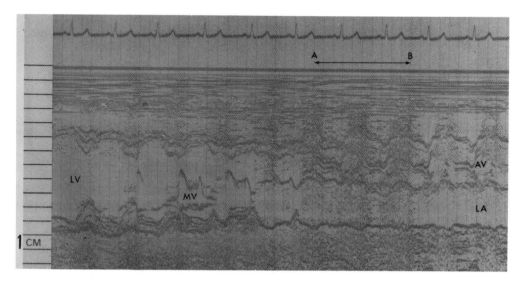

Fig. 2-24. A 52-year-old female patient with aortic insufficiency. The scan was from the left ventricle to the aorta. Area A↔B was recorded at identical amplification used to record ventricular wall echoes. The visualization of the aortic root and the valvular motion improved when the gain was decreased. LV, left ventricle; MV, mitral valve; AV, aortic valve; LA, left atrium.

If the patient's heart is positioned vertically within the chest, the transducer must be angled more cephalad than usual. Horizontal cardiac placement requires exaggerated medial transducer angulation. Horizontal cardiac placement should be expected in patients with unusual elevation of the diaphragm, massive ascites, obesity, pregnancy, or increased thoracic diameter.

Motion

Mechanical filling and emptying of the left atrium is probably most responsible for the anterior-posterior displacement of the aortic root.[6] A normal aortic root shows four patterns of movement throughout a cardiac cycle (Fig. 2–25). Rapid anterior movement toward the transducer occurs at the onset of mechanical systole, corresponding to left atrial filling and ventricular ejection. A short time after aortic valve closure, rapid posterior displacement occurs coincident with rapid left atrial emptying and ventricular filling. Passive movement, being neither anterior nor posterior, corresponds to the conduit phase of left atrial emptying. Further posterior displacement occurs during atrial contraction and left atrial emptying. Systolic amplitude of the anterior aortic wall often exceeds that of the posterior wall and may be due to slight expansion of the aortic root during ejection[7] (Table 2–7).

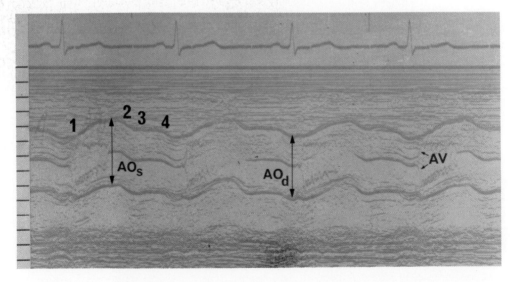

Fig. 2–25. A 47-year-old male patient with renal disease. The characteristic motion of the aortic root is: 1, anterior displacement at the onset of systole; 2, posterior displacement coincident with left atrial emptying; 3, mid-diastolic conduit phase; 4, posterior displacement coincident with atrial contraction. AO_s, end-systolic aortic root dimension; AO_d, diastolic aortic root dimension; AV, aortic valve motion.

Table 2-7.
Effect of Position of the Patient upon the Diastolic and Systolic Aortic Root Dimensions

Patient	Age (yr)	BSA (m^2)	Supine AO$_d$ (mm)	Supine AO$_s$ (mm)	LL AO$_d$ (mm)	LL AO$_s$ (mm)	Subxiphoid AO$_d$ (mm)	Subxiphoid AO$_s$ (mm)
A	53	1.66	25	30	26	30	22	25
B	58	1.72	30	30	—	—	33	33
C	41	1.64	25	25	—	—	30	33
D	56	1.71	35	35	34	36	32	34
E	57	1.66	31	32	31	32	34	35
F	55	1.96	32	33	33	33	35	38
G	43	2.14	35	37	35	38	32	37
H	62	1.89	—	—	30	31	29	32
I	61	2.03	—	—	30	33	30	30
J	41	1.91	28	29	30	32	31	32

Abbreviations: BSA, body surface area (per square meter); AO$_d$, diastolic dimension of aortic root; AO$_s$, systolic dimension of aortic root; LL, left lateral decubitus (partial).

Measurement

The aortic root dimension is obtained by measuring perpendicularly from the top of the anterior aortic root echo to the top of the posterior aortic root echo, coincident with the onset of ventricular depolarization on the electrocardiogram (Fig. 2–25). Although this measurement does not represent the true external or internal root dimension, it does provide definite reference points unaffected by amplification. Root dimension does not seem to be significantly influenced by the patient's position during examination (Table 2–7).

Relationship of Aortic Root with Transducer

Scans from the left ventricle and the mitral valve to the aortic root are useful to identify the transducer's relationship with these structures.[8] When the diastolic position of the anterior aortic wall and the diastolic position of the left septum are equidistant from the transducer, then the transducer has been positioned most perpendicularly over the ventricular base (Fig. 2–26). If the difference between these two measurements, aorta–transducer and left septum–transducer, exceeds 1 cm, then the transducer has been located closer to the apical portion of the left ventricle (Fig. 2–27). Greater cephalad angulation is required to obtain echoes from the aortic root when the transducer is in this position.

Scanning serves an additional purpose of establishing septal-aortic continuity. Apparent discontinuity may be achieved by positioning the transducer *above* the left ven-

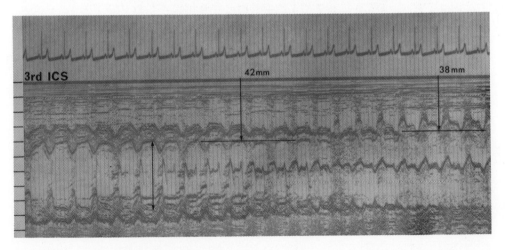

Fig. 2–26. A 24-year-old female patient with a kidney stone. The diastolic left septum was 42 mm from the transducer and the diastolic aortic wall was 38 mm from the transducer. The difference between these two measurements equaled less than 1 cm; this distance indicated that the transducer was relatively equidistant from the ventricular base and the aorta.

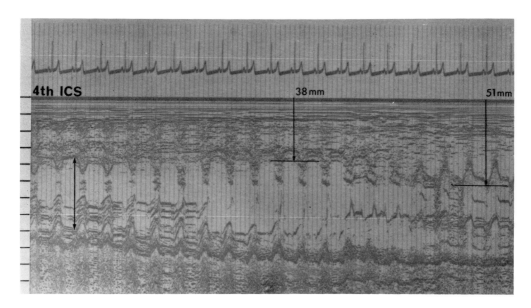

Fig. 2–27. Scan from patient in Figure 2–26. The transducer was moved one intercostal space lower and slightly laterally on the chest. The diastolic septum was 38 mm from the transducer; the diastolic anterior aortic wall was 51 mm from the transducer. The difference between these measurements exceeded 1 cm; this difference indicated that the transducer was in closer proximity to the cardiac apex. Echoes from the aorta were obtained only after extraordinary angulation superiorly toward this structure.

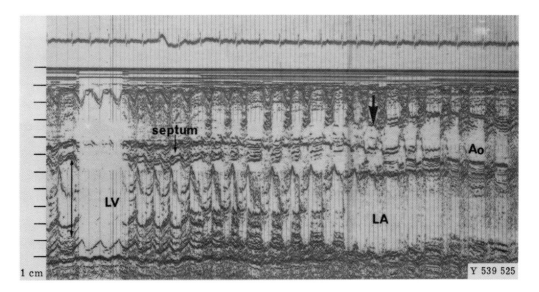

Fig. 2–28. A 51-year-old female patient with mitral insufficiency. The transducer was positioned in the second intercostal space and was angled from the left ventricle to the aorta. The aorta appeared to override both ventricles. No ventricular septal defect was identified during catheterization for evaluation of mitral regurgitation. Moderate pericardial effusion and a dilated left atrium were present. LV, left ventricle; Ao, Aorta; LA, left atrium; bold arrow, anterior aortic wall.

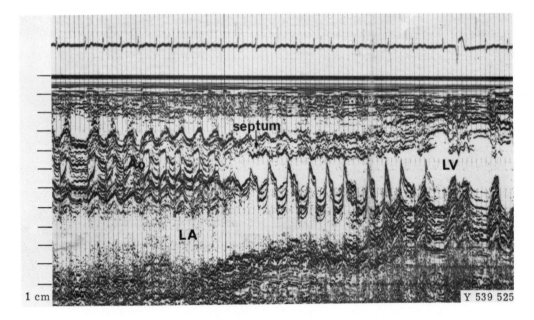

Fig. 2–29. Scan from the aorta to the left ventricle from the patient in Figure 2–28. Tracing from the third intercostal space showed a continuity between the anterior aorta and the septum. Ao, aorta; LV, left ventricle; LA, left atrium.

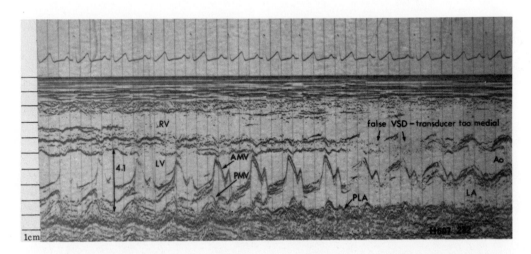

Fig. 2–30. A 13-year-old male patient with mild aortic stenosis and moderate mitral insufficiency. Selective dye curves revealed no evidence of intracardiac shunting. The loss of echoes in the membranous septum was due to excessive medial angulation of transducer during the scan from the left ventricle to the aorta. RV, right ventricle; LV, left ventricle; AMV, anterior mitral valve; PMV, posterior mitral valve; PLA, posterior left atrial wall; VSD, ventricular septal defect; Ao, aorta; LA, left atrium.

tricular base. The aorta appears to override the ventricular septum, even though no anatomic overriding exists (Fig. 2–28). Positioning the transducer in a lower intercostal space eliminates this artifact (Fig. 2–29). Parasternal, long-axis, two-dimensional echocardiography is the preferred method to establish the presence of an overriding aorta (see Fig. 8–1).

Loss of echoes in the area of the membranous septum suggests the presence of a ventricular septal defect. Morphologically incorrect tracings may be achieved from normal persons by angling the transducer too medially while scanning from the ventricle to the aorta (Fig. 2–30). Multiple scans from several intercostal spaces should be performed when the patient is supine and when in a partially left lateral position. If echoes cannot be recorded from the membranous septal area from several intercostal spaces, then a large, membranous ventricular septal defect is probably present (Figs. 2–31 and 2–32). Compatibility of clinical findings with the echocardiographic evidence is essential.

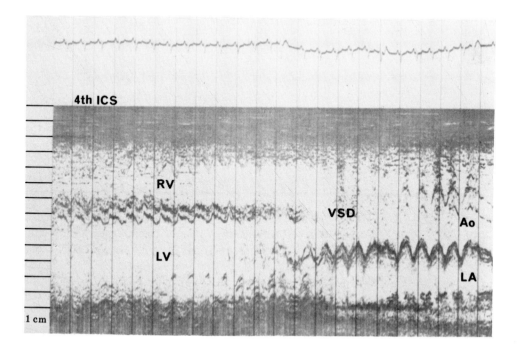

Fig. 2–31. A 44-year-old male patient with tetralogy of Fallot. Note the loss of echoes from the area of the membranous septum and the overriding septum (septal-aortic discontinuity). RV, right ventricle; LV, left ventricle; VSD, ventricular septal defect; Ao, aorta; LA, left atrium.

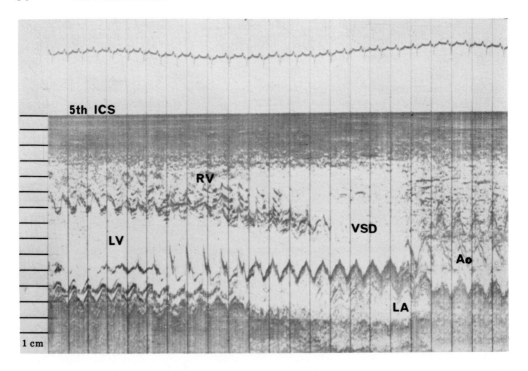

Fig. 2–32. Scan from the apex to the left atrium from the patient in Figure 2–31. The discontinuity between the septum and the anterior aorta persisted from the lower intercostal space. The complete absence of echoes from the membranous septum suggested a large ventricular septal defect. The anterior aorta did not appear to override from this new examination site. LV, left ventricle; RV, right ventricle; VSD, ventricular septal defect; LA, left atrium; Ao, aorta.

Catheter Artifact

Although reflections from a catheter often display greater intensity than the surrounding tissue, this is not always true. Swan-Ganz catheters positioned in the pulmonary artery can be mistaken for anterior aortic root motion (Fig. 2–33). To identify catheter motion, one should correlate the movement with an electrocardiogram and motion of the posterior aortic root. Whereas aortic root motion shows anterior displacement with the onset of systole, catheter motion is discordant. We have observed discordant aortic wall motion in patients with aortic root aneurysm secondary to Marfan's syndrome. In these cases, the aortic root was abnormally widened.

NORMAL AORTIC VALVE

Normal aortic valve tissue returns echoes of less intensity than do the walls of the aortic root (Fig. 2–34). Echoes returned from an anterior right coronary cusp and the posterior noncoronary cusp exhibit systolic patterns of motion resem-

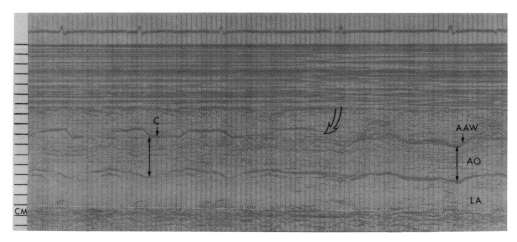

Fig. 2–33. A 32-year-old female patient with Pickwickian syndrome and congestive heart failure. The structure initially thought to be an anterior aortic root was a Swan-Ganz catheter (C). The systolic motion was discordant with the posterior aortic root motion. The tracing was obtained by angling the transducer medially to record the motion of the catheter, then rotated slightly cephalad to record the true anterior aortic wall motion. Open arrow, discontinuity between these 2 structures; AAW, anterior aortic wall motion; AO, aorta, LA, left atrium. (Tracing recorded by Julie Arthur, Medical College of Ohio, Toledo, Ohio.)

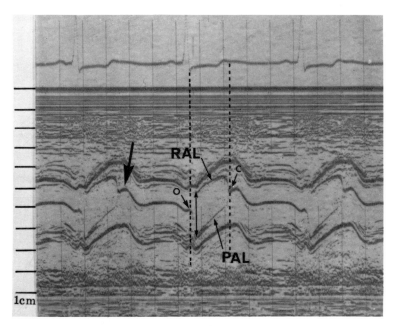

Fig. 2–34. A normal 23-year-old male. Normal aortic root and leaflet motion during sinus rhythm are shown. Bold arrow, anterior motion of aortic root and leaflets probably related to continued left atrial filling against closed mitral leaflets during isovolumic relaxation; RAL, right anterior leaflet motion; PAL, posterior noncoronary leaflet motion, o, open; c, closed.

bling a box. The shape of this box is dependent upon the patient's heart rate, stroke volume, and the pliability and size of the leaflets. Motion from the left anterior leaflet is usually not recorded, since its plane of systolic movement is away from the sound beam.

Shortly after ventricular depolarization, ejection of blood forces the leaflets to open widely toward the peripheral walls of the aortic root. Some systolic vibration of the leaflets is common and assists differentiation of leaflet tissue from the walls of the aortic root (Fig 2–35). Maximum cusp separation occurs in early systole with diminishing separation throughout mid-to-late systole. Rapid aortic valve closure begins with the onset of isovolumic left ventricular relaxation. Leaflet closure occurs simultaneously with the second heart sound. Following leaflet closure, the valve and aortic root continue a slight

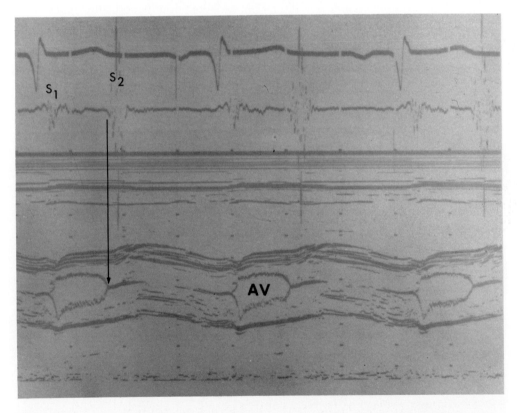

Fig. 2–35. A 24-year-old male illicit drug user with a malfunction of Bjork-Shiley tilting disc valve in the mitral position, congestive heart failure, and massive tricuspid insufficiency. Mild systolic fluttering of the aortic leaflets is a common phenomenon of no known clinical significance. The posterior cusp showed marked, early systolic rebound movement consistent with decreased flow through the valve. The end-systolic leaflet closure occurred simultaneously with the onset of the second heart sound (S$_2$). AV, motion of anterior and posterior aortic cusps during diastole and systole.

anterior movement toward the transducer. This movement, of short duration, may be related to continued left atrial filling against a closed mitral valve during isovolumic relaxation (Fig. 2–34).

Recording Technique

An electrocardiographic "Q" wave and echographic aortic leaflet opening and closing movements must be recorded simultaneously. Aortic leaflet motion is best recorded when the sound beam transects the sinuses of Valsalva. If the sound beam is not angled superiorly enough above the fibrous mitral-aortic junction, the posterior aortic cusp's movement will not be seen. One should use a simultaneous phonocardiogram to identify the end of mechanical systole when aortic leaflet closure cannot be achieved. Excessive reflection of echoes from aortic leaflets during diastole suggests leaflet thickening (Fig. 2–36). Parasternal, long-axis, two-dimensional echocardiography is then necessary to show the normal curvature of the closed aortic cusps as a potential source of the multiple echoes (Figs. 2–37 and 8–1).

If one wishes to measure systolic time intervals from the aortic echogram, the paper recording speed should be 100 mm/sec and never less than 50 mm/sec. If time lines are available, they should be spaced 40 msec apart.

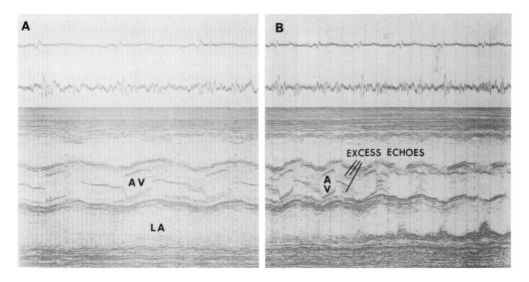

Fig. 2–36. A 58-year-old male patient with acute inferior myocardial infarction. *A,* The normal appearance of an aortic valve echogram during diastole and systole. *B,* The transducer angulation was altered slightly and the amplification was slightly increased. There appeared to be increased echo-reflectiveness from the aortic leaflets during diastole (see Fig. 2–37). AV, aortic valve motion; LA, left atrium.

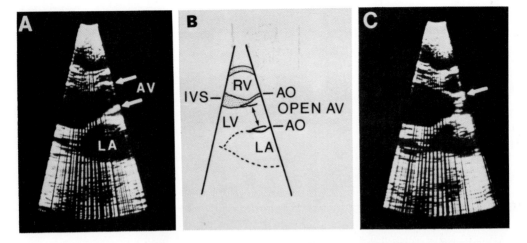

Fig. 2–37. Single frames of a long-axis, two-dimensional echogram of the aortic valve from the patient in Figure 2–36. A, B, Early systolic position of anterior aortic leaflet and posterior noncoronary aortic leaflet. C, Diastolic position of these leaflets. The leaflets curve inward toward the left ventricular outflow tract. Sound reflected from these curved surfaces produced multiple diastolic echoes recorded on the aortic valve M-mode echogram shown in Figure 2–36. AV, aortic valve; LA, left atrium; RV, right ventricle; LV, left ventricle; IVS, interventricular septum; Ao, aorta; single arrow in C, closed and centrally positioned aortic leaflets.

Systolic Time Intervals

Movement of the aortic leaflets provides an attractive method to achieve systolic time intervals when carotid arterial pulses are not suitable for evaluation or cannot be obtained.[9] Combining echographic systolic time intervals with M-mode and two-dimensional echocardiographic evaluation of left ventricular function permits an effective, noninvasive evaluation of the patient's cardiac status.

Measurement of Pre-ejection Period (PEP). The pre-ejection period represents the time needed to generate enough pressure to move blood from the left ventricle into the aorta. This time interval is measured from the onset of the electrocardiographic "Q" wave to the initial aortic leaflet separation (Fig. 2–38). Although we are not sure precisely when blood begins to enter the aorta, the onset of leaflet separation is a consistent point of reference for measurement. In some patients, the aortic leaflets separate rapidly. In other patients, the aortic leaflets separate slowly, with increasing acceleration occurring 10 to 20 msec later (Fig. 2–39).

If time lines are not available on the recording equipment, systolic time intervals can still be calculated as follows: Measure the distance between the "Q" wave and the onset of aortic leaflet opening with fine-pointed calipers and read to the nearest 0.25 mm on a graduated ruler. Divide by the paper

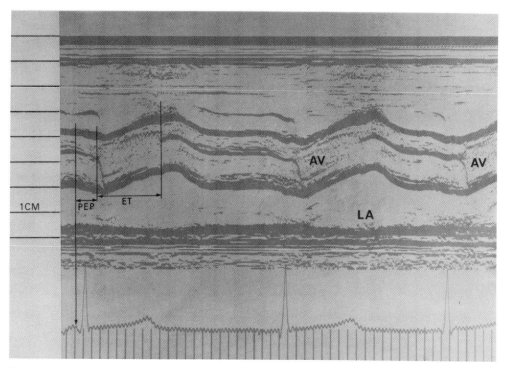

Fig. 2–38. A nine-year-old male patient with a wandering atrial pacemaker. The pre-ejection time (PEP) was measured from the electrocardiographic "Q" to the initial aortic leaflet opening. The ejection time (ET) was measured from the initial aortic leaflet opening to the end-systolic leaflet closure. Pre-ejection time may also be obtained by subtracting the ejection time from the total electromechanical systole (PEP + ET). AV, aortic valve motion; LA, left atrium.

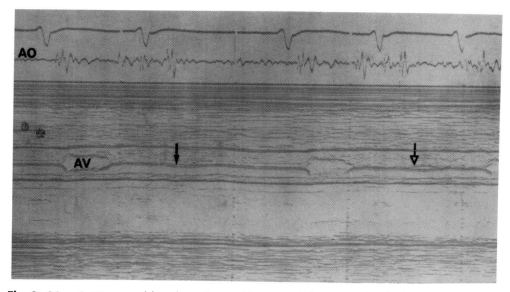

Fig. 2–39. A 41-year-old male patient with severe left ventricular dysfunction following mitral valve replacement. The aortic leaflets exhibited diminished opening excursion, drifting toward a closed position throughout systole and consistent with a poorly sustained flow through the valve during systole. Arrows, aortic leaflets that failed to open during systole; AO, phonocardiogram recorded from third right intercostal space; AV, aortic leaflet motion.

recording speed in mm/sec, also read to the nearest 0.25 mm. Multiply the quotient by 1000 to express this time interval in milliseconds.

Measurement of Ejection Time (ET). The left ventricular ejection time represents the duration of sustained blood flow through the aortic leaflets. Ejection time is measured from the initial onset of aortic leaflet opening to complete leaflet closure or the onset of the second heart sound (Fig. 2–38).

If time lines are not available on the recording equipment, this time interval may also be calculated by the same method used to calculate the pre-ejection time interval. Measure the distance between aortic leaflet opening and aortic leaflet closure with fine-pointed calipers and read to the nearest 0.25 mm on a graduated ruler. Divide the paper recording speed in mm/sec, also read to the nearest 0.25 mm. Multiply the quotient by 1000 to express this time interval in milliseconds.

Pre-ejection and ejection time intervals are influenced by age and heart rate. Whereas the systolic time interval ratio (PEP/ET) is affected by neither of these variables, normal ratios can be obtained from abnormal time intervals. In these cases, each time interval must be corrected for heart rate.[10] Normal values and clinical application of systolic time intervals may be found in a review of this method.[11]

NORMAL RIGHT VENTRICLE

The thin, anterior, right ventricular wall is the first moving structure encountered by the ultrasonic beam as it passes through the left or right parasternal chest wall[12] (Fig. 2–40). In the adult, right ventricular epicardial and endocardial interfaces are often poorly defined (Fig. 2–41). Lower-frequency transducers (3.5 MHz and 2.25 MHz) and higher-gain settings are required to record motion of cardiac structures deeper in the adult chest. These conditions are not favorable for visualization of the right ventricular wall. Second, the transducer is seldom perpendicular to the epicardium and endocardium of the right ventricle when septal and posterior left ventricular wall motion are recorded. The resultant tracings of right ventricular wall motion are incomplete throughout a cardiac cycle or show poor movement.

Recording Technique

Epicardial and endocardial interfaces are not immediately obvious during cursory examination along the left parasternum. Scanning from the left ventricle to the aorta helps to localize these structures (Fig. 2–42). The paper recording speed should be increased to facilitate analysis of wall thickness and motion (Fig. 2–43).

Technically adequate right ventricular wall thickness could not be recorded from the left parasternum or through the

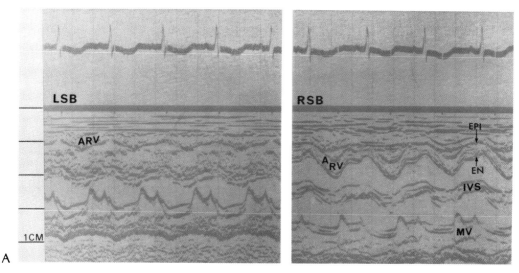

Fig. 2–40. A normal 12-hour-old male infant, supine and asleep. The anterior right ventricular epicardium (EPI) and endocardium (EN) recorded from the right and left sternal borders demonstrated different systolic wall excursion. *A* (LSB), left sternal border; *B* (RSB), right sternal border; ARV, anterior right ventricular wall; IVS, interventricular septum; MV, mitral valve motion. (From Chang, S., Roberts, S., Chang, J., Kleinberg, M., and Torres, R.: Technique of echographic examination of right ventricular wall thickness from the right sternal border. Jpn. Heart J., *20*: 289, 1979.)

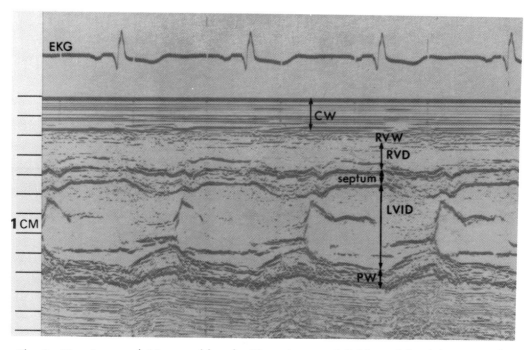

Fig. 2–41. A normal 18-year-old male. There is poor definition of the right ventricular wall thickness in contrast to the signals returned from the left ventricular walls. CW, chest wall; RVW, right ventricular wall; RVD, right ventricular cavity; LVID, left ventricular cavity; PW, posterior left ventricular wall.

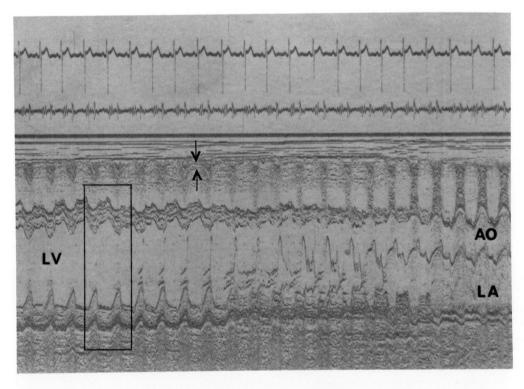

Fig. 2–42. A normal 22-year-old female. In this compressed scan from the left ventricle to the aorta, the right ventricular epicardial and endocardial interfaces (arrows) were poorly visualized until the sound beam transected the right and left ventricles at the level of mitral chordae tendineae. LV, left ventricle; AO, Aorta; LA, left atrium; enclosed box, location of left ventricular echoes recorded in Figure 2–43.

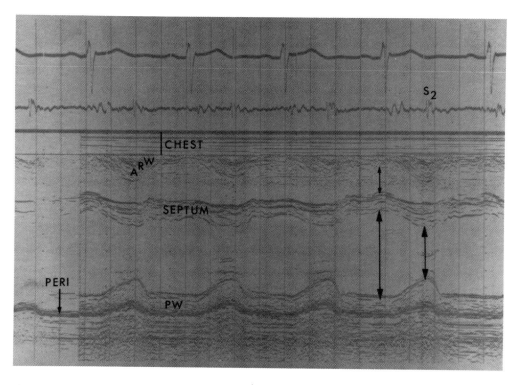

Fig. 2–43. The paper recording speed increased while monitoring the segment of right and left ventricular wall motion shown in the "box" in Figure 2–42. The right ventricular endocardium was well defined throughout the cardiac cycle. During diastole, the right ventricular epicardial interface was poorly seen and the wall thickness was not measured. ARV, anterior right ventricular wall; PERI, pericardium; PW, posterior left ventricular wall; S_2, second heart sound, and termination of mechanical systole.

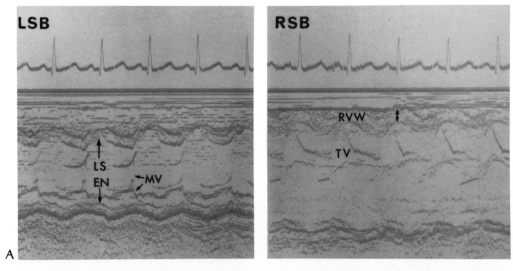

Fig. 2–44. A 10-year-old female patient with a small ventricular septal defect, QpQs ratio, 1.2:1. The peak right ventricular systolic pressure was 20 mm Hg. *A* (LSB), the right ventricular wall's motion could not be identified from the left sternal border. *B*(RSB), the patient was turned to a partial right lateral decubitus position and the transducer, located along the right sternal border, was angled medially toward the tricuspid valve. LS, left septum; EN, endocardial surface of posterior left ventricular wall; RVW, right ventricular wall; LSB, left sternal border; RSB, right sternal border; TV, tricuspid valve motion.

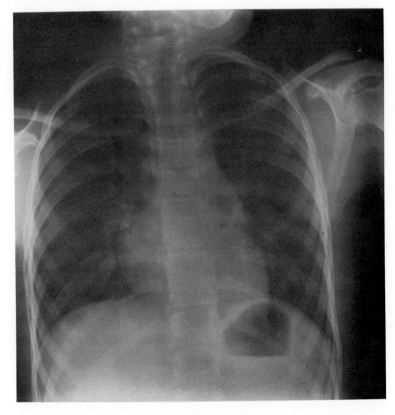

Fig. 2–45. A chest film of the patient in Figure 2–44.

sternum in some pediatric patients (Fig. 2–44). This phenomenon has been seen more often in children whose hearts have shifted or have rotated rightward (Fig. 2–45). In these cases, the transducer has been relocated along the right parasternum (Fig. 2–46).

If the adult heart is shifted or is rotated rightward, an examination of right ventricular wall thickness and motion should be attempted along the right parasternum. Tracings may not be achieved in every patient because of increased lung overlay in this region. Examination is easier if the patient is turned to a partial or steep right lateral decubitus position. A pillow tucked behind the patient's back aids comfort and stability.

Recumbent infants and children under two years of age can be examined from the right parasternum without difficulty. Children over the age of two years are more easily examined when the heart is rotated toward the right sternum. The transducer should be angled medially toward the tricuspid valve or the mitral valve with little superior or inferior angulation. Tricuspid or mitral valve motion is a reproducible landmark for comparative serial study of the right ventricular wall thickness. Measurements are derived from tracings showing maximum systolic wall motion (Fig. 2–47).

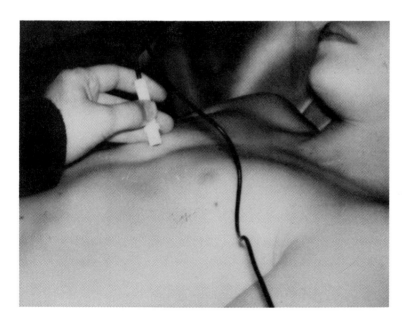

Fig. 2–46. The relation of the transducer to the chest wall during examination from the right sternal border. This individual required only minimal right lateral positioning for optimal recording of right ventricular wall motion.

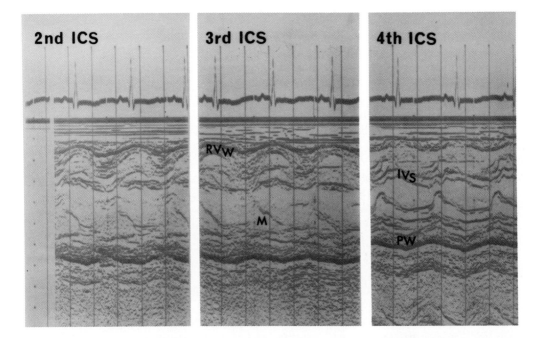

Fig. 2–47. A four-month-old female patient with acyanotic tetralogy of Fallot. The right ventricular wall motion and thickness were only obtained from different intercostal spaces along the *right* parasternum. RVW, right ventricular wall; M, mitral valve motion; IVS, interventricular septum; PW, posterior left ventricular wall. (From Chang, S., Roberts, S., Chang, J., Kleinberg, M., and Torres, R.: Technique of echographic examination of right ventricular wall thickness from the right sternal border. Jpn. Heart J., *20*: 289, 1979.) (Tracing recorded by Susan Roberts, Medical College of Ohio, Toledo, Ohio.)

Instrumentation. Right ventricular epicardial and endocardial interfaces were more readily identified with little reject, moderate damping, and higher-frequency transducers ranging from 3.5 to 7.0 MHz for premature infants. Infants with small right ventricular cavities were examined without depth compensation. Infants with dilated right ventricular cavities, and older children and adults with more developed right ventricles, permitted the use of depth compensation and low amplification of reflections from the anterior wall (Fig. 2–48).

Measurement and Evaluation of Right Ventricular Wall

Right ventricular wall thickness was measured from the top of the epicardial echo to the top of the endocardial echo, coincident with the electrocardiographic "Q" wave (see Fig. 2–40). Measurements of the right ventricular wall thickness were similar when epicardial and endocardial interfaces were identified from both sides of the sternum (Table 2–8).

Occasionally, the anterior right ventricular wall separates from the inner chest wall during systole. This minor separa-

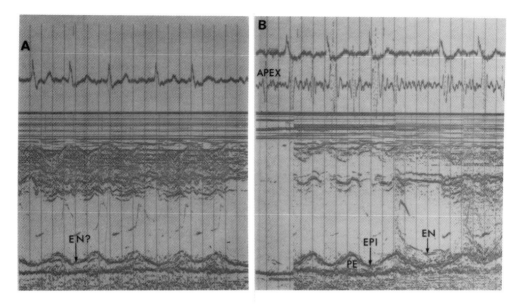

Fig. 2-48. A 65-year-old female patient with pericardial effusion. *A,* Echoes from the right ventricular wall and the septum were over-amplified, obscuring blood-tissue interfaces of these structures. The echo designated *EN?* was initially thought to originate from the left ventricular endocardium. *B,* Low-intensity echoes from the myocardium and the endocardium were amplified. *EN?* was actually the epicardial interface of the posterior left ventricular wall. Amplification of echoes near the chest wall was decreased to show the right ventricular wall and septal motion. EPI, epicardium; EN, endocardium; PE, pericardial effusion.

tion between a stationary structure (chest wall) and a dynamic structure (right ventricular wall) does not represent significant anterior pericardial effusion in the absence of other clinical or echographic findings. In fact, this separation can be used to differentiate right ventricular wall tissue from chest wall tissue (Fig. 2-48).

Normal right ventricular wall thickness exceeds wall thickness of the left ventricle during the immediate postnatal period. Some right ventricular atrophy should occur during the first months of life, resulting in a loss of right ventricular wall thickness.[13,14] This thickness is regained slowly from infancy to adulthood. Persistent or increasing right ventricular wall thickness in the pediatric patient can indicate chronic pressure elevation in the right heart or in the pulmonary system.

Adult right ventricular wall thicknesses ranged from 3.0 to 9.0 mm, averaging 5.0 mm when recorded with 2.25 MHz transducers (Table 2-9). Using the subcostal approach, the right ventricular wall measurement tends to be thicker than wall measurements obtained from the left parasternum (Table 2-9). Subcostal right ventricular wall thickness has been

Table 2–8.
Measurement of Right Ventricular Wall Thickness by Echocardiography

Patient	Age	BSA (m²)	Wall Thickness (mm)		Wall Amplitude (mm)		RVp (mm Hg)	Diagnosis
			RSB	LSB	RSB	LSB		
Endocardial and epicardial motion recorded at right and left sternal borders								
A	72 hr	0.20	2.4	2.3	1.8	1.9	NC	Normal
B	21 days	0.19	2.6	2.6	2.7	2.3	NC	Normal
C*	49 days	0.23	3.0	2.4	4.2	1.0	NC	Normal
D	10 mo	0.32	6.7	6.4	5.7	7.3	92/0	Taussig-Bing syndrome
E†	3 yr	0.69	6.0	6.2	4.1	4.8	88/8	ECD, PA banding, age 1 yr
F	4 yr	0.77	3.9	3.7	4.0	3.5	NC	AS, mild, congenital
G	5 yr	0.66	5.4	6.5	5.4	3.4	67/9	PS
Epicardium seen at right sternal border only; endocardium seen at right and left sternal borders								
H	24 hr	0.18	6.2	3.6	4.6	5.2	51/10	ECD
I	96 hr	0.19	3.2	3.0	3.8	2.5	NC	Normal
J	2 mo	0.30	3.6	2.6	4.8	4.1	NC	VSD
K	5 mo	0.24	3.8	3.3	3.1	1.3	22/9	PDA
L	13 mo	0.38	4.1	3.3	6.3	4.9	24/4	PDA
M	13 mo	0.46	6.5	5.4	5.9	3.8	106/18	VSD + PS
N	5 yr	0.82	3.7	3.1	6.1	3.3	NC	AS, mild, congenital
O	6 yr	0.68	5.3	3.5	4.9	4.2	23/4	Coarctation of aorta
P	6 yr	0.81	5.1	3.0	6.0	4.1	30/4	PS
Q	12 yr	1.34	7.6	5.6	6.8	4.9	84/7	PS

* Died at home; right ventricular wall thickness at autopsy was 2.0 mm (10% formalin fixation, 18 days).
† Died after ECD repair; right ventricular wall thickness at autopsy was 6.0 mm (fresh specimen).
Abbreviations: BSA, body surface area (per square meter); RSB, right sternal border; LSB, left sternal border; RVp, right ventricular pressure; NC, no catheterization; ECD, endocardial cushion defect; PA, pulmonary artery; AS, aortic stenosis; PS, pulmonic stenosis; VSD, ventricular septal defect.
(Modified with permission from Chang, S., et al.: Technique of echographic examination of right ventricular wall thickness from the right sternal border. Jpn. Heart J., 20:289, 1979.)

Table 2-9.
Right Ventricular Wall Thickness in 20 Persons Without Evidence of Cardiovascular Disease

Patient	Sex	Age (yr)	BSA (m²)	Supine (mm)	Position LL (mm)	Subxiphoid (mm)	Tobacco use (yr)
A	M	41	1.99	5	6	6	10
B	F	41	1.39	4	4	5	17
C	F	41	1.91	5	5	8	0
D	M	41	1.67	3	3	6	0
E	M	41	2.05	5	6	9	18
F	M	42	2.00	5	5	7	0
G	F	42	1.64	5	5	7	21
H	M	43	2.14	3	5	8	18
I	M	44	2.10	5	5	8	5
J	M	44	2.00	4	5	6	0
K	F	45	1.58	3	4	4	0
L	M	45	2.02	3	5	6	10
M	F	46	1.53	3	4	7	26
N	F	46	1.90	5	5	5	20
O	M	46	2.04	5	5	9	25
P	M	48	2.02	6	7	6	33
Q	F	48	1.77	3	3	5	0
R	M	50	1.80	5	5	8	32
S	M	50	1.80	3	5	5	30
T	F	51	1.67	4	4	6	34

Abbreviations: BSA, body surface area (per square meter); LL, left lateral decubitus.

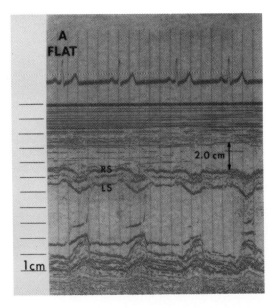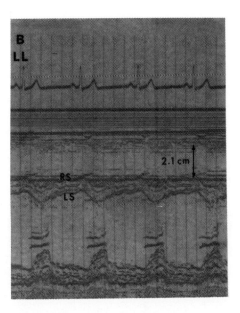

Fig. 2–49. A normal 29-year-old male. *A* and *B*, The right ventricular dimension was essentially unchanged as the patient was rotated from a supine position to a left lateral decubitus position. RS, right side of septum; LS, left side of septum. (From Chang, S.: The representative septum. Med. Ultrasound, *0(8):7*, 1976.)

shown to be comparable to that obtained from the left parasternum if recorded simultaneously with the tricuspid valve.[15]

Measurement and Evaluation of Right Ventricular Dimension

Right ventricular dimensions obtained from an M-mode echocardiogram are not representative of the dimension of this chamber, since the majority of the right ventricular cavity lies under the sternum. The measurement represents only that portion of the right ventricle that is anterior to the left ventricle along the left parasternum. A dimension is obtained by drawing a perpendicular line from the right ventricular endocardium to the right side of the interventricular septum at the onset of the electrocardiographic "Q" wave (Fig. 2–49).

Generally, the right ventricular dimension does not change dramatically when the patient is rotated from a supine to a left lateral position (Table 2–10). However, a few patients exhibit excessive clockwise rotation of the heart when they are changed from a recumbent to a left lateral decubitus position (Fig. 2–50). Before assigning "right ventricular enlargement" to these persons, all other variables on the echocardiogram should be examined and correlated with the patient's clinical findings to exclude a disorder that would cause the right heart to enlarge.

Table 2–10.
**Effect of Positional Change upon the Right Ventricular Dimension in
24 Normal Persons**

Patient	Age (yr)	BSA (m²)	Sex	RV DIMENSION (mm) Supine	LL	Subxiphoid
A	40	2.31	M	24	26	12
B	41	2.05	M	22	31	27
C	41	1.67	M	18	24	20
D	44	2.10	M	23	30	7
E	45	2.02	M	29	24	7
F	46	1.90	M	21	23	18
G	50	1.80	M	19	21	7
H	55	1.68	M	13	29	8
I	57	1.87	M	10	23	12
J	58	2.03	M	20	19	4
K	61	2.03	M	10	10	14
L	62	2.12	M	12	22	22
M	42	1.84	F	21	23	6
N	45	1.58	F	20	21	5
O	46	1.53	F	10	16	19
P	48	1.77	F	18	18	10
Q	51	1.67	F	13	17	8
R	55	1.67	F	16	20	19
S	55	1.74	F	11	10	16
T	56	1.64	F	6	16	3
U	56	1.71	F	20	24	13
V	57	1.52	F	19	17	10
W	57	1.70	F	15	20	13
X	60	1.70	F	12	18	20

Abbreviations: BSA, body surface area (per square meter); RV, right ventricle; LL, partial left lateral decubitus.

Right ventricular dimensions are occasionally influenced by respiratory changes. The right ventricle enlarges during inspiration as more blood is returned to the right heart. The dimension decreases to normal values during expiration, and it is at this time that measurements should be taken (Fig. 2–51). Marked changes in the right ventricular dimension, with labored breathing and pericardial effusion or pericardial thickening, are consistent with cardiac tamponade. Correlation with clinical data is essential.

NORMAL LEFT VENTRICLE

The muscular, high-pressure chamber of the left ventricle lies directly behind, and is partially enveloped by, the right ventricle. The primary function of this chamber is to receive blood from the left atrium and to expel it again into the aorta. Our ability to analyze the pumping efficiency or function of the left ventricle is limited with M-mode echocardiography.

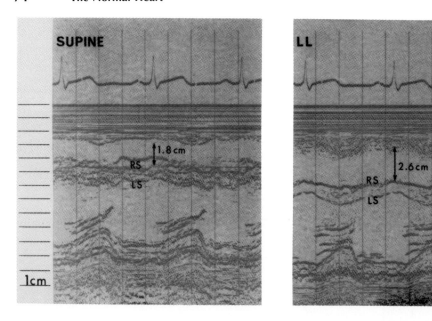

Fig. 2–50. A normal 21-year-old male professional hockey player. The right ventricular dimension and systolic septal excursion increased after rotation of the supine patient to the left lateral decubitus position (LL). RS, right side of septum; LS, left side of septum. (From Chang, S.: The representative septum. Med. Ultrasound, *0(8)*:7, 1976.)

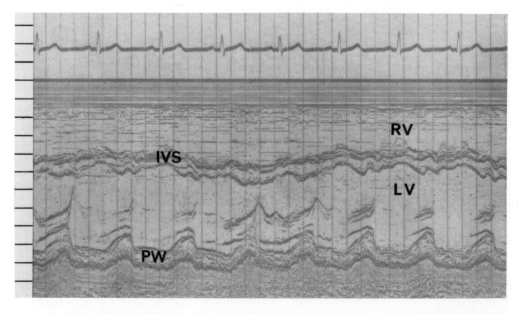

Fig. 2–51. A normal 38-year-old female. The undulating septal motion was due to respiration. The right ventricular dimension increased with inspiration and decreased with expiration. The dimension of the right ventricle should be measured during quiet expiration. IVS, interventricular septum; RV, right ventricle; LV, left ventricle; PW, posterior left ventricular wall.

This limitation is due to the small segments of ventricular muscle motion seen in "ice-pick" views through the heart (Fig. 2–52). Although "ice-pick" views from several intercostal spaces and subcostally enlarge our mental image of left ventricular size and quality of contraction, data from isolated planes of examination should not be used to *assume* overall ventricular shape and performance. Segmental motion does not necessarily represent intracardiac dimension, wall thickness, and function in other areas that cannot be monitored. Two-dimensional echocardiography is more suitable to provide spatial information concerning left ventricular shape

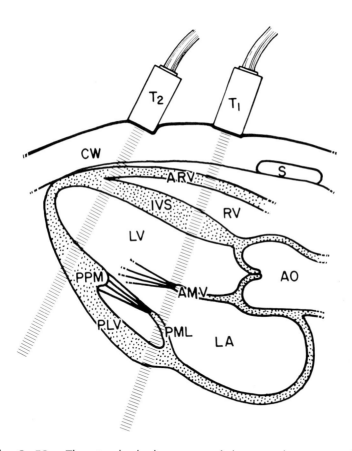

Fig. 2–52. The standard placement of the transducer over the heart for routine examination of the mitral valve, the base of left ventricle, the aorta, and the left atrium (T₁). The left ventricular wall motion and the dimension at the level of papillary muscles was obtained by moving the transducer one intercostal space lower and slightly laterally (T₂). CW, chest wall; PPM, posterior papillary muscle; LV, left ventricle; ARV, anterior right ventricular wall; RV, right ventricle; AMV, anterior mitral valve; PML, posterior mitral valve; LA, left atrium; AO, aorta; S, sternum; PLV, posterior left ventricular wall; IVS, interventricular septum.

and regional contraction. Systolic time intervals are useful, but not infallible, for assessment of overall left ventricular contraction.

A technically adequate left ventricular study requires simultaneous echographic motion of the right septum, left septum, free edges of the mitral valve, and endocardial, epicardial, and pericardial interfaces of the posterior left ventricular wall (Fig. 2–53). The plane from which one may record all these structures simultaneously is nearly identical in serial studies.[16] In addition to being reproducible, a technically satisfactory left ventricular study must be representative of the function of that segment of the heart being examined (Fig. 2–54).

Recording Technique

Site of Examination. Cursory examination of several intercostal spaces along the left sternal border may be necessary to localize the strongest reflected signals from the mitral leaflets. Then, by directing the transducer inferiorly and laterally, strong reflected signals should no longer be received from the mitral leaflets. Instead, the sound beam becomes more per-

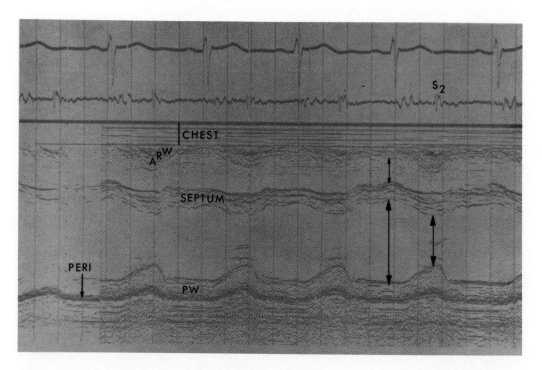

Fig. 2–53. A representative echogram of normal left ventricular walls just below the free edges of mitral leaflets. The right and left ventricular diastolic dimensions were measured simultaneously with the electrocardiographic "R" wave. It is now more desirable to measure these dimensions at the onset of left ventricular depolarization. The systolic dimension was measured at the onset of the second heart sound (S_2). ARV, anterior right ventricular wall; PERI, parietal pericardium; PW, posterior left ventricular wall.

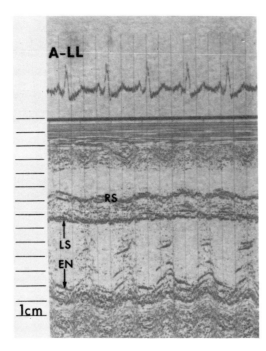
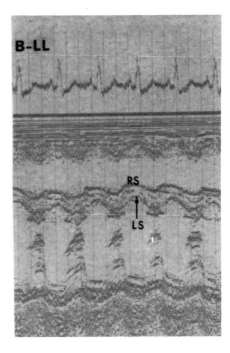

Fig. 2–54. A 61-year-old female with a murmur of aortic regurgitation four months following a Bjork-Shiley aortic valve replacement. *A,* The hypokinetic septum was not compatible with the patient's clinical findings. *B,* The slightest lateral angulation of the transducer in the same examination site showed normal septal motion. RS, right septum; LS, left septum; EN, endocardial surface of posterior left ventricular wall. (From Chang, S.: The representative septum. Med. Ultrasound, *0(8):7,* 1976.)

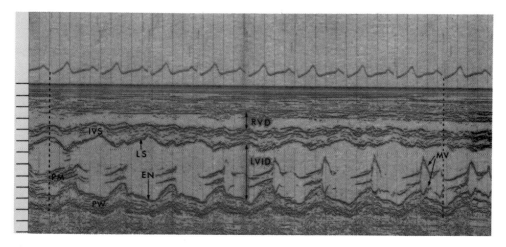

Fig. 2–55. An 18-year-old male patient with uremia. This was a normal scan from deep in the left ventricle to the mitral valve. The systolic septal excursion decreased as the transducer was angled superiorly and medially from posterior papillary muscle (PM) toward the mitral valve (MV). IVS, interventricular septum; LS, left septum; EN, endocardial surface of posterior left ventricular wall; RVD, diastolic right ventricular dimension; LVID, diastolic left ventricular dimension.

pendicular to the anterior septum and the posterior left ventricular wall at the level of the chordae tendineae. The systolic amplitude of the ventricular wall motion should increase. The right and left sides of the septum should move synchronously (Fig. 2–55). Variables of left ventricular function are routinely obtained from this region.

Position of the Patient. Initially, an echocardiographic examination is begun when the patient is supine with 20 to 30° elevation of the head and torso. However, most technically satisfactory tracings are achieved when the patient is rotated to a partial or steep left lateral decubitus position. As the patient is turned, the heart rotates clockwise and shifts laterally as the left lung is displaced (Fig. 2–56).

The intrathoracic position of the heart varies with the body habitus and the position of the patient.

The interventricular septum of tall, thin patients is often *vertically* oriented. The septum lies on a plane almost parallel to the ultrasound beam. This type of individual should be turned to an extreme left lateral decubitus position on a flat bed. One should relocate the transducer close to the left sternum and direct the beam laterally. Examination from several intercostal spaces may be necessary to locate maximum septal motion. The transducer can also be located at the right parasternum, directing the sound beam medially toward the sternum and the atrioventricular valves. If this examination site is used, the heart should be rotated further to

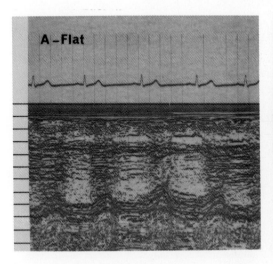
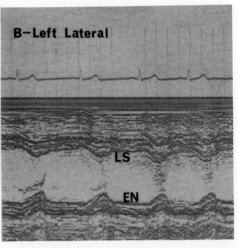

Fig. 2–56. A normal 19-year-old female. *A,* The left ventricular echogram from the supine patient. The quality of the record was technically unsuitable to evaluate septal thickness. *B,* The septal echogram improved after the patient was rotated to the left lateral position. The transducer was held in the same location on the chest at the left parasternum during the position change. The amplification was reduced slightly. LS, left septum; EN, endocardial interface of posterior left ventricular wall.

the right by turning the patient toward a right lateral decubitus position. The heart shifts rightward as the right lung is displaced. Left ventricular tracings may be achieved from the subcostal examination site (see Chap. 3). Often, this is the only source of septal echoes exhibiting maximum systolic movement.

A *horizontally positioned* heart causes many technical problems. When it is oriented with the cardiac apex directed toward the chest wall and the atria directed toward the spine, M-mode recordings of mitral valve and ventricular wall motion are fragmented, except near the apex or the aorta. This type of orientation is found in the patient with an increased thoracic diameter.

Other patients have horizontally positioned hearts, but the orientation is different. The cardiac apex is directed laterally toward the left rib cage and the atria are located midthoracically and medially. This orientation is found in obese patients, women in the third trimester of their pregnancy, or in patients with elevated diaphragms secondary to ascites. Elevation of the torso to a more upright or a sitting position may help to lower the horizontally positioned apex. The transducer has to be angled more medially to locate the aortic root and valvular motion and more laterally to record posterior left ventricular wall motion. The septum may display abnormal motion attributable to the peculiar relation of the septum to the sound beam. However, abnormal septal motion could be due to septal perfusion defects, or to right ventricular volume overloads, if accompanied by a dilated right ventricle and other appropriate clinical findings. Clinical correlation with the echocardiogram is necessary for accurate evaluation of the patient's true cardiac status.

Position of the Transducer. Positioning the transducer too laterally on the chest allows interference from the lung to preclude satisfactory studies (Fig. 2–57). To avoid excessive respiratory interference, one should rotate the patient toward a left lateral decubitus position and slide the transducer closer to the left parasternum. Examination may be necessary at another intercostal space. If nothing else works, the patient should hold his breath following quiet expiration.

Compressed scanning[8] is useful to determine whether the transducer is positioned more perpendicularly to the ventricular base or to the ventricular apex. Compressed scans are obtained by reducing the paper recording speed to approximately 10 mm/sec while the echocardiographer maintains constant transducer angulation changes from one area of the heart to another. Recording is continued nonstop throughout the entire scan.

The relationship of the transducer to the mitral valve becomes obvious when compressed scanning is used. If the

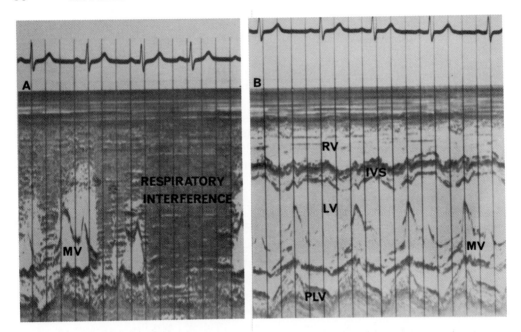

Fig. 2–57. *A,* The transducer was positioned along the left parasternum in the third intercostal space. Only the diastolic mitral valve motion could be recorded. *B,* The transducer was relocated at the fourth intercostal space to obtain motion from the left ventricular walls. RV, right ventricle; LV, left ventricle; MV, mitral valve motion; IVS, interventricular septal motion; PLV, posterior left ventricular wall.

transducer has been positioned perpendicular to the mitral valve's plane of movement, the diastolic distance between the left septum and the transducer is comparable to the distance between the anterior aorta and the transducer (see Fig. 2–26). Patterns of septal movement are unbroken throughout the cardiac cycle.

Relocation of the transducer closer to the papillary muscles reveals a compressed scan with different characteristics. The distances between the aorta and the transducer and the left septum and the transducer are no longer equivalent (see Fig. 2–27). The diastolic position of the anterior aortic wall appears to be posteriorly displaced when compared with the diastolic position of the left septum. In addition, the right and left sides of the septum do not exhibit continuous motion throughout the cardiac cycle. The pattern of motion is fragmented as the septum intermittently passes in and out of the sound beam. Motion from the posterior left ventricular wall and from the posterior mitral leaflet is poorly demonstrated. Ventricular wall thickness and mobility are best at the level of the papillary muscles and not at the desired level of the mitral chordae tendineae.

Measurements

Figure 2–58 is a representative echogram, showing the source of routine left ventricular measurements.

Septal Wall Thickness. Diastolic septal wall thickness is measured at the onset of electrical depolarization, from the top of the right septal-blood interface to the top of the left septal-blood interface. The uneven, trabeculated surface of the right septum is much more echo-reflective than is the smooth surface of the left septum.[17] Echoes from muscle bundles or tricuspid valve tissue can cause the right septum to appear heavily echo-reflective and can lead to an erroneous measurement of septal thickness.[18,19] Diastolic septal wall thickness varies with the position of the patient as the septum is rotated toward a better plane with respect to the interrogating sound beam. Measurements of septal thickness should remain within the normal limits (Table 2–11). Septal wall

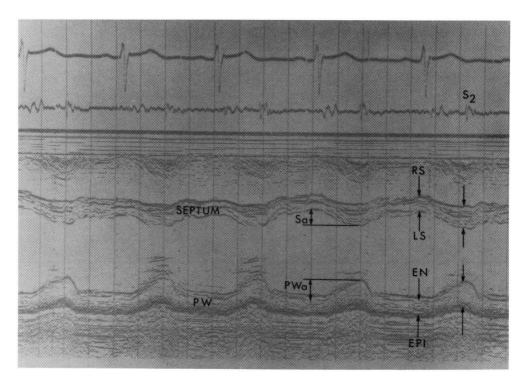

Fig. 2–58. A representative tracing exhibiting ventricular wall thickness and systolic excursion. The diastolic septal wall thickness was measured from the top of the right septum (RS) to the top of the left septal echo (LS). The diastolic posterior wall thickness was measured from the top of the endocardium to the top of the epicardium (EPI). Unmarked arrows, systolic wall thickness; PW, posterior left ventricular wall; Sa, systolic septal amplitude (excursion); PWa, systolic posterior left ventricular wall amplitude (excursion); S_2, second heart sound and termination of mechanical systole.

Table 2–11.
Effects of Position of the Patient on the Diastolic Left Ventricular Dimension and Wall Thickness in 20 Persons Without Cardiovascular Disease

Patient	Sex	Age (yr)	BSA (m²)	$LVID_d$ (mm)			PW_t (mm)			IVS_t (mm)		
				S	LL	Subx	S	LL	Subx	S	LL	Subx
A	F	41	1.39	45	42	40	8	8	8	8	8	8
B	F	46	1.53	40	40	38	7	8	7	8	7	9
C	F	45	1.58	41	43	45	10	10	10	10	10	10
D	F	52	1.62	44	42	42	9	9	10	9	8	9
E	F	58	1.63	41	39	38	10	8	10	9	8	10
F	F	41	1.64	41	45	43	10	10	10	8	8	10
G	M	57	1.66	43	43	38	9	8	10	9	9	10
H	M	41	1.67	44	42	42	10	9	10	8	9	10
I	F	45	1.70	41	45	48	8	8	7	8	8	10
J	M	56	1.71	48	41	50	9	9	9	9	9	9
K	F	50	1.72	45	50	47	10	10	9	9	7	9
L	F	55	1.74	48	47	50	10	11	9	9	10	9
M	F	48	1.77	47	50	47	10	10	11	10	10	10
N	F	50	1.80	44	46	41	10	9	9	8	9	9
O	F	42	1.84	43	40	42	10	11	11	10	11	11
P	M	57	1.87	49	43	48	11	10	10	8	10	10
Q	M	46	1.90	46	46	45	11	11	11	9	9	11
R	M	44	2.00	53	50	50	11	12	12	11	11	11
S	M	62	2.12	48	53	50	10	11	10	9	10	11
T	M	40	2.31	50	50	49	8	8	9	8	8	9

Abbreviations: BSA, Body surface area (per square meter); S, supine, 20° elevation of thorax and head; LL, left lateral position, 20° elevation of thorax and head; subx, subxiphoid; $LVID_d$, left ventricular internal dimension, diastole; PW_t, posterior wall thickness; IVS_t, interventricular septal wall thickness, diastole.

thickness should be comparable to posterior wall thickness in the absence of disease that could cause asymmetrical wall thickening.

Systolic septal wall thickness should be measured coincident with the second heart sound, or when the septum has reached its nadir of posterior displacement, or at the end of ventricular repolarization on the electrocardiogram. This last method may not be accurate if there is abnormally early or late ventricular repolarization.

Posterior Left Ventricular Wall Thickness. The posterior ventricular endocardial surface is trabeculated and thus is more echo-reflective. If the resolution of the echograph and its recorder is superb, it might be difficult to distinguish the true endocardial surface from the trabeculations. For practical purposes, this problem is solved by choosing those echoes that exhibit maximum mobility and synchrony of movement with other myocardial echoes arising from intramuscular inclusions and the epicardium.

Diastolic left ventricular wall thickness is measured at the onset of electrical ventricular depolarization, from the top of the endocardial echo to the top of the epicardial echo. If the epicardial echo is not well defined, then one should measure from the top of the pericardial echo. The thickness of the septum and the posterior wall thickness are similar in the normal person (Tables 2–11 and 2–12).

Systolic left ventricular wall thickness should be measured coincident with the onset of the second heart sound. If one is unable to record simultaneous heart sounds, the end of systole may be estimated by measuring wall thickness coincident with the end of ventricular repolarization on the electrocardiogram. Maximum anterior displacement of the wall can be used to determine the end of systole. However, this point may be abnormally late in the presence of cardiomyopathy, perfusion defects, and abnormal repolarization of the posterior left ventricular wall.

Diastolic Left Ventricular Dimension. Most left ventricular filling occurs during early diastole. The ventricular walls move rapidly away from each other as the chamber becomes distended with inflowing blood. The diameter of the filled chamber is measured at the onset of ventricular depolarization. Averaging dimensions from five or more sequential beats minimizes respiratory influences upon ventricular filling. Similar diameters of a left ventricle's minor axis can be obtained from the parasternal and subcostal examination sites (Table 2–11). Abnormally large or small ventricles are more detectable if the ventricular diameters are corrected for the body size (see Fig. Appendix–1). Diastolic left ventricular dimensions should not exceed 3.2 cm/M^2 in a person of normal body weight and height. This corrected value does not apply

Table 2–12.
Diastolic Left Ventricular Dimension and Wall Thickness in 26 Morbidly Obese Patients Without Cardiovascular Disease Prior to Ileobypass Operations

Patient	Age (yr)	HT (cm)	WT (kg)	BSA (m²)	BP (mm Hg)	LVID (cm)	LVID (cm/m²)	PW_t (mm)	IV_t (mm)
A	46	157	77.3	1.78	110/70	4.8	2.7	10	10
B	44	155	93.2	1.92	175/100	4.2	2.2	10	10
C	54	157	96.3	1.97	150/80	4.9	2.5	11	11
D	42	157	104.0	2.02	160/100	4.6	2.3	10	10
E	32	160	103.2	2.04	—	4.8	2.4	10	10
F	42	155	113.6	2.08	130/80	4.6	2.2	11	10
G	32	157	110.9	2.08	170/110	4.4	2.1	12	12
H	21	160	112.7	2.12	126/76	4.3	2.0	9	9
I	43	163	108.2	2.12	190/130	4.3	2.0	11	8
J	31	155	120.9	2.14	190/100	4.9	2.3	10	10
K	25	157	116.8	2.14	—	4.4	2.1	10	11
L	32	164	115.7	2.18	—	5.1	2.3	10	10
M	23	163	121.3	2.23	152/108	4.5	2.0	10	10
N	38	166	119.0	2.24	150/95	4.5	2.0	10	10
O	38	163	127.5	2.25	130/85	5.0	2.2	10	10
P	34	173	116.8	2.28	130/70	5.0	2.2	11	10
Q	26	169	127.7	2.32	160/98	5.0	2.2	12	12
R	21	170	131.4	2.32	160/110	4.3	1.9	12	12
S	30	165	133.2	2.34	—	4.3	1.8	10	10
T	22	165	137.5	2.36	—	5.3	2.2	10	10
U	28	173	132.7	2.39	—	4.5	1.9	11	11
V	27	165	154.1	2.45	160/100	5.8	2.4	10	10
W	30	178	138.2	2.50	160/90	4.4	1.8	10	10
X	19	180	143.6	2.60	140/80	5.1	2.0	11	10
Y	22	175	172.7	2.72	—	5.3	1.9	10	9
Z	34	175	190.0	2.84	—	5.3	1.9	12	12
RANGE	19–54			1.78–2.84		4.2–5.8	1.8–2.7	9–12	8–12
MEAN	32			2.25		4.7	2.1		
SD						±0.90	±0.24		

Abbreviations: BSA, body surface area (per square meter); BP, blood pressure; LVID, left ventricular internal dimension; PW, posterior left ventricular wall thickness; IV, interventricular septal wall thickness; SD, standard deviation.

to the obese patient. For this reason, echograms were obtained from 26 morbidly obese patients scheduled for ileobypass operations (Table 2–12). In this group, the mean diastolic left ventricular dimension, corrected for body size, was 2.1 ± 0.24 cm/M^2.

Systolic Left Ventricular Dimension. The minimum distance between the septum and the posterior left ventricular wall is achieved before or is coincident with the onset of the second heart sound. Five or more sequential beats should be averaged to obtain a more representative dimension.

Systolic Ventricular Wall Excursion. Systolic wall excursion is the amount of perpendicular displacement of each wall from its diastolic position to its position at the end of systole. Within 40 msec of the onset of ventricular depolarization, the anterior septum begins to move posteriorly away from the chest wall. The posterior left ventricular wall moves anteriorly toward the chest wall. This wall motion continues until the end of ejection. The quantity of wall displacement is a combination of wall thickening and decreasing intracavitary size during ventricular ejection. The change in volume allows the ventricular walls to move inward toward each other. Systolic wall displacement can occur without wall thickening, but this situation does not occur in the normal heart.

REFERENCES

1. Ranganathan, N., et al.: Morphology of the human mitral valve. II. The valve leaflets. Circulation, 41:459, 1970.
2. Konecke, L., et al.: Abnormal mitral valve motion in patients with elevated left ventricular diastolic pressures. Circulation, 47:989, 1973.
3. Schabelman, S., et al.: Comparison of four two-dimensional echocardiographic views for measuring left atrial size. Am. J. Cardiol., 41:391, 1978 (Abstr.).
3a. Goldberg, B.,: Ultrasonic measurement of the aortic arch, right pulmonary artery and left atrium. Radiology, 101:383, 1971.
4. Allen, H., et al.: Suprasternal notch echocardiography: assessment of its clinical utility in pediatric cardiology. Circulation, 55:605, 1977.
5. McAlpine, W.: Heart and Coronary Arteries. New York, Springer-Verlag, 1975, p. 2 (illus. 6); p. 18 (illus. 5 and 6); p. 22 (illus. 5); p. 32 (illus. 2 and 3).
6. Strunk, B., et al.: The posterior aortic wall echocardiogram: its relationship to left atrial volume change. Circulation, 54:744, 1976.
7. Brewer, R., et al.: The dynamic root: its role in aortic valve function. J. Thorac. Cardiovasc. Surg., 72:413, 1976.
8. Chang, S., et al.: Condensed M-mode echocardiographic scan of the symmetrical left ventricle. Chest, 68:93, 1975.
9. Stefadourous, M., et al.: Systolic time intervals by echocardiography. Circulation, 51:114, 1975.
10. Lewis, R., et al.: Systolic time intervals. In Noninvasive Cardiology. Edited by A.M. Weissler. New York, Grune & Stratton, 1974, p. 310 and Table 6–2.
11. Lewis, R., et al.: A critical review of the systolic time intervals. Circulation, 56:146, 1977.
12. Chang, S., et al.: Technique of echographic examination of right ventricular wall thickness from the right sternal border. Jpn. Heart J., 20:289, 1979.

13. Hort, W.: The normal heart of the fetus and its metamorphosis in the transition period. *In* The Heart and Circulation in the Newborn Infant. Edited by D.E. Cassels. New York, Grune & Stratton, 1966, p. 210.
14. Oda, T., et al.: Developmental aspects of pulmonary circulation; clinical implications of postnatal maturation of right heart system. Jpn. Circ. J., 38:887, 1974.
15. Matsukubo, H., et al.: Echocardiographic measurement of right ventricular wall thickness: A new application of subxiphoid echocardiography. Circulation, 56:278, 1977.
16. Stefadourous, M., et al.: Reproducibility of echocardiographic estimates of left ventricular dimension. Br. Heart J., 39:390, 1977.
17. McAlpine, W.: Heart and Coronary Arteries. New York, Springer-Verlag, 1975, p. 20 (illus. 3); p. 32 (illus. 1).
18. Roelandt, J., et al.: Resolution problems in echocardiology: a source of interpretation errors. Am. J. Cardiol., 37:256, 1976.
19. Allen, J., et al.: Problems in ultrasonic estimation of septal thickness. Am. J. Cardiol., 42:89, 1978.

BIBLIOGRAPHY

AORTA

Age-related Dimension

Allen, H., et al.: A quantitative echocardiographic study of champion childhood swimmers. Circulation, 55:142, 1977.
Epstein, M., et al.: Great vessel, cardiac chamber and wall growth patterns in nine children. Circulation, 51:1123, 1975.
Gerstenblith, G., et al.: Echocardiographic assessment of a normal adult aging population. Circulation, 56:273, 1977.
Henry, W., et al.: Echocardiographic measurements in normal subjects: Growth-related changes that occur between infancy and early adulthood. Circulation, 57:278, 1978.
Lortscher, R., et al.: Echocardiographic determinations of dimensions of normal newborns at 5, 280 feet elevation. J. Clin. Ultrasound, 2:51, 1975.

Anatomic Relationships, Technique, Measurement

Francis, G., et al.: Accuracy of echocardiography for assessing aortic root diameter. Br. Heart J., 37:376, 1975.
Furukawa, K., et al.: Proceedings: measurement of aortic root diameter by echocardiography. Jpn. Circ. J., 39:868, 1975.
Furukawa, K., et al.: Echocardiographic measurement of aortic root diameter. Jpn. Heart J., 17:465, 1976.
Gramiak, R., et al.: Echocardiography of the aortic root. Invest. Radiol., 3:356, 1968.
Nanda, N.: Echocardiography of the aortic root. Am. J. Med., 62:836, 1977.
Story, W., et al.: Echocardiographic criteria for the diagnosis of mitral semilunar valve continuity. Am. Heart J., 93:575, 1977.
Strunk, B., et al.: Echocardiographic recognition of the mitral valve—posterior aortic wall relationship. Circulation, 51:594, 1975.

Influence of Atrial, Ventricular Volume

Akgün, G., et al.: Aortic root and left atrial wall motion. Br. Heart J., 39:1082, 1977.
Burggraf, G., et al.: Aortic root motion determined by ultrasound: relation to cardiac performance in man. Cathet. Cardiovasc. Diagn., 4:29, 1978.
Lalani, A., et al.: Echocardiographic measurement of cardiac output using the mitral valve and aortic root echo. Circulation, 54:738, 1976.
Pratt, R., et al.: The influence of left ventricular stroke volume on aortic root motion; an echocardiographic study. Circulation, 53:947, 1976.
Strunk, B., et al.: The posterior aortic wall echocardiogram: its relationship to left atrial volume change. Circulation, 54:744, 1976.

Miscellaneous

Ambrose, J.: Hemodynamic correlates of late diastolic posterior motion of the aortic root. Am. Heart J., 100:433, 1980.

Atsuchi, Y., et al.: Echocardiographic manifestation of annuloaortic ectasia; its "paradoxical" motion of the aorta and premature systolic closure of the aortic valve. Am. Heart J., 93:428, 1977.

Charuzi, Y., et al.: Echocardiographic interpretation in the presence of Swan-Ganz intracardiac catheters. Am. J. Cardiol., 40:989, 1977.

Manouguian, S., et al.: Patch enlargement of the aortic valve ring by extending the aortic incision into the anterior mitral leaflet. New operative technique. J. Thorac. Cardiovasc. Surg., 78:402, 1979.

Tye, K., et al.: Relation between apexcardiographic a wave and posterior aortic wall motion. Am. J. Cardiol., 43:24, 1979.

Wasserman, A., et al.: The relationship of pulmonary wedge pressure to the posterior aortic wall echocardiogram in patients free of obstructive mitral valve disease. Am. Heart J., 100:500, 1980.

AORTIC VALVE

Anastassiades, P., et al.: Aortic valve closure: echocardiographic, phonocardiographic and hemodynamic assessment. Am. Heart J., 91:228, 1976.

Feizi, O., et al.: Echocardiography of normal and diseased aortic valve. Br. Heart J., 35:560, 1973.

Feizi, O., et al.: Echocardiography of the aortic valve. Studies of normal aortic valve, aortic stenosis, aortic regurgitation and mixed aortic valve disease. Br. Heart J., 36:341, 1974.

Gramiak, R., et al.: Echocardiography of the normal and diseased aortic valve. Radiology, 96:1, 1970.

Hernberg, J., et al.: The ultrasonic recording of aortic valve motion. Radiology, 94:361, 1970.

Hirschfeld, S., et al.: Intracardiac pressure-sound correlates of echographic aortic valve closure. Circulation, 55:602, 1977.

Laniado, S., et al.: Hemodynamic correlates of the normal aortic valve echogram. A study of sound, flow and motion. Circulation, 54:729, 1976.

Mills, P., et al.: Echocardiographic and hemodynamic relationships of ejection sounds. Circulation, 56:430, 1977.

Sakamoto, T., et al.: Echocardiogram in pulsus paradoxus. Respiration dependent cyclic changes in mitral and aortic valve motion: a case report. Jpn. Heart J., 18:883, 1977.

Shah, P.: Echocardiography of the aortic and pulmonary valves. Prog. Cardiovasc. Dis., 20:451, 1978.

Thubrikar, M., et al.: Normal aortic valve function in dogs. Am. J. Cardiol., 40:563, 1977.

CONTRAST ECHOCARDIOGRAPHY

Bove, A., et al.: Ultrasonic detection of in vivo cavitation and pressure. Effects of high-speed injections through catheters. Invest. Radiol., 4:236, 1969.

Gramiak, R., et al.: Ultrasound cardiography: contrast studies in anatomy and function. Radiology, 92:939, 1969.

Seward, J., et al.: Echocardiographic contrast studies: initial experience. Mayo Clin. Proc., 50:163, 1975.

Seward, J., et al.: Peripheral venous contrast echocardiography. Am. J. Cardiol., 39:202, 1977.

Wang, X., et al.: Contrast echocardiography with hydrogen peroxide. I. Experimental study. Chin. Med. J. (Engl.), 92:595, 1979.

Wang, X., et al.: Contrast echocardiography with hydrogen peroxide. II. Clinical application. Chin. Med. J. (Engl.), 92:693, 1979.

LEFT ATRIUM

Biancaniello, T., et al.: Left atrial size in childhood. J. Electrocardiol., 13:11, 1980.

Chandraratna, P.: Determination of zero reference level for left atrial pressure by echocardiography. Am. Heart J., 89:159, 1975.

Ewy, G., et al.: Response of atrial fibrillation to therapy: role of etiology and left atrial diameter. J. Electrocardiol., 13:119, 1980.

Francis, G., et al.: Echocardiographic criteria of normal left atrial size in adults. Circulation (Suppl.), 50:76, 1974 (Abstr.).

Hagan, A., et al.: Echocardiographic criteria for the normal newborn infants. Circulation, 48:1221, 1973.

Hirata, T., et al.: Estimation of left atrial size using ultrasound. Am. Heart J., 78:43, 1969.

Lundstrom, N., et al.: Clinical applications of echocardiography in infants and children. II. Estimation of aortic root diameter and left atrial size. A comparison between echocardiography and angiography. Acta Paediatr. Scand., 63:33, 1974.

Raizada, V., et al.: Simultaneous left atrial echocardiography and aortic blood velocity during right ventricular pacing in man. Chest, 73:532, 1978.

Sasse, L.: Echocardiography of left atrial wall. J.A.M.A. 228:1667, 1974.

Schuilenburg, R., et al.: Further observations on the ventricular echo phenomenon elicited in the human heart: is the atrium part of the echo pathway? Circulation, 45:629, 1972.

Solinger, R., et al.: Echocardiography in the normal neonate. Circulation, 47:108, 1973.

TenCate, F., et al.: Dimensions and volumes of left atrium and ventricle determined by single beam echocardiography. Br. Heart J., 36:737, 1974.

Yabek, S., et al.: Echocardiographic determination of left atrial volumes in children with congenital heart disease. Circulation, 53:268, 1976.

Yoshikawa, J., et al.: Study of posterior left atrial wall motion by echocardiography and its clinical application. Jpn. Heart J., 16:683, 1975.

LEFT VENTRICLE

Dimension

Belenkie, I.: Beat-to-beat variability of echocardiographic measurements of left ventricular end-diastolic diameter and performance. J. Clin. Ultrasound, 7:263, 1979.

Bennett, D., et al.: Test of reliability of echocardiographic estimation of left ventricular dimensions and volumes. Br. Heart J., 38:1133, 1976.

Bhatt, D., et al.: Accuracy of echocardiography in assessing left ventricular dimensions and volume. Circulation, 57:699, 1978.

Brenner, J., et al.: Effect of phasic respiration on left ventricular dimension and performance in a normal population. Circulation, 57:122, 1978.

Chang, S., et al.: Condensed M-mode echocardiographic scan of the symmetrical left ventricle. Chest, 68:93, 1975.

Cohen, J., et al.: The heart of a dancer: noninvasive cardiac evaluation of professional ballet dancers. Am. J. Cardiol., 45:959, 1980.

Conetta, D., et al.: Echocardiographic analysis of systolic and diastolic left ventricular wall motion in normal man. Chest, 76:76, 1979.

Cooperberg, P., et al.: Estimation of cardiac chamber size by routine chest radiography and echocardiography. Radiology, 119:193, 1976.

DeMaria, A., et al.: Systemic correlation of cardiac chamber size and ventricular performance determined with echocardiography and alterations in heart rate in normal persons. Am. J. Cardiol., 43:1, 1979.

Feigenbaum, H., et al.: Identification of ultrasound echoes from the left ventricle using intracardiac injections of indocyanine green. Circulation, 41:615, 1970.

Feigenbaum, H., et al.: Ultrasound measurements of the left ventricle: a correlative study with angiography. Arch. Intern. Med., 129:461, 1972.

Felner, J., et al.: Sources of variability in echocardiographic measurements. Am. J. Cardiol., 45:995, 1980.

Fiedler, V., et al.: Determination of left ventricular dimensions with ultrasound. J. Pharmacol. Methods., 3:201, 1980.

Gibson, D.: Estimation of left ventricular size by echocardiography. Br. Heart J., 35:128, 1973.

Gibson, D., et al.: Measurement of instantaneous left ventricular dimension and filling rate in man using echocardiography. Br. Heart J., 35:1141, 1973.

Lerman, B., et al.: Reciprocal changes in ventricular dimensions related to respiration. Arch. Intern. Med., 140:685, 1980.

Manoli, S.: An intraventricular ultrasound method for measurement of left ventricular dimensions. Biomed. Eng., 21:333, 1974.

Manoli, S.: An ultrasonic gauge for measurement of ventricular dimensions. Ultrasound Med. Biol., 3:247, 1977.

Marsh, J., et al.: Left ventricular end-systolic pressure-dimension and stress-length relations in normal human subjects. Am. J. Cardiol., 44:1311, 1979.

Mashiro, I., et al.: Comparison of measurement of left ventricle by echography and cineangiography. Jpn. Circ. J., 39:23, 1975.

Nieminen, M.: Normal left echoventriculography. Ann. Clin. Res., 7:1, 1975.

Popp, R., et al.: Effect of transducer placement on echocardiographic measurement of left ventricular dimensions. Am. J. Cardiol., 35:537, 1975.

Sandler, H., et al.: Determination of left ventricular size and shape. Circ. Res., 40:1, 1974.

Schieken, R., et al.: Measurement criteria for group echocardiographic studies. Am. J. Epidemiol., 110:504, 1979.

Stefadourous, M., et al.: Reproducibility of echocardiographic estimates of left ventricular dimensions. Br. Heart J., 39:390, 1977.

Sullivan, J., et al.: The effect of diet on echocardiographic left ventricular dimensions in normal man. Am. J. Clin. Nutr., 32:2410, 1979.

TenCate, F., et al.: The plain chest film as an unreliable method to determine left ventricular size. Jpn. Heart J., 18:878, 1977.

Vignola, P., et al.: Interobserver variability in echocardiography. J. Clin. Ultrasound, 5:238, 1977.

Wröblewski, T., et al.: Left ventricular wall motion determined by echocardiography in elderly subjects. Acta Physiol. Pol., 31:47, 1980.

Wall Thickness and Mass

Allen, J., et al.: Problems in ultrasonic estimates of septal thickness. Am. J. Cardiol., 42:89, 1978.

Bahler, A., et al.: Correlations of electrocardiography and echocardiography in determination of left ventricular wall thickness: study of apparently normal subjects. Am. J. Cardiol., 39:189, 1977.

Bennett, D., et al.: Correlation of left ventricular mass determined by echocardiography with vectorcardiographic and electrocardiographic voltage measurements. Br. Heart J., 36:981, 1974.

Devereux, R., et al.: Echocardiographic determination of left ventricular mass in man. Anatomic validation of the method. Circulation, 55:613, 1977.

Feigenbaum, H., et al.: Left ventricular wall thickness measured by ultrasound. Arch. Intern. Med., 121:391, 1968.

Fowles, R., et al.: Apparent asymmetric septal hypertrophy due to angled interventricular septum. Am. J. Cardiol., 46:386, 1980.

Grossman, W., et al.: Wall thickness and diastolic properties of the left ventricle. Circulation, 49:129, 1974.

Gaasch, W., et al.: The effect of acute changes in coronary blood flow on left ventricular end-diastolic wall thickness. Circulation, 56:593, 1977.

Horton, J., et al.: Distance correction for precordial electrocardiographic voltage in estimating left ventricular mass: an echocardiographic study. Circulation, 55:509, 1977.

Larkin, H., et al.: Anatomical accuracy of echocardiographically assessed left ventricular wall thickness. Clin. Sci., 57 (Suppl. 5):55, 1979.

Monoson, P., et al.: Measurements of left ventricular wall thickness and systolic thickening by M-mode echocardiography: interobserver and intrapatient variability. J. Clin. Ultrasound, 6:252, 1978.

Maron, B., et al.: Comparison of echocardiographic and necropsy measurements of ventricular wall thicknesses in patients with and without disproportionate septal thickening. Circulation, 55:341, 1977.

Osakada, G., et al.: The analysis of left ventricular wall thickness and shear by an ultrasonic triangulation technique in the dog. Circ. Res., 47:173, 1980.

Roelandt, J., et al.: Resolution problems in echocardiology: a source of interpretation errors. Am. J. Cardiol., 37:256, 1976.

Sasayama, S., et al.: Dynamic changes in left ventricular wall thickness and their use in analyzing cardiac function in the conscious dog. Am. J. Cardiol., 38:870, 1976.

Sawaya, J., et al.: Echocardiographic interventricular septal wall motion and thickness: a study in health and disease. Am. Heart J., 87:681, 1974.

Sjögren, A.: Left ventricular wall thickness determined by ultrasound in 100 subjects without heart disease. Chest, 60:341, 1971.

Sjögren, A., et al.: Ultrasonic measurements of left ventricular wall thickness. Chest, 57:37, 1970.

Tanaka, H., et al.: Diastolic bulging of the interventricular septum toward the left ventricle. An echocardiographic manifestation of negative interventricular pressure gradient between left and right ventricles during diastole. Circulation, 62:558, 1980.

Traill, T., et al.: Study of left ventricular wall thickness and dimension changes using echocardiography. Br. Heart J., 40:162, 1978.

Troy, B., et al.: Measurement of left ventricular wall thickness and mass by echocardiography. Circulation, 45:602, 1972.

Winsberg, F., et al.: Echo patterns of cardiac posterior wall. Invest. Radiol., 4:173, 1969.

Pediatric

Epstein, M., et al.: Great vessel, cardiac chamber and wall growth patterns in nine children. Circulation, 51:1123, 1975.

Hagan, A., et al.: Echocardiographic criteria for normal newborn infants. Circulation, 48:1221, 1973.

Henry, W., et al.: Echocardiographic measurements in normal subjects. Growth-related changes that occur between infancy and early adulthood. Circulation, 57:278, 1978.

Lortscher, R., et al.: Echocardiographic determinations of dimensions of normal newborns at 5, 280 feet elevation. J. Clin. Ultrasound, 2:51, 1975.

Lundstrom, N., et al.: Ultrasoundcardiography in infants and children. Acta Paediatr. Scand., 60:117, 1971.

Sapire, D., et al.: Neonatal echocardiography. Cardiovasc. Clin., 9:229, 1978.

Solinger, R., et al.: Echocardiography in the normal neonate. Circulation, 47:108, 1973.

Warburton, D., et al.: Anatomic confirmation of echocardiographic measurements in neonatal hearts. Pediatrics, 64:468, 1979.

MITRAL VALVE

Arrhythmia

Chandraratna, P., et al.: Abnormal mitral valve motion during ventricular extrasystoles. Am. J. Cardiol., 34:783, 1974.

DeMaria, A., et al.: Echographic assessment of atrial transport, mitral movement and ventricular performance following electroversion of supraventricular arrhythmias. Circulation, 51:273, 1975.

Fujii, J., et al.: Dual echocardiographic determination of atrial contraction sequency in atrial flutter and other related atrial arrhythmias. Circulation, 58:314, 1978.

Garbor, G., et al.: Motion of mitral valves in cardiac arrhythmias. Invest. Radiol., 5:273, 1975.

Greenberg, M., et al.: Mitral valve closure in atrial flutter. Circulation, 59:902, 1979.

Iwa, T., et al.: Localization and interruption of accessory conduction pathway in the Wolff-Parkinson-White syndrome. J. Thorac. Cardiovasc. Surg., 80:271, 1980.

Okumura, M., et al.: Non-invasive localization of the pre-excitation site in patients with the Wolff-Parkinson-White syndrome. Vectorcardiographic and echocardiographic correlations. Jpn. Heart J., 21:157, 1980.

Olsson, S., et al.: Spontaneous reversion from long-lasting atrial fibrillation to sinus rhythm. Acta Med. Scand., 2071:5, 1980.

Prabhu, R., et al.: Echocardiographic correlates of atrial contraction in normal and abnormal atrial rhythm. Prog. Cardiovasc. Dis., 20:463, 1978.

Procacci, P., et al.: Dissimilar atrial rhythms diagnosed by echocardiography. Chest, 73:429, 1978.

Zoneraich, O., et al.: Atrial flutter; electrocardiographic, vectorcardiographic and echocardiographic correlation. Am. Heart J., 96:286, 1978.

Zoneraich, S., et al.: Echocardiographic findings in atrial flutter. Circulation, 52:455, 1975.

Effect of Pressure

Ambrose, J., et al.: The influence of left ventricular late diastolic filling on the A-wave of the left ventricular pressure trace. Circulation, 60:510, 1979.

Konecke, L., et al.: Abnormal mitral valve motion in patients with elevated left ventricular diastolic pressures. Circulation, 47:989, 1973.

Quinnones, M., et al.: Reduction in the rate of diastolic descent of the mitral valve echogram in patients with altered left ventricular diastolic pressure-volume relations. Circulation, 49:246, 1974.

Tsakiris, A., et al.: Relation of mitral valve opening and closure to left atrial and ventricular pressures in the intact dog. Am. J. Physiol., 3:146, 1978.

Vignola, P., et al.: Alteration of the left ventricular pressure-volume relationship in man and its effect on the mitral echocardiographic early diastolic closure slope. Circulation, 56:586, 1977.

Normal

Bodenheimer, M., et al.: Echocardiography of the mitral valve. Md. State Med. J., 20:50, 1971.

Buyukozturk, K., et al.: The influences of heart rate, age and sex on the movements of mitral valve. Acta Cardiol., 27:427, 1972.

Chakorn, S., et al.: Study of normal and abnormal movements of mitral valve ring using reflected ultrasound. Br. Heart J., 34:480, 1972.

Dale, G., et al.: Different incidences of echographic investigation of the mitral apparatus. J. Radiol. Electrol. Med. Nucl., 54:189, 1973.

DeMaria, A., et al.: Mitral valve early diastolic closing velocity in the echocardiogram: relation to sequential diastolic flow and ventricular compliance. Am. J. Cardiol., 37:693, 1976.

Derman, U.: Changes of the mitral echocardiogram with aging and the influence of atherosclerotic risk factors. Atherosclerosis, 15:349, 1972.

Emerson, R., et al.: Maximal instantaneous mitral valve velocities measured with a digital echocardiographic tracing system. IEEE Trans. Biomed. Eng., 24:71, 1977.

Fenichel, N., et al.: The effect of respiratory motion on the echocardiogram. Chest, 69:655, 1976.

Laiken, S., et al.: Instantaneous transmitral blood flow and anterior mitral leaflet motion in man. Circulation, 59:476, 1979.

Laniado, S., et al.: A study of the dynamic relations between the mitral valve echogram and phasic mitral flow. Circulation, 51:104, 1975.

Laniado, S., et al: Simultaneous recording of mitral valve echogram and transmitral flow. In The Mitral Valve. Edited by D. Kalmanson. Acton, Mass., Publishing Sciences Group, 1976, pp. 155–162.

Layton, C., et al.: Diastolic closure rate of normal mitral valve. Br. Heart J., 35:166, 1973.

Little, R.: The mechanism of closure of the mitral valve: a continuing controversy. Circulation, 59:615, 1979.

Luisada, A., et al.: Correlates of the echographic waves of the mitral valve in normal subjects of various ages. J. Am. Geriatr. Soc., 23:216, 1975.

McAlpine, W.: Heart and Coronary Arteries. New York, Springer-Verlag, 1975.

Marzilli, M., et al.: Role of the papillary muscle in opening and closure of the mitral valve. Am. J. Physiol., 238:348, 1980.

Parisi, A., et al.: Echocardiographic evaluation of the Valsalva maneuver in healthy subjects and patients with and without heart failure. Circulation, 54:921, 1976.

Pohost, G., et al.: The echocardiogram of the anterior leaflet of the mitral valve: correlation with hemodynamic cineroentgenographic studies in dogs. Circulation, 51:88, 1975.

Ranganathan, N., et al.: Morphology of the human mitral valve. II. The valve leaflets. Circulation, 41:459, 1970.

Robertson, D., et al.: The effect of the Valsalva maneuver on echographic dimensions in man. Circulation, 55:596, 1977.

Rodger, J., et al.: Measurement of diastolic closure rate of normal mitral valve. Br. Heart J., 37:504, 1975.

Rothbaum, D., et al.: Diastolic heart sound produced by mid-diastolic closure of the mitral valve. Am. J. Cardiol., 34:367, 1974.

Rubenstein, J., et al.: The echocardiographic determination of mitral valve opening and closure: correlation with hemodynamic studies in man. Circulation, 51:98, 1975.

Upton, M., et al.: Instantaneous mitral valve leaflet velocity and its relation to left ventricular wall movement in normal subjects. Br. Heart J., 38:51, 1976.

Wharton, C., et al.: Mitral valve movement: a study using an ultrasound technique. Br. Heart J., 32:344, 1970.

Ziady, G., et al.: Diastolic closure rate of mitral valve as determined by ultrasound. Br. Heart J., 35:560, 1973.

Phono-Echo Correlations

Burggraf, G., et al.: The first heart sound in complete heart block. Circulation, 50:17, 1974.

Chandraratna, P., et al.: Echocardiographic observations on the mechanism of production of the second heart sound. Circulation, 51:292, 1975.

Craige, E.: Echocardiography in studies of the genesis of heart sounds and murmurs. In Progress in Cardiology. Vol. 4. Edited by P. Yu and J. Goodwin. Philadelphia, Lea & Febiger, 1975.

Fortuin, N., et al.: Echocardiographic studies of genesis of mitral diastolic murmurs. Br. Heart J., 35:75, 1973.

Letham, A., et al.: Observations on relation between heart sounds and valve movements by simultaneous echo and phonocardiography. Br. Heart J., 37:557, 1975.

Luisada, A., et al.: Changing views on the mechanism of the first and second heart sounds. Am. Heart J., 88:503, 1974.

Mehl, S. , et al.: Audible atrial sounds in atrial flutter modulating an aortic regurgitant murmur. Echocardiographic and phonocardiographic correlates. Chest, 73:101, 1978.

Mills, P., et al.: Echo-phonocardiographic studies of the contribution of the atrioventricular valves to the first heart sound. Circulation, 54:944, 1976.

Parisi, A., et al.: Relation of mitral valve closure to the first heart sound in man. Am. J. Cardiol., 32:779, 1973.

Prakash, R., et al.: First heart sound: a phono-echocardiographic correlation with mitral, tricuspid and aortic valvular events. Cathet. Cardiovasc. Diagn., 2:281, 1976.

Reddy, P., et al.: Sound-pressure correlates of the Austin Flint murmur: an intracardiac sound study. Circulation, 53:210, 1976.

Rothbaum, D., et al.: Diastolic heart sound produced by mid-diastolic closure of mitral valve. Am. J. Cardiol., 34:367, 1974.

Sakamoto, T., et al.: Genesis of the third heart sound. Jpn. Heart J., 17:150, 1976.

Toutouzas, P., et al.: Mechanism of diastolic rumble and pre-systolic murmur in mitral stenosis. Br. Heart J., 36:1096, 1974.

Towne, W., et al.: Pseudoatrial gallop with atrioventricular block: demonstration of a possible mechanism by echocardiography. Am. J. Med., 57:299, 1974.

Waider, W., et al.: First heart sound and ejection sounds. Echocardiographic and phonocardiographic correlation with valvular events. Am. J. Cardiol., 35:346, 1975.

RIGHT VENTRICLE

Dimension

Epstein, M., et al.: Great vessel, cardiac chamber and wall growth patterns in normal children. Circulation, 51:1124, 1975.

Hagan, A., et al.: Echocardiographic criteria for normal newborn infants. Circulation, 48:1221, 1973.

Lundstrom, N., et al.: Clinical applications of echocardiography in infants and children. III. Estimation of left and right ventricular size: a comparison between echocardiography and angiocardiography. Acta Paediatr. Scand., 63:257, 1974.

Popp, R., et al.: Estimation of right and left ventricular size by ultrasound. A study of the echoes from the interventricular septum. Am. J. Cardiol., 24:523, 1969.

Solinger, R., et al.: Echocardiography in the normal neonate. Circulation, 47:108, 1973.

Wall Thickness

Arcilla, R., et al.: Right ventricular mass estimation by angio-echocardiography. Cathet. Cardiovasc. Diagn., 2:125, 1976.

Chang, S., et al.: Technique of echographic examination of right ventricular wall thickness from the right sternal border. Jpn. Heart J., 20:289, 1979.

de la Cruz, M., et al.: A qualitative and quantitative study of the ventricles and great vessels of normal children. Am. Heart J., 60:675, 1960.

Eckner, F., et al.: Dimensions of normal human hearts. Arch. Pathol., 88:497, 1969.

Epstein, M., et al.: Great vessel, cardiac chamber and wall growth patterns in normal children. Circulation, 51:1124, 1975.

Hagan, A., et al.: Echocardiographic criteria for normal newborn infants. Circulation, 48:1221, 1973.

Matsukuko, H., et al.: Echocardiographic measurement of right ventricular wall thickness: a new application of subxiphoid echocardiography. Circulation, 56:278, 1977.

Prakash, R.: Determination of right ventricular wall thickness in systole and diastole. Echocardiographic and necropsy correlation in 32 patients. Br. Heart J., 40:1257, 1978.

Prakash, R., et al.: Determination of right ventricular wall thickness by echocardiogram. J.A.M.A., 239:638, 1978.

Prakash, R., et al.: Diagnosis of right ventricular hypertrophy: an echocardiographic study of 81 patients with autopsy correlation in 25 subjects. Am. J. Cardiol., 41:437, 1978.

Rowlatt, U., et al.: The quantitative anatomy of the normal child's heart. Pediatr. Clin. North Am., 10:499, 1963.

Schulz, D., et al.: Hearts of infants and children. Arch. Pathol., 74:464, 1962.

Solinger, R., et al.: Echocardiography in the normal neonate. Circulation, 47:108, 1973.

SUPRASTERNAL ECHOCARDIOGRAPHY

Allen, H., et al.: Suprasternal notch echocardiography: assessment of its clinical utility in pediatric cardiology. Circulation, 55:605, 1977.

Goh, T., et al.: Scanning suprasternal echocardiography. Br. Heart J., 43:148, 1980.

Goldberg, B.: Suprasternal ultrasonography. J.A.M.A., 215:245, 1971.

Goldberg, B.: Ultrasonic measurement of the aortic arch, right pulmonary artery and left atrium. Radiology, 101:383, 1971.

Kasper, W., et al.: Wall motion characteristic of the right pulmonary artery in the suprasternal echocardiogram. J. Clin. Ultrasound, 8:201, 1980.

Mortera, C., et al.: Contrast echocardiography and the suprasternal approach in infants and children. Eur. J. Cardiol., 9:437, 1979.

SYSTOLIC TIME INTERVALS

Oberhänsli, I., et al.: Growth patterns of cardiac structures and changes in systolic time intervals in the newborn and infant. A longitudinal echocardiographic study. Acta Paediatr. Scand., 69:239, 1980.

Hedvall, G.: Systolic time intervals in newborn infants. Acta Paediatr. Scand., 64:839, 1975.

Hirschfeld, S., et al.: Measurement of right and left ventricular systolic time intervals by echocardiography. Circulation, 51:304, 1975.

Lewis, R., et al.: Systolic time intervals. In Noninvasive Cardiology. Edited by A. M. Weissler. New York, Grune & Stratton, 1974, p. 301.

Lewis, R., et al.: A critical review of the systolic time intervals. Circulation, 56:146, 1977.

Spitaels, S., et al.: The influence of heart rate and age on the systolic and diastolic time intervals in children. Circulation, 49:1107, 1974.

Stefadouros, M., et al.: Systolic time intervals by echocardiography. Circulation, 51:114, 1975.

3

Subcostal Echocardiography

An echocardiographic examination is technically unsatisfactory when no useful information can be obtained. Through the use of the subcostal examination, "technically unsatisfactory" becomes merely "technically difficult," whereby some useful information is obtained from patients with increased thoracic diameters, chronic obstructive lung disease, cor pulmonale, and depressed diaphragms. Two-dimensional echocardiographic examinations of the intra-atrial septum for secundum and primum atrial septal defects are most accurate when recorded subcostally. Left ventricular shape and size have been readily identified in the presence of the hypoplastic left heart syndrome. Ascites, obesity, pregnancy, or hepatomegaly may preclude satisfactory studies from the subcostal examination site.

RECORDING TECHNIQUE

The best records are obtained when the heart lies at or below the fourth intercostal space. One should place the adult patient in a supine position with a 20° to 30° elevation of the head and thorax to relax the abdominal muscles. If necessary, the patient may draw the knees upward with the soles of the feet placed flat on the bed to aid abdominal relaxation. A small cushion could be placed behind the back.[1] Infants and children can remain supine without elevation of the torso.

One should palpate the abdomen 1 or 2 cm to the right of and below the xiphoid process to locate an area of soft tissue. Then one should place the transducer in this region and gently, but firmly, push the probe toward the spine while tilting upward toward the throat (Fig. 3–1). The transducer should not be jabbed into the subcostal tissue. This is painful for the patient and does not help to correct the probe's position. If there is significant leftward displacement of the heart, the transducer may have to be positioned to the left of the patient's xiphoid process. By placing one's hand *over* the transducer, maximum pressure may be exerted upon the probe, with a minimum of finger fatigue. The angulation of the probe in any direction is unimpeded by the examiner's hand (Fig. 3–2).

The cardiac structures to be examined lie in a sector between the throat and the left shoulder (Fig. 3–3). With the

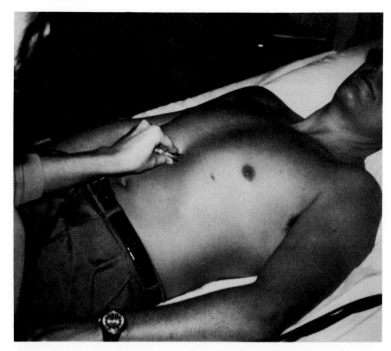

Fig. 3–1. Side view of a subcostal examination. The probe positioning is easier if the abdominal muscles are relaxed by elevating the patient's head and thorax to 20° to 30°. The echographic ventricular septal motion improves when the transducer is positioned toward the patient's right, with the sound beam directed laterally toward the left shoulder.

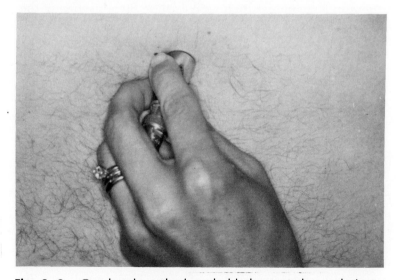

Fig. 3–2. Overhand method to hold the transducer during a subcostal examination. This method allows the maximum pressure to be exerted on the probe with a minimum of finger fatigue. Angulation of the probe in any direction is unimpeded by the examiner's hand.

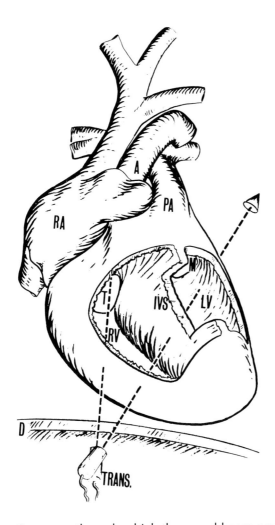

Fig. 3–3. Structures through which the sound beam passes when the transducer is positioned subcostally and is arced in sector-scan from the right heart to the left heart. A, aorta; D, diaphragm; IVS, interventricular septum, inferomedial aspect; LV, left ventricle; RV, right ventricle; RA, right atrium; T, tricuspid valve orifice; M, mitral valve orifice; PA, pulmonary artery; Trans, transducer. (From Chang, S., and Feigenbaum, H.: Subxiphoid echocardiography. J. Clin. Ultrasound, *1*: 14, 1973.)

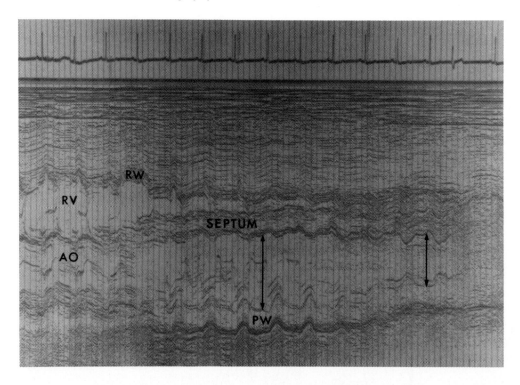

Fig. 3–4. A 62-year-old male patient with diabetes, hypertension, and chest pain. The transducer was positioned subcostally. A slow, continuous paper recording was maintained while the transducer was angled in a sector-scan from the right heart to the left heart (compressed scan). The echoes reflected between the transducer and the right ventricular wall (RW) originated from skin, muscle, fatty tissue, and liver. RV, right ventricle with some tricuspid leaflet motion; AO, aortic leaflet motion; PW, posterolateral left ventricular wall; arrows denote diastolic intracavitary dimension of the left ventricle at levels of the mitral valve and the apex.

transducer directed toward the throat, the sound beam passes through skin, muscle, fatty tissue, liver, diaphragm, right ventricular wall, tricuspid valve, and aortic root (Fig. 3–4). Angulation of the transducer laterally and dorsally toward the left midclavicular line permits visualization of the infero-medial septum, mitral valve, left ventricular cavity, and posterolateral left ventricular wall (Fig. 3–4). Left ventricular apical wall motion, at the level of the papillary muscles, may be recorded by continued lateral angulation of the transducer while simultaneously angling the transducer ventrally or dorsally to align the sound beam most perpendicularly with the maximum plane of wall movement.

Instrumentation

Because the sound beam must traverse a much greater distance to be reflected from cardiac tissue, more tissue depth must be displayed on the preview monitor. One should

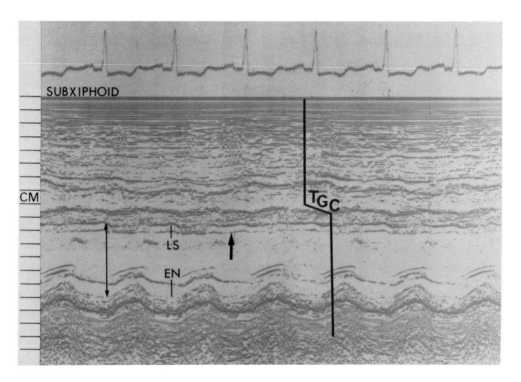

Fig. 3–5. A 60-year-old female patient with coronary artery disease. With the transducer positioned subcostally, the septum was far away from the transducer. Depth compensation (TGC) was positioned at the right septum with reduced amplification of echoes between the transducer and the septum. Bold arrow, a low-intensity echo posterior to the left septum (LS) was excluded from the measurement of septal wall thickness. (See Fig. 3–6.) EN, endocardial-blood interface of posterolateral left ventricular wall.

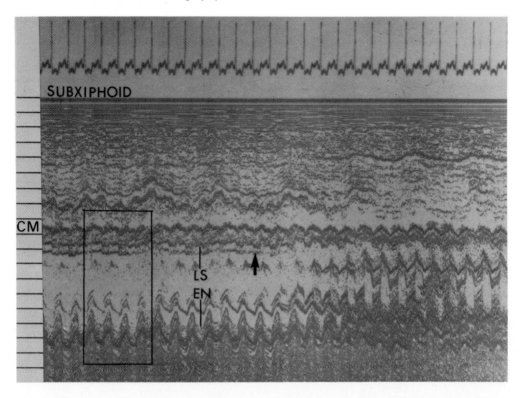

Fig. 3–6. A compressed scan from the patient in Figure 3–5. The box encloses the site of the tracing shown in Figure 3–5. The bold arrow indicates a phantom echo that disappeared as the probe was angled from the left ventricle toward the mitral valve. The compressed scans assist the identification of wall thickness and establish spatial relationships between ventricular chambers and valves. LS, left inferomedial septum; EN, endocardial interface of posterolateral left ventricular wall.

increase the rate of compensation to end in the vicinity of mitral valve motion and amplify reflections from the posterolateral left ventricular wall. Depth compensation must be positioned at the right septal-blood interface (Fig. 3–5). Echoes reflected from the right ventricular wall and right septum do not require much signal amplification. Tracing analysis is easier when the paper's recording speed is 50 mm/sec, but a slow recording speed (10 mm/sec) allows easier visual appreciation of ventricular wall and valve relationships (Fig. 3–6).

Mechanically oscillating two-dimensional echocardiographic transducers should be used only briefly in the subcostal position on infants who have just eaten. Breathing rhythms and heart rate may change with stimulation of the diaphragm, particularly in infants with respiratory distress.

USING RESPIRATION TO FIND HEART

Occasionally, even the subcostal approach seems to be unable to provide access to the heart (Fig. 3–7). However, if the patient inhales deeply, the heart will descend with the diaphragm. This brings the heart into closer proximity to the transducer. One should proceed with the examination as previously described, maintaining the selected transducer position, and record during the patient's slow expiration. When maximum motion of the septal and posterolateral left ventricular wall are seen, the patient should hold his breath while records are obtained (Fig. 3–7).

If echoes from the right ventricular wall and septum are poorly differentiated, the patient should inhale slowly and deeply while one constantly monitors intracardiac motion. Figures 3–8 and 3–9 show the right ventricular wall and septum as inspiration-augmented right ventricular filling.

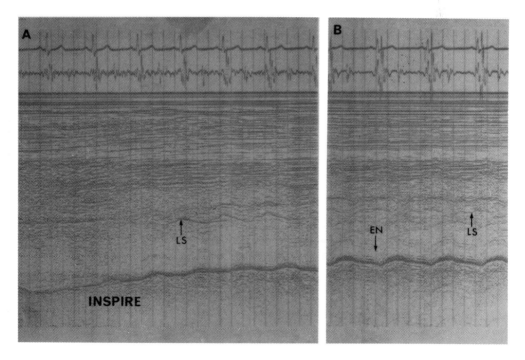

Fig. 3–7. A male patient with chronic obstructive lung disease. The transducer was positioned subcostally. *A,* The left ventricular walls appeared passive until the patient inhaled slowly and deeply. The heart and the diaphragm descended into the range of the sound beam with inspiration. *B,* The patient held his breath following deep inspiration until the maximum ventricular wall motion could be identified and recorded. LS, left inferomedial septal wall motion; EN, endocardial interface of posterolateral left ventricular wall.

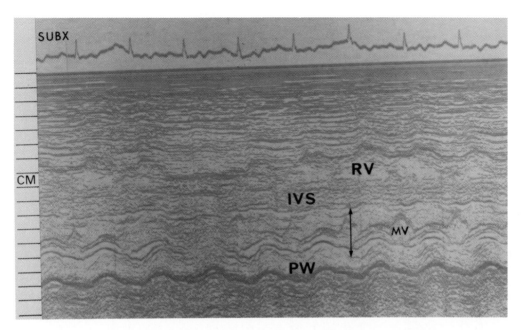

Fig. 3–8. A 76-year-old male patient with chronic obstructive lung disease, coronary artery disease, and congestive heart failure. The sleeping patient's head and thorax were elevated 70° to assist respiration. The right ventricular wall separated from the septum during deep inspiration (snoring). RV, right ventricle; IVS, inferomedial septum; PW, posterolateral left ventricular wall; MV, mitral valve motion.

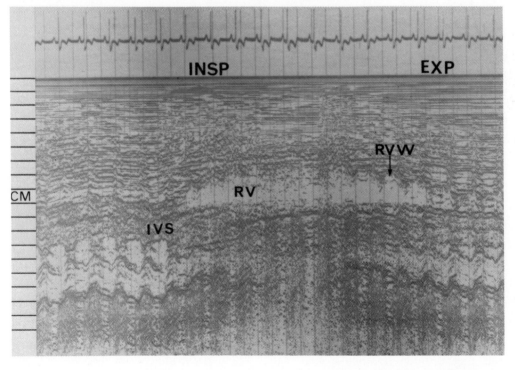

Fig. 3–9. A 57-year-old male patient with coronary artery disease. The transducer was positioned subcostally. Echoes from the right ventricular wall and the septum were poorly differentiated until the patient was instructed to inhale slowly and deeply. Insp, inspiration; Exp, expiration; RVW, right ventricular wall; RV, right ventricle; IVS, inferomedial septum.

PULMONARY TRUNK VERSUS LEFT ATRIUM

The literature does not show conclusive proof of whether the echo-free space behind the aortic root is the left atrium or the pulmonary trunk. Motion of a Swan-Ganz catheter was recorded in the right ventricle and in an area presumed to be the pulmonary trunk (Fig. 3–10). More experience and personal communications with another investigator lead me to believe that catheter motion in the presumed pulmonary trunk may actually have originated from reverberations from the catheter located in the right ventricle.[1] Two-dimensional echocardiography with contrast studies can probably answer this anatomic puzzle.

Pulmonary valve motion has been recorded from the subcostal examination site (Fig. 3–11).[2] This recording was accomplished by directing the transducer toward the throat and dorsally to obtain aortic valve motion. Then the transducer was angled *ventrally* so the sound beam was nearly parallel to the anterior chest wall. Slight medial or lateral angulation was necessary to obtain leaflet motion. Echoes from the pulmonary valve were consistently more distant from the transducer than were echoes from the aortic valve. The valves' opening and closing relationships were comparable to similar time intervals obtained from the parasternum.

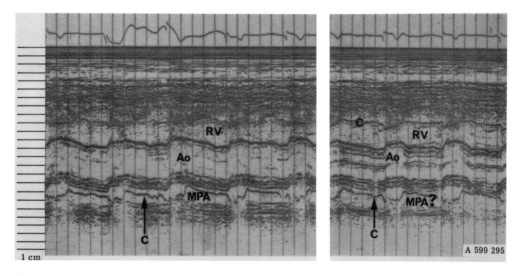

Fig. 3–10. A 71-year-old male patient with coronary artery disease. A Swan-Ganz catheter was positioned in the main pulmonary artery. Reflections from the catheter (C) were seen in the right ventricle and in the presumed pulmonary artery (MPA). However, recent studies[1] indicate that the catheter echo in the presumed pulmonary artery is probably a reverberation of the right ventricular catheter. The presumed main pulmonary artery is probably the left atrium.[2] More definitive studies are required with two-dimensional echocardiography and contrast agents.

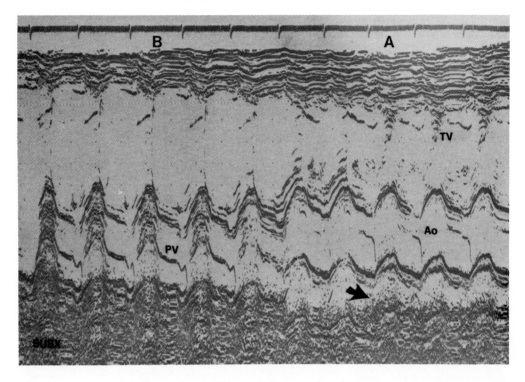

Fig. 3–11. A subcostal scan from the pulmonary valve (PV) to the aorta (Ao). The pulmonary valve motion was obtained by positioning the transducer at the costal-xiphoid arch. The sound beam was nearly parallel with the anterior chest wall. Slight dorsal and lateral angulation recovered the aortic valve motion. Arrow, presumed left atrial cavity[1]; TV, tricuspid valve motion. (From Gullace, G.: Subxiphoid M-mode echocardiography. *In* Recent Advances in Ultrasound Diagnosis, Vol. II. (International Congress Series, No. 498. Proceedings of International Symposium on "Recent Advances in Ultrasound Diagnosis, 1979.") Edited by A. Kurjak. Amsterdam, Excerpta Medica, 1980.)

QUALITY CONTROL OF A SUBCOSTAL ECHOCARDIOGRAM

Tracings obtained from the subcostal examination site must meet the same criteria used to judge the quality of a tracing obtained from the parasternum. The aortic valve must be confined by synchronously moving aortic walls. Systolic time intervals can be measured only if the aortic valve opening is recorded. A simultaneously recorded second heart sound can be used to identify aortic valve closure. Motion of the right and left sides of the interventricular septum and the endocardium and epicardium of the posterolateral wall must be recorded just below the level of the mitral valve. Maximum septal motion must be recorded. The posterolateral left ventricular wall should show wall excursion comparable to that obtained from the parasternum. When the left ventricular base is symmetrically shaped and without contraction abnormalities, subcostal intracardiac dimensions, wall thicknesses,

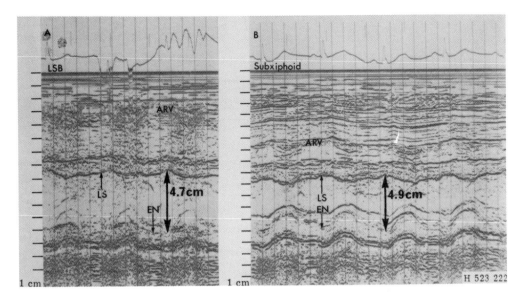

Fig. 3–12. A 64-year-old male patient with hypertension. *A,* A tracing from the left parasternum (LSB). This tracing was technically satisfactory for evaluation of the right and left ventricular dimensions, wall thickness, and wall excursion. *B,* A technically satisfactory subcostal study from the same patient showing the left ventricular dimension comparable to the dimension obtained at left parasternum. ARV, inferomedial right ventricular wall; LS, inferomedial left septum; EN, endocardial-blood interface of posterolateral left ventricular wall.

and ventricular function are comparable to similar measurements obtained from the parasternum[3] (Fig. 3–12).

APPLICATION OF SUBXIPHOID EXAMINATION

Technically unsatisfactory echocardiographic studies along the left parasternum are salvaged by the use of the subcostal approach (Figs. 3–13 to 3–15).

Although it is impossible to exaggerate ventricular wall motion artificially by angulation of the transducer or by the position of the patient, it is always possible to produce hypokinetic or passive wall motion (Fig. 3–16). When the observed wall motion is incompatible with the patient's clinical findings, a subcostal examination should disclose more representative wall movement (Figs. 3–17 and 3–18).

Mitral valve prolapse is rarely recorded from the subxiphoid plane of examination because the sound beam's line of incidence is oblique to the direction of leaflet movement. However, if prolapse of the mitral leaflets can be recorded from the subxiphoid examination site, the motion is comparable to that seen at the left parasternum (Fig. 3–19). Mitral stenosis may also be appreciated by the subcostal approach (Figs. 3–20 and 3–21).

(Text continues on page 113.)

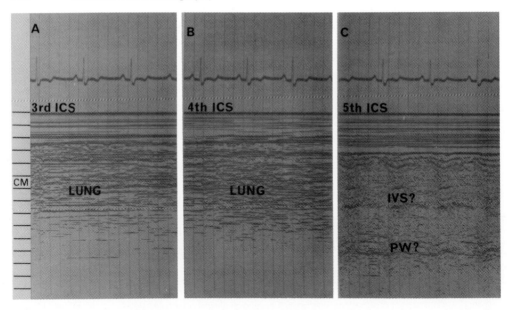

Fig. 3–13. A 57-year-old male patient with coronary artery disease. The transducer was positioned along the left parasternum at several intercostal spaces (ICS). Superimposition of lung precluded any satisfactory recordings of cardiac motion. IVS, motion *may* originate from interventricular septum; PW, motion *may* originate from posterior left ventricular wall. (See Fig. 3–14.)

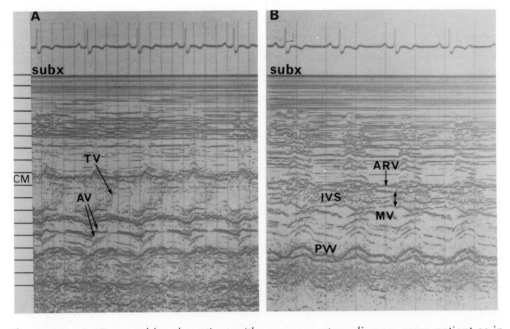

Fig. 3–14. A 57-year-old male patient with coronary artery disease; same patient as in Figure 3–13. *A,* The transducer was placed subcostally and directed toward the throat. The sound beam passed through the tricuspid valve (TV) and the aortic valve (AV). *B,* The transducer was angled laterally, toward the left shoulder, and tilted dorsally. The sound beam passed through the right ventricular wall (ARV), the inferomedial septum (IVS), some portion of mitral valve apparatus (MV), and the posterolateral left ventricular wall (PW).

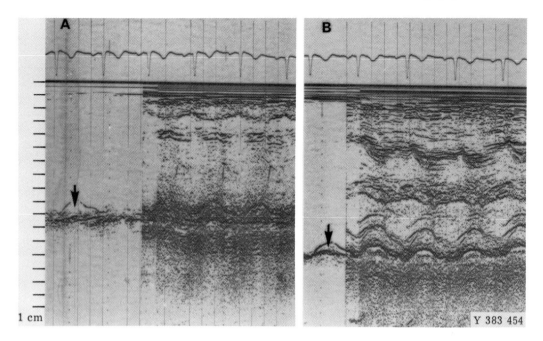

Fig. 3–15. A 76-year-old female patient with hypertensive cardiomyopathy. *A*, A technically unsatisfactory left ventricular study from the left parasternum. *B*, A technically satisfactory left ventricular study using the subcostal approach. The "septal thickness" at the left parasternum and subcostal examination sites is different. A differential diagnosis of primary cardiomyopathy versus burned-out hypertensive-ischemic heart disease with cardiomegaly was never resolved.

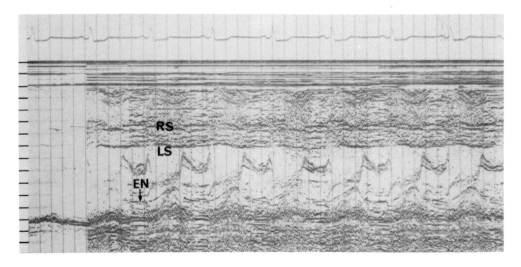

Fig. 3–16. A 54-year-old male patient with severe calcific aortic stenosis, mild aortic insufficiency, and chronic obstructive lung disease. Hypokinesis of the anterior septum could be due either to coronary artery disease or to improper relationship between septum and interrogating sound beam. (See Fig. 3–17.) RS, right septum; LS, left septum; EN, endocardial interface of posterior left ventricular wall.

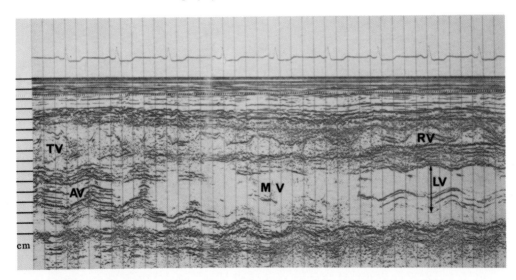

Fig. 3–17. A subcostal tracing from the patient in Figure 3–16. The transducer was arced in a sector-scan from the tricuspid and aortic valve area toward the left ventricular apex. More motion was exhibited by the septum from this examination site. Cineangiography disclosed normal coronary arteries. TV, tricuspid valve motion; MV, mitral valve motion; AV, aortic valve motion; RV, right ventricle; LV, left ventricle.

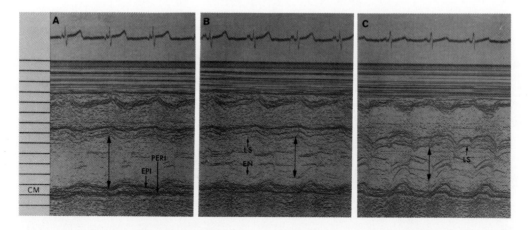

Fig. 3–18. A 52-year-old female patient with rheumatic heart disease and coronary artery disease. *A,* The patient was supine during examination. The coarse gain was too low, eliminating echoes from the posterior left ventricular wall endocardium. The intracavitary dimension was erroneous. *B,* The coarse gain was increased to receive echoes from the left ventricular endocardium and the myocardium. The systolic motion of the anterior septum was within normal limits. *C,* The transducer was relocated to the subcostal examination site. The posterolateral left ventricular wall was well defined with a paradoxical inferomedial septal motion. In each illustration, there was a persistent echo-reflective space between the epicardium (EPI) and the pericardium (PERI) that represented a small, nonhomogeneous pericardial exudate, or a fat pad. The patient did not have any clinical findings for pericarditis. LS, left septum; EN, endocardial surface of posterior left ventricular wall.

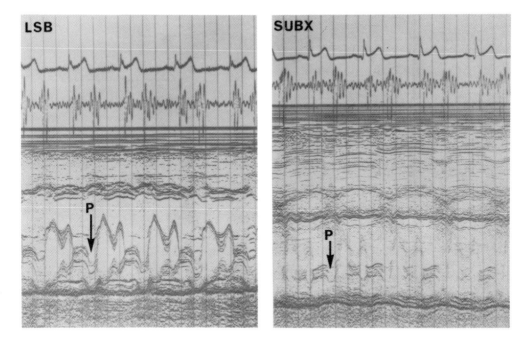

Fig. 3–19. A 21-year-old male patient. Midsystolic prolapse of the mitral valve (P) was identified at *A*, left parasternum (LSB), and *B*, subcostal (SUBX) examination sites.

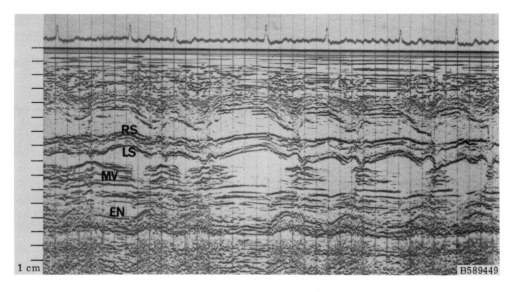

Fig. 3–20. A subcostal echocardiogram from a patient with mitral stenosis. The mitral valve's excursion was the least accurate measurement owing to the oblique opening of the valve in relation to the sound beam. (See Fig. 3–21.) RS, right septum; LS, left septum; MV, mitral valve motion; EN, endocardial-blood interface of posterolateral left ventricular wall.

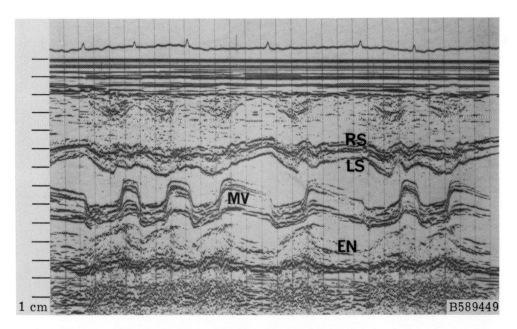

Fig. 3–21. A recording obtained along the left parasternum from the patient in Figure 3–20. The excursion of the obstructed mitral leaflet was greater from this examination site. RS, right septum; LS, left septum; MV, mitral leaflet motion; EN, endocardial-blood interface of posterior left ventricular wall.

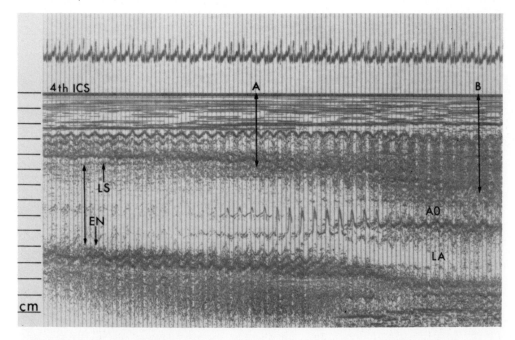

Fig. 3–22. A 61-year-old female patient with coronary artery disease. The transducer was located in closer proximity to the left ventricular apex, as indicated by the nearness of septum-to-transducer (A), in contrast to the distance of the anterior aortic wall-to-transducer (B). Paper recording speed was slow and continuous while the angle of the transducer was directed superiorly toward the aorta (AO), resulting in a "compressed scan." Passive septal motion was evident below the mitral valve. (See Fig. 3–23.) LS, left septum; EN, endocardial surface of posterior left ventricular wall; LA, left atrium. (From Chang, S.: The representative septum. Med. Ultrasound, *0(8):* 7, 1976.)

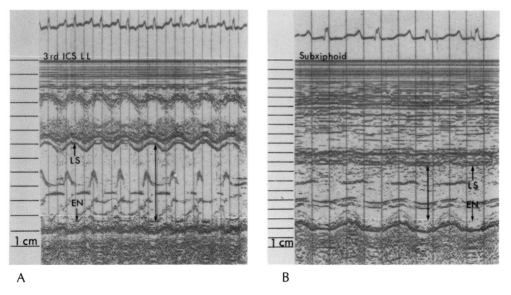

A   B

Fig. 3–23. A tracing from the patient in Figure 3–22. A, With the transducer positioned at the third intercostal space, the quality of septal motion was more representative of basilar contraction than was seen in Figure 3–22. B, Relocation of the transducer to the subcostal examination site disclosed akinetic septal movement. Cineangiography disclosed severe and diffuse contraction abnormalities of the entire heart with only the anterobasilar segment of left ventricle contracting with any vigor. LS, left septum; EN, endocardial-blood interface of posterior left ventricular wall. (From Chang, S.: The representative septum. Med. Ultrasound, *0(8)*: 7, 1976.)

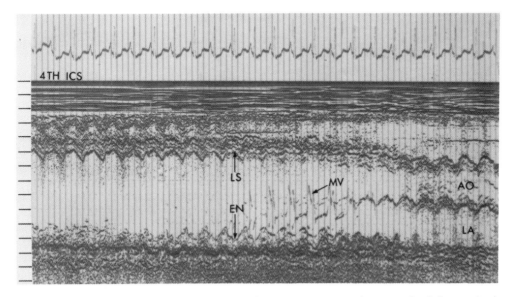

Fig. 3–24. A 48-year-old male patient with coronary artery disease. The left ventricular study could not be obtained from the third intercostal space. The maximum anterior septal motion, below mitral valve, was recorded from a lower intercostal space shown here. The posterior left ventricular wall motion was diminished below the level of the mitral valve (See Fig. 3–25.) LS, left septum, EN, endocardial surface of posterior left ventricular wall: MV, mitral valve motion; AO, aorta; LA, left atrium.

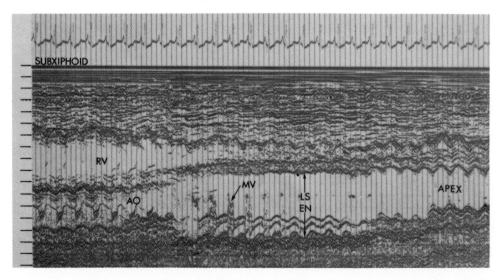

Fig. 3–25. A subcostal tracing from the patient in Figure 3–24. The basilar inferomedial septum was passive, with better motion closer to the apex. At catheterization, the apical septum was well supplied with collateral vessels filling retrograde from the left coronary system. The right coronary artery was totally occluded. RV, right ventricle; AO, aorta; MV, mitral valve; LS, left septum; EN, endocardial surface of posterolateral wall.

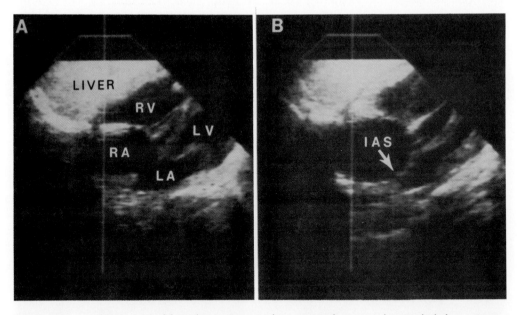

Fig. 3–26. A three-year-old male patient with a secundum atrial septal defect, QpQs ratio, 1.14:1, right-to-left shunt. Pulmonary vascular resistance was elevated at 22 units. A, A subcostal, two-dimensional echocardiogram showed a large septal defect. B, A slight upward angulation of the transducer showed an apparently intact atrial septum (arrow); this difference indicates the necessity for careful examination and cautious interpretation. The intra-atrial septum (IAS) appeared to bulge toward the left atrium. The mean atrial pressures were nearly equal: right atrium (RA), 8 mm Hg; left atrium (LA), 9 mm Hg. Other catheterization data: right ventricle, 112/4 mm Hg; pulmonary artery, 85/53 mm Hg; aorta, 114/80 mm Hg. (See Fig. 3–27.) RV, right ventricle; LV, left ventricle.

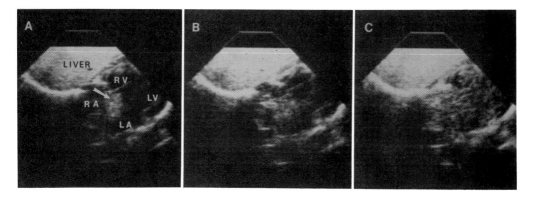

Fig. 3–27. The same patient as in Figure 3–26; sequential single frames from two-dimensional echocardiogram. *A,* Right atrium, arrow, showed initial entry of hand-injected D₅W solution through a peripheral venous catheter. *B,* The entry of the contrast agent into the left atrium indicates either preferential streaming or significant right-to-left shunting through the patent foramen ovale or the atrial septal defect. *C,* The contrast agent filled all intracardiac chambers. RA, right atrium; LA, left atrium; RV, right ventricle; LV, left ventricle.

The subcostal approach is most useful in the M-mode echocardiographic evaluation of left ventricular dimensions and wall motion in patients with coronary artery disease. Abnormally contracting segments monitored at the left parasternum may not represent the quality of systolic wall contraction available to subcostal examination. The combined records from both examination sites provide more information than do data derived from a single plane of examination (Figs. 3–22 to 3–25).

Whereas the sensitivity and specificity of subcostal two-dimensional echocardiographic detection of atrial septal defects have not been conclusively established, this method shows promise of increased accuracy. By aligning a wide-angle sector of sound with the intra-atrial septum, large defects in this structure have been identified (Fig. 3–26). When feasible, contrast studies assist in the evaluation of left-to-right or right-to-left shunting across the defect (Fig. 3–27).

REFERENCES

1. Gullace, G.: Contrast studies of the pulmonary artery from subxiphoid position. Personal communication.
2. Gullace, G.: Subxiphoid versus standard M-mode echocardiography. *In* Echocardiology. Edited by C. T. Lancee. The Hague, Martinus Nijhoff, 1979, pp. 73–76.
3. Starling, M., et al.: Accuracy of subxiphoid echocardiography for assessing left ventricular size and performance. Circulation, *61*: 367, 1980.

BIBLIOGRAPHY

Bierman, F., et al.: Subxiphoid two-dimensional imaging of the interatrial septum in infants and neonates with congenital heart disease. Circulation, *60*: 80, 1979.

Chang, S., et al.: Subxiphoid echocardiography. J. Clin. Ultrasound, *1*: 14, 1973.

Chang, S., et al.: Subxiphoid echocardiography: a review. Chest, *68*: 233, 1975.

Direttore, E.: Subxiphoid echocardiography. G. Ital. Cardiol., 8: 238, 1978.

Gullace, G.: L'esplorazione echocardiografica per via subxifoidea. G. Ital. Cardiol., *9*: 817, 1979.

Lange, L., et al.: Subxiphoid cross-sectional echocardiography in infants and children with congenital heart disease. Circulation, *59*: 513, 1979.

Matsukubo, H., et al.: Echocardiographic measurement of right ventricular wall thickness: a new application of subxiphoid echocardiography. Circulation, *56*: 278, 1977.

Rusconi, C., et al.: Echocardiografia subxifoidea: arteria polmonare od aorta? G. Ital. Cardiol., 7: 870, 1977.

Starling, M., et al.: Accuracy of subxiphoid echocardiography for assessing left ventricular size and performance. Circulation, *61*: 367, 1980.

Tajik, A., et al.: Two-dimensional real-time ultrasonic imaging of the heart and great vessels. Mayo. Clin. Proc., *53*: 271, 1978.

Weyman, A., et al.: Negative contrast echocardiography: a new method for detecting left-to-right shunts. Circulation, *59*: 498, 1979.

4

The Big Heart

Cardiomegaly is secondary to isolated or combined ventricular wall thickening, atrial or ventricular chamber enlargement, and pericardial effusion. Symptoms appearing on echocardiographic requisitions include chest pain, shortness of breath, orthopnea, palpitations, heart murmurs, dizziness, fatigue, congestive heart failure, arrhythmias, cyanosis, myocardial ischemia or infarction, hypertension, and diabetes. The echocardiographer must perform a complete examination of the heart, including two-dimensional echocardiography, to seek the cause of cardiac enlargement and its extent.

VENTRICULAR HYPERTROPHY

Left Heart

Adult and pediatric patients with systemic hypertension, coarctation of the aorta, or aortic stenosis require higher systolic pressure to eject blood from the left ventricle into the aorta. This increased work load often leads to thickening of the left ventricular walls (Fig. 4–1). Chronic renal disease and

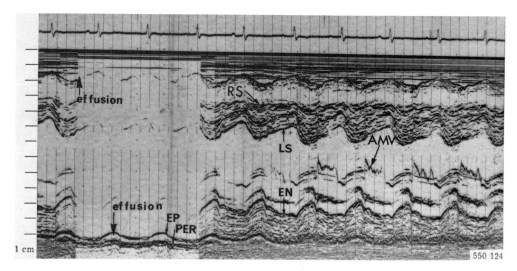

Fig. 4–1. A 67-year-old female patient with systemic hypertension and severe aortic regurgitation. The left ventricle has thickened without decreasing the size of the ventricular cavity. A small, posterior pericardial effusion was present. AMV, anterior mitral leaflet motion; EN, endocardial surface of posterior left ventricular wall; LS, left septum; RS, right septum; EP, epicardial surface of posterior left ventricular wall; PER, pericardium.

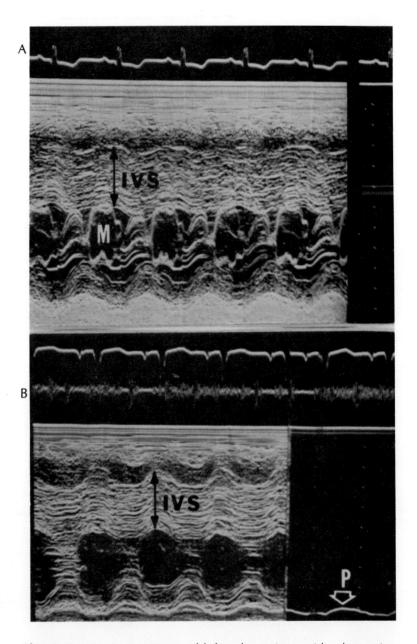

Fig. 4–2. *A*, A seven-year-old female patient with obstructive idiopathic cardiomyopathy, also present in *B*, her 17-year-old brother. The brother's clinical symptoms were more severe, requiring an operation. The septums were markedly thickened in contrast to the posterior left ventricular walls. The tracings were recorded on Polaroid film from Sanyo videotape. The camera was set at f-stop 5.6, "B" exposure time, and the foot pedal was plugged into a camera input jack. The shutter opened when the foot pedal was pressed at the beginning of the M-mode presentation on the preview monitor. The shutter closed when the foot pedal was released at the end of the presentation. IVS, interventricular septum; P, pericardium; M, diastolic mitral valve motion. During systole, the mitral valve coapted with the septum.

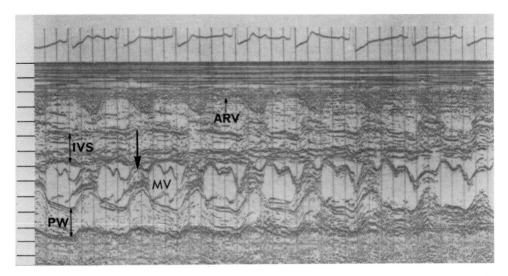

Fig. 4–3. A 31-year-old female patient with severe, hypertrophic subaortic stenosis. The ventricular walls were thickened at the expense of cavity size. IVS, interventricular septum; ARV, anterior right ventricular wall; PW, posterior left ventricular wall; MV, mitral leaflet motion; bold arrow, systolic anterior displacement of mitral valve apparatus. (From Feigenbaum, H.: Echocardiography. Philadelphia, Lea & Febiger, 1976.)

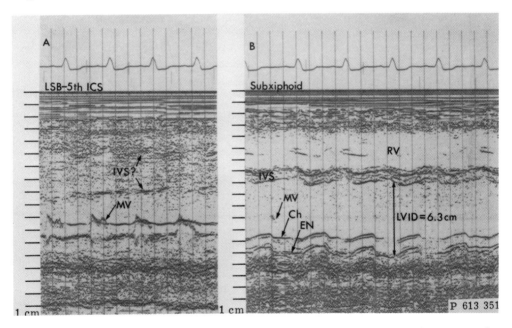

Fig. 4–4. A 76-year-old female patient with hypertensive cardiomyopathy. *A,* A technically unsatisfactory tracing of the left ventricle from the left parasternum. Evaluations of septal thickness, posterior wall thickness, and ventricular dimensions were not attempted. *B,* The technical quality of the septum and the posterolateral left ventricular wall improved when recorded from the subcostal examination site. IVS, interventricular septum; MV, mitral leaflet motion; Ch, chordae tendineae; EN, endocardial surface of posterior left ventricular wall; RV, right ventricle; LVID, left ventricular internal dimension during diastole.

glycogen storage disease may produce echographic tracings similar to those in Figure 4–1. However, patients with chronic renal failure may have a combination of thickened left ventricular walls and cavity dilatation, whereas patients with Pompe's disease or amyloidosis exhibit only ventricular wall hypertrophy. Localized thickening of the septum is most often associated with hypertrophic cardiomyopathy (Fig. 4–2), but concentric hypertrophy can also occur in this disease (Fig. 4–3).

Normal adult left ventricular wall thickness ranged from 7 to 12 mm (see Table 2–11). The left ventricular wall thickness of 26 morbidly obese patients ranged from 8 to 12 mm (see Table 2–12). Wall thickness exceeding 12 mm is evidence of myocardial hypertrophy in the adult.

Positive identification of the septum and posterior left ventricular wall must be established when tracings are recorded. Echoes from structures lying in close proximity to the right septum can lead to erroneous measurement of the septal thickness (Figs. 4–4 A and 4–5). Mistakes can be avoided by additional examination from other intercostal spaces or from the subcostal examination site (Fig. 4–4 B). Continuous recording, while changing the transducer's angulation, should

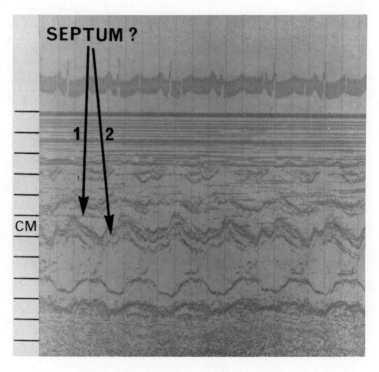

Fig. 4–5. A 35-year-old female patient with mitral stenosis. Identification of the true septum was difficult without a scan to relate the septum to other cardiac structures. (See Fig. 4–6.)

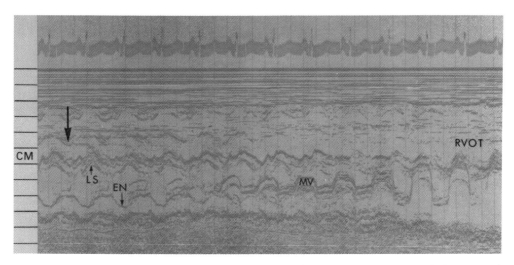

Fig. 4–6. A scan from the patient in Figure 4–5. The transducer was angled superiorly from the left ventricle toward the aorta. The bold arrow indicates echoes reflected from the right-sided structure, which was not an integral part of the septum. LS, left septum; EN, endocardial surface of posterior left ventricular wall; MV, stenotic mitral leaflet motion; RVOT, dilated right ventricular outflow tract.

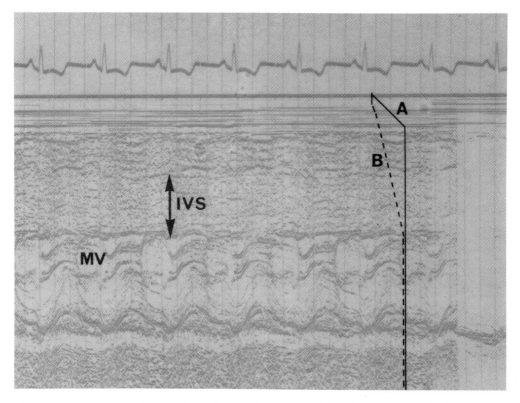

Fig. 4–7. A 44-year-old female patient with hypertrophic subaortic stenosis. The septum was markedly thickened and poorly distinguished from the right ventricular wall. To minimize the erroneous selection of the right septal wall, depth compensation was moved anteriorly to chest wall (A) and the "rate" of compensation was decreased (B). Thus, all echoes reflected between the chest wall and the left septum were recorded. IVS, interventricular septum; MV, mitral leaflet motion.

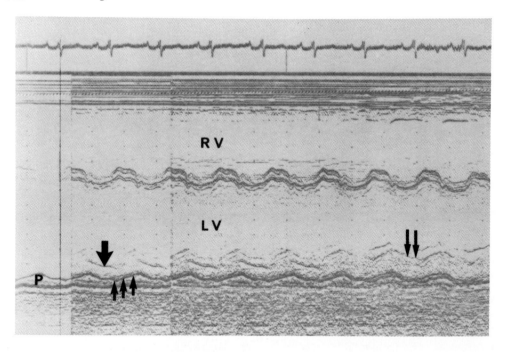

Fig. 4–8. A 51-year-old male patient with alcoholic cardiomyopathy. Single arrow, excessive damping of echoes reflected from the posterior left ventricular wall allowed erroneous identification of endocardial surface; double arrows, the true endocardial surface. (See Fig. 4–9.) Minimal pericardial effusion was present (P). Triple arrows, epicardial interface; RV, right ventricle; LV, left ventricle.

reveal "signal drop-out" of echoes unrelated to the septum (Fig. 4–6). One may avoid selective elimination of the right side of a thickened septum through proper use of the controls. When a thick septum is suspected, one should move the "depth compensation" forward to the crystal artifact (Fig. 4–7 A). The "rate" of compensation should be extended over 6 or 7 cm of tissue depth to allow gradual signal suppression between the right ventricular wall and the left septum (Fig. 4–7 B). Excessive signal attenuation eliminates weak signals reflected from the posterior endocardial surface and could result in erroneous left ventricular wall thickness measurements (Figs. 4–8 and 4–9).

Right Heart

Unusual thickening of the right ventricular wall is consistent with chronically elevated right ventricular systolic pressure (Fig. 4–10). This type of hypertrophy commonly occurs secondary to congenital heart disease: valvular and subvalvular pulmonary stenosis, transposition of the great arteries, tetralogy of Fallot, Taussig-Bing syndrome, persistent truncus arteriosus, and double-outlet right ventricle. Patients with

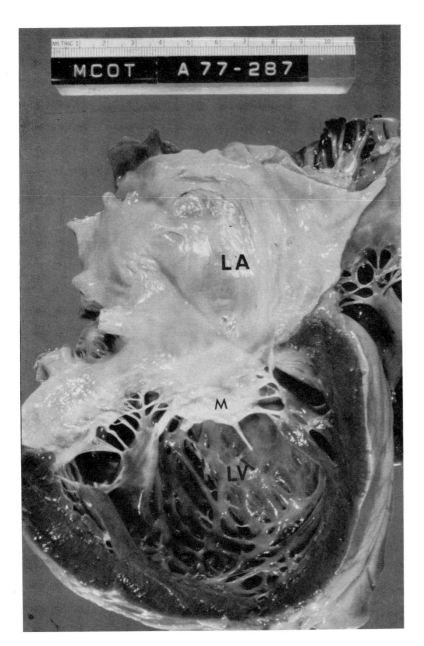

Fig. 4–9. A necropsy specimen of the left ventricle from the patient in Figure 4–8. The pericardium was smooth, containing 150 ml of clear, yellow fluid. The epicardial surface was smooth and translucent. The left ventricular wall thickness measured 15 mm. The mitral leaflets exhibited nodular thickening. The left atrial walls were thickened and opaque. LA, left atrium; M, mitral leaflet, anterior; LV, left ventricle.

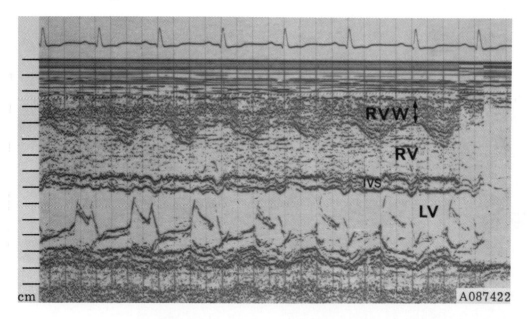

Fig. 4–10. A 29-year-old male patient with tetralogy of Fallot. The pressure gradient across the pulmonary valve exceeded 75 mm Hg. The right ventricle (RV) was dilated and the anterior right ventricular wall was markedly thickened. LV, left ventricle; IVS, interventricular septum. (From Feigenbaum, H.: Echocardiography. Philadelphia, Lea & Febiger, 1976.)

pulmonary hypertension secondary to cystic fibrosis, ventricular septal defect, chronic obstructive lung disease, coarctation of the aorta, and mitral stenosis can show progressive thickening of the right ventricular wall on serial echocardiograms.

Before measuring right ventricular wall thickness, one should be sure that both epicardial and endocardial echoes have been recorded. Examination from the right parasternum has been helpful to identify these right ventricular structures in children. Diastolic wall thickness should be measured coincident with the onset of ventricular depolarization (Fig. 4–11). Adult right ventricular wall thickness usually does not exceed 6 mm. Using 2.25-MHz and 3.5-MHz transducers, right ventricular wall thicknesses up to 9 mm were recorded from 20 persons without clinical evidence of cardiovascular disease (see Table 2–9). Right ventricular wall thickness exceeding 10 mm is consistent with chronically elevated right ventricular systolic pressure. However, clinical correlation is necessary.

Pediatric right ventricular wall thickness should not exceed 4 mm before the age of 10 years, averaging about 3 mm from one month of age to 7 years. Premature and full-term infants commonly have increased right ventricular wall thicknesses exceeding 4 mm secondary to fetal circulation. This wall thickness should diminish within the first 3 months of life.

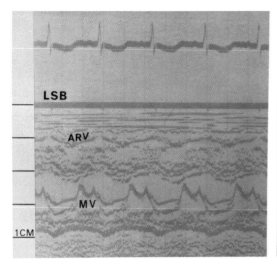 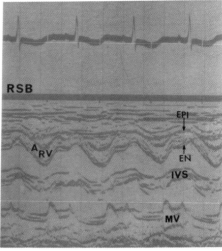

Fig. 4–11. A normal, 12-hour-old male infant. The echographic quality of the anterior right ventricular wall thickness and motion improved when recorded at the right parasternum (RSB). Right ventricular hypertrophy is common in newborn infants. Wall thickness should diminish within the first three months of life and should not exceed 4 mm before ten years of age. LSB, left sternal border; ARV, anterior right ventricular wall; EPI, epicardium; EN, endocardial surface of right ventricular wall; IVS, interventricular septum; MV, mitral leaflet motion. (From Chang, S., Roberts, S., Chang, J., Kleinberg, M., and Torres, R.: Techniques of echographic examination of right ventricular wall thickness from the right sternal border. Jpn. Heart J., 20: 289, 1979.)

Failure to do so should cause one to suspect persistently elevated right heart pressures. (See Chap. 2, "Normal Right Ventricle.")

VENTRICULAR VOLUME OVERLOAD

Left Heart

Overfilling of the left ventricle results from aortic or mitral regurgitation and from congenital heart defects such as patent ductus arteriosus or ventricular septal defect. Left ventricular enlargement often occurs with pregnancy, chronic renal failure, and severe anemia. A left ventricular dimension equaling or exceeding 3.2 cm/m^2 is evidence of cavitary enlargement in the adult patient.

A compensated ventricle is capable of pumping a large volume of blood forward into the aorta with each heartbeat. A failing ventricle contracts poorly and allows an abnormal quantity of blood to remain in the chamber following each heartbeat. This excess contributes to progressive ventricular dilatation. The global size and shape of the enlarged left ventricle is best appreciated with apical, two-dimensional echocardiography (Figs. 4–12 to 4–14).

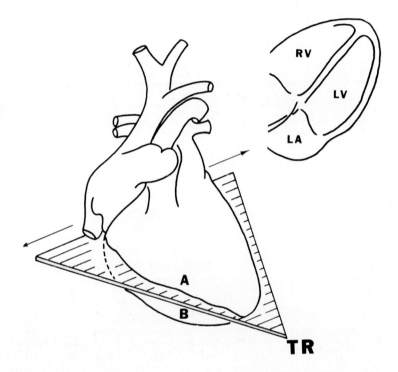

Fig. 4-12. Schematics for two-dimensional examination of the heart from the left ventricular apex (apical four-chamber view). The transducer is located in the vicinity of the "point of maximal impulse" and is directed toward the crux of the heart, where atrial and ventricular septa meet. Sound beams bisect the heart through a long axis from right to left. Inset: the diagram shows section (A) lifted from section (B) to a fully opened position. This is the presentation of the heart on an echograph monitor during examination of the left ventricle and other chambers from the apex.

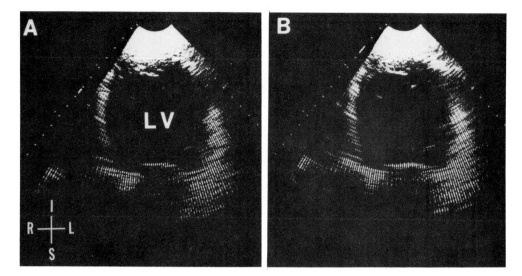

Fig. 4–13. A 47-year-old male patient with congestive cardiomyopathy; two-dimensional echocardiogram, apical four-chamber view of the left ventricle (LV). *A*, Four superimposed frames show massive diastolic dilatation of the left ventricle. *B*, Four superimposed frames show insignificant systolic change in cavity size owing to generalized hypokinetic wall movement. I, inferior or cardiac apex; S, superior or cardiac base; R, right, near sternum; L, left or lateral.

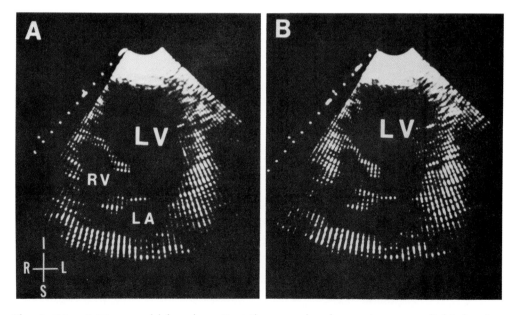

Fig. 4–14. A 71-year-old female patient three weeks after acute myocardial infarction; two-dimensional echocardiogram of the left ventricle (LV) using the apical approach. *A*, A single frame shows the left ventricular shape coincident with the electrocardiographic "R" wave; *B*, A single frame shows the left ventricular shape during systole. The contractile movement was seen only near the base of the ventricle with vigorous right ventricular wall movement. The left ventricular apex was markedly distended and totally akinetic. RV, right ventricle; LA, left atrium.

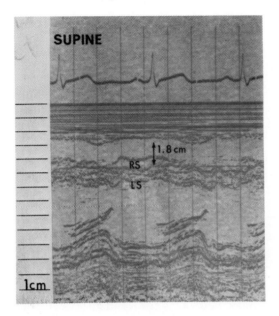
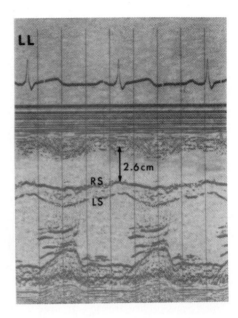

Fig. 4–15. A normal 21-year-old male professional hockey player. *A,* The tracing was recorded from the recumbent individual. *B,* An increased right ventricular dimension was due to cardiac displacement and rotation as the patient was turned to a partial left lateral decubitus position. RS, right septum; LS, left septum. (From Chang, S.: The representative septum. Med. Ultrasound, *0(8):* 7, 1976.)

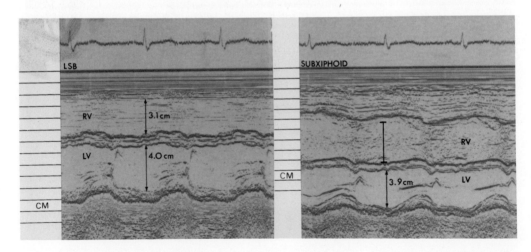

Fig. 4–16. A 50-year-old female patient with a secundum atrial septal defect, QpQs ratio, 2.5:1. The patient was recumbent throughout the examination. The right ventricular dimension was increased at *A,* the left parasternum (LSB) and *B,* the subxiphoid examination site. Septal movement was dyskinetic, moving anteriorly following ventricular depolarization. At catheterization, the mean pulmonary artery pressure was 24 mm Hg. RV, right ventricle; LV, left ventricle.

Right Heart

Atrial septal defect, tricuspid and pulmonary regurgitation, and anomalous pulmonary venous return produce chronic overfilling of the right ventricle and lead to enlargement of this chamber, with abnormal septal motion.

The right ventricular dimension should be measured at the onset of ventricular depolarization, on tracings obtained from a supine patient to exclude "positional dilatation" (Fig. 4–15). In the adult only, one may measure from the inner chest wall to the right side of the septum and subtract 5 mm to exclude an "estimated" right ventricular wall thickness from the right ventricular cavity dimension (Fig. 4–16). Right ventricular enlargement is suggested when its dimension exceeds 1.4 cm/m^2 in the supine patient or 1.7 cm/m^2 in the left-laterally positioned patient. Clinical correlation is necessary.

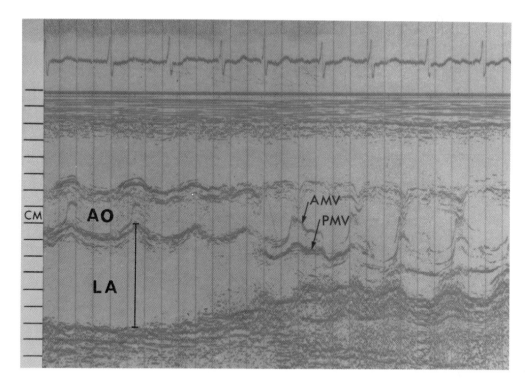

Fig. 4–17. A 64-year-old male patient with mitral stenosis and ruptured mitral chordae; scan from the aorta (AO) and left atrium (LA) inferior to the mitral valve. The diameter of the enlarged left atrial chamber was measured at end-systole from the top of the posterior aortic wall echo to the top of the posterior left atrial wall echo. AMV, anterior mitral valve motion; PMV, posterior mitral valve motion. (From Chang, S., and Chang J.: Mitral stenosis and ruptured mitral chordae: an unusual echocardiographically detectable combination. Med. Ultrasound, 2: 27, 1978.)

LEFT ATRIAL DILATATION

Left atrial enlargement can be expected in the presence of chronic, idiopathic atrial fibrillation, congestive heart failure, patent ductus arteriosus, ventricular septal defect, chronic mitral regurgitation, and mitral stenosis (Fig. 4–17). Enlargement is usually not evident with acute mitral regurgitation. An adult left atrial dimension exceeding 2.2 cm/m² is evidence of atrial enlargement. Normal left atrial dimension should not exceed 1.72 cm/m² in the morbidly obese individual (see Table 2–6). Measurements should be taken at the onset of the second heart sound or at the end of ventricular repolarization from the top of the posterior aortic root echo to the top of the posterior left atrial wall echo.

BIBLIOGRAPHY

CARDIOMEGALY

Abbasi, A., et al.: Left ventricular hypertrophy diagnosed by echocardiography. N. Eng. J. Med., 289: 118, 1973.
Abbasi, A.: Echocardiography in the differential diagnosis of the large heart. Am. J. Med., 60: 677, 1976.
Anderson, J., et al.: Postpartum cardiac failure—heart failure due to volume overload? Am. Heart J., 97: 613, 1979.
Browne, P., et al.: The echocardiographic correlates of left ventricular hypertrophy diagnosed by electrocardiography. J. Electrocardiol., 10: 105, 1977.
Browne, P., et al.: Hypertrophy or dilatation? a vectorial analysis of echocardiographically determined left ventricular enlargement. J. Electrocardiol., 11: 117, 1978.
Crawford, M., et al.: The athlete's heart. Adv. Intern. Med., 24: 311, 1979.
Gibson, D., et al.: Echocardiographic features of secondary left ventricular hypertrophy. Br. Heart J., 41: 54, 1979.
Katz, R., et al.: Effects of natural volume overload state (pregnancy) on left ventricular performance in normal human subjects. Circulation, 58: 434, 1978.
Luboshitzki, R., et al.: The heart in acromegaly: correlation of echocardiographic and clinical findings. Isr. J. Med. Sci., 16: 378, 1980.
McFarland, T., et al.: Echocardiographic diagnosis of left ventricular hypertrophy. Circulation, 57: 1140, 1978.
Martins, J., et al.: Cardiac size and function in acromegaly. Circulation, 56: 863, 1977.
Morganroth, J., et al.: Electrocardiographic evidence of left ventricular hypertrophy in otherwise normal children: clarification by echocardiography. Am. J. Cardiol., 35: 278, 1975.
Rees, A., et al.: Echocardiographic evidence of outflow tract obstruction in Pompe's disease (glycogen storage disease of heart). Am. J. Cardiol., 37: 1103, 1976.
Rees, A., et al.: Left ventricular performance in children with homozygous sickle cell anemia. Br. Heart J., 40: 690, 1978.
Rubler, S., et al.: Cardiac size and performance during pregnancy estimated with echocardiography. Am. J. Cardiol., 40: 534, 1977.
Sanderson, J., et al.: Postpartum cardiac failure—heart failure due to volume overload. Am. Heart J., 97: 613, 1979.
Schieken, R., et al.: Cardiac manifestations of the mucopolysaccharidoses. Circulation, 52: 700, 1975.
Seides, S., et al.: Echocardiographic findings in isolated, surgically created tricuspid insufficiency. Am. J. Cardiol., 35: 679, 1974.
Smallridge, R., et al.: Acromegaly and the heart. An echocardiographic study. Am. J. Med., 66: 22, 1979.

Yoshikawa, J., et al.: Reappraisal of jugular phlebogram in the diagnosis of tricuspid regurgitation. Relationship between echocardiographic interventricular septal motion and jugular phlebogram. Jpn. Heart J., *18*: 31, 1977.

CARDIOMYOPATHY

Abbasi, A., et al.: Ultrasound in the diagnosis of primary congestive cardiomyopathy. Chest, *63*: 937, 1973.

Acquatella, H., et al.: M-mode and two-dimensional echocardiography in chronic Chagas' heart disease. A clinical and pathologic study. Circulation, *62*: 787, 1980.

Burch, G., et al.: Echocardiographic detection of abnormal motion of the interventricular septum in ischemic cardiomyopathy. Am. J. Med., *57*: 293, 1974.

Chew, C., et al.: Primary restrictive cardiomyopathy: nontropical endomyocardial fibrosis and hypereosinophilic heart disease. Br. Heart J., *39*: 399, 1977.

Chiaramida, S., et al.: Real-time, cross-sectional echocardiographic diagnosis of infiltrative cardiomyopathy due to amyloid. J. Clin. Ultrasound, *8*: 58, 1980.

Child, J., et al: Echocardiographic manifestations of infiltrative cardiomyopathy: a report of seven cases due to amyloid. Chest, *70*: 726, 1976.

Corya, B., et al.: Echocardiographic features of congestive cardiomyopathy compared with normal subjects and patients with coronary artery disease. Circulation, *49*: 1153, 1974.

Fortuin, N.: The enlarged heart. Dilated-type cardiomyopathy. Med. Times, *108*: 66, 1980.

Giles, T., et al.: Echocardiographic findings in amyloid cardiomyopathy. South. Med. J., *71*: 1393, 1978.

Gutgesell, H., et al.: Characterization of the cardiomyopathy in infants of diabetic mothers. Circulation, *61*: 441, 1980.

Hern'andez-Pieretti, O.: Echocardiographic diagnosis and evaluation of cardiomyopathies: idiopathic hypertrophic subaortic stenosis, Chagas' heart disease and endomyocardial fibrosis. Postgrad. Med. J., *53*: 533, 1977.

Kansal, S., et al.: Interventricular septal thickness and left ventricular hypertrophy. An echocardiographic study. Circulation, *60*: 1058, 1979.

Levisman, J.: Echocardiographic diagnosis of mitral regurgitation in congestive cardiomyopathy. Am. Heart J., *93*: 33, 1977.

Mason, J., et al.: Cardiac biopsy evidence for a cardiomyopathy associated with symptomatic mitral valve prolapse. Am. J. Cardiol., *42*: 557, 1978.

Mintz, G., et al.: Echocardiographic features of cardiomyopathy. Cardiovasc. Clin., *9*: 123, 1978.

Mir, M.: Evidence for non-infiltrative cardiomyopathy in acute leukaemia and lymphoma. A clinical and echocardiographic study. Br. Heart J., *40*: 725, 1978.

Morganroth, J., et al.: Noninvasive diagnosis of the cardiomyopathies. Med. Clin. North Am., *64*: 33, 1980.

Nimura, Y., et al.: An unusual pattern of the mitral echocardiogram observed in cases of congestive cardiomyopathy and other myocardial diseases. Jpn. Heart J., *16*: 500, 1975.

Oakley, C.: Clinical definitions and classifications of cardiomyopathies. Postgrad. Med. J., *48*: 703, 1972.

Przybojewski, J., et al.: Primary cardiac amyloidosis: a case presentation. S. Afr. Med. J., *57*: 774, 1980.

Przybojewski, J., et al.: Primary cardiac amyloidosis: a review of the literature. S. Afr. Med. J., *57*: 831, 1980.

Puigb'o, J., et al.: Diagnosis of Chagas' cardiomyopathy. Noninvasive techniques. Postgrad. Med. J., *53*: 527, 1977.

Santos, A., et al.: Echocardiographic characterization of the reversible cardiomyopathy of hypothyroidism. Am. J. Med., *68*: 675, 1980.

Schipperheyn, J., et al.: Hypokalaemic periodic paralysis and cardiomyopathy. Acta Neurol. Scand., *58*: 374, 1978.

Ziady, G., et al.: Proceedings. Primary restrictive cardiomyopathy. Br. Heart J., *37*: 556, 1975.

LEFT ATRIAL ENLARGEMENT

Bartall, H., et al.: Echocardiographic left atrial enlargement. Comparison of vectorcardiogram and electrocardiogram for detection. J. Electrocardiol., *11*: 355, 1978.

Brown, O., et al.: An improved method for echographic detection of left atrial enlargement. Circulation, *50*: 58, 1974.

Chandraratna, P.: Echocardiographic study of the effects of acute left atrial hypertension on left atrial size. J. Clin. Ultrasound, *4*: 15, 1976.

Chirife, R., et al.: Electrocardiographic detection of left atrial enlargement. Correlation of P wave with left atrial dimension by echocardiography. Br. Heart J., *37*: 1281, 1975.

Henry, W., et al.: Relation between echocardiographically determined left atrial size and atrial fibrillation. Circulation, *53*: 273, 1976.

Hirata, T., et al.: Estimation of left atrial size using ultrasound. Am. Heart J., *78*: 43, 1969.

Ikram, H., et al.: The noninvasive recognition of left atrial enlargement. Comparison of electro- and echocardiographic measurements. Postgrad. Med. J., *53*: 356, 1977.

Josephson, M., et al.: Electrocardiographic left atrial enlargement. Electrophysiologic, echocardiographic and hemodynamic correlates. Am. J. Cardiol., *39*: 967, 1977.

Kronzon, I., et al.: Giant left atrium. Chest, *65*: 677, 1974.

Lemire, F., et al.: Asymmetric left atrial enlargement; an echocardiographic observation. Chest, *69*: 779, 1976.

Morganroth, J., et al.: Relationship of atrial fibrillatory wave amplitude to left atrial size and etiology of heart disease. An old generalization reexamined. Am. Heart J., *97*: 184, 1979.

Ratshin, R., et al.: Possible false-positive diagnosis of pericardial effusion by echocardiography in presence of large left atrium. Chest, *65*: 112, 1974.

Rubler, S., et al.: Comparison of left atrial size and pulmonary capillary pressure with P wave on electrocardiogram. Am. Heart J., *92*: 73, 1976.

Sherrid, M., et al.: Echocardiographic analysis of left atrial size before and after operation in mitral valve disease. Am. J. Cardiol., *43*: 171, 1979.

TenCate, F., et al.: Dimensions and volumes of left atrium and ventricle determined by single beam echocardiography. Br. Heart J., *36*: 737, 1974.

Termini, B., et al.: Echocardiographic and electrocardiographic criteria for diagnosing left atrial enlargement. South. Med. J., *68*: 161, 1975.

Waggoner, A., et al.: Left atrial enlargement: echocardiographic assessment of electrocardiographic criteria. Circulation, *54*: 553, 1976.

LEFT VENTRICULAR PRESSURE OVERLOAD

Aortic Stenosis

Abbasi, A., et al.: Left ventricular hypertrophy diagnosed by echocardiography. N. Engl. J. Med., *289*: 118, 1973.

Aziz, K., et al.: Echocardiographic assessment of the relation between left ventricular wall and cavity dimensions and peak systolic pressure in children with aortic stenosis. Am. J. Cardiol., *40*: 775, 1977.

Bennett, D., et al.: Echocardiographic left ventricular dimensions in pressure and volume overload. Their use in assessing aortic stenosis. Br. Heart J., *37*: 971, 1975.

Blackwood, R., et al.: Aortic stenosis in children. Experience with echocardiographic prediction of severity. Circulation, *57*: 263, 1978.

Broderick, T., et al.: Critical aortic stenosis in neonates. Radiology, *129*: 393, 1978.

Chang, S., et al.: Aortic stenosis: echocardiographic cusps separation and surgical description of aortic valve in 22 patients. Am. J. Cardiol., *39*: 499, 1977.

Dawkins, P.: Aortic stenosis with coronary artery disease: dilemma of management. Chest, *67*: 90, 1975.

Feigenbaum, H.: Clinical applications of echocardiography. Prog. Cardiovasc. Dis., *14*: 531, 1972.

Feizi, O., et al.: Echocardiography of the aortic valve. I: studies of normal aortic valve, aortic stenosis, aortic regurgitation and mixed aortic valve disease. Br. Heart J., 36: 341, 1974.

Fowles, R., et al.: Two-dimensional echocardiographic features of bicuspid aortic valve. Chest 75: 434, 1979.

Gewitz, M., et al.: Role of echocardiography in aortic stenosis: pre- and postoperative studies. Am. J. Cardiol., 43: 67, 1979.

Glanz, S., et al.: Echocardiographic assessment of the severity of aortic stenosis in children and adolescents. Am. J. Cardiol., 38: 620, 1976.

Gramiak, R., et al.: Echocardiography of the normal and diseased aortic valve. Radiology, 96: 1, 1970.

Hernberg, J., et al.: The ultrasonic recording of aortic valve motion. Radiology, 94: 361, 1970.

Hess, P., et al.: Echocardiographic features of combined membranous subaortic stenosis and acquired calcific aortic valvulopathy. Am. Heart J., 94: 349, 1977.

Johnson, G., et al.: Left ventricular function by echocardiography in children with fixed aortic stenosis. Am. J. Cardiol., 38: 611, 1976.

McDonald, I.: Echocardiographic assessment of left ventricular function in aortic valve disease. Circulation, 53: 860, 1976.

Morgan, D., et al.: Occult aortic stenosis as cause of intractable heart failure. Br. Med. J., 1: 784, 1979.

Nanda, N., et al.: Echocardiographic recognition of the congenital bicuspid aortic valve. Circulation, 49: 870, 1974.

Nanda, N., et al.: Echocardiography in the diagnosis of IHSS co-existing with aortic valve disease. Circulation, 50: 752, 1974.

Radford, D., et al.: Echocardiographic assessment of bicuspid aortic valves: angiographic and pathological correlates. Circulation, 53: 80, 1976.

Raj, M., et al.: Coexistence of asymmetric septal hypertrophy and aortic valve disease in adults. Thorax, 34: 91, 1979.

Schwartz, A., et al.: Echocardiographic estimation of aortic valve gradient in aortic stenosis. Ann. Intern. Med., 89: 329, 1978.

Shah, P., et al.: Diagnosis and treatment of aortic valve stenosis. Curr. Probl. Cardiol., 2: 1, 1977.

Sheppard, J., et al.: Distinctive echocardiographic pattern of posterior wall endocardial motion in aortic stenosis. Am. Heart J., 96: 9, 1978.

Vukas, M., et al.: Preliminary observations on interventricular septum vibrations: an echocardiographic sign in aortic valvular stenosis. Acta Med. Scand., 202: 363, 1977.

Weyman, A., et al.: Cross-sectional echocardiography in assessing the severity of valvular aortic stenosis. Circulation, 52: 828, 1975.

Weyman, A., et al.: Cross-sectional echocardiographic assessment of the severity of aortic stenosis in children. Circulation, 55: 773, 1977.

Yeh, H., et al.: Echocardiographic aortic valve orifice dimension; its use in evaluating aortic stenosis and cardiac output. J. Clin. Ultrasound, 1: 182, 1973.

Coarctation of Aorta

Graham, T., et al.: Right and left heart size and function in infants with symptomatic coarctation. Circulation, 56: 641, 1977.

Sahn, D., et al.: Real-time cross-sectional echocardiographic diagnosis of coarctation of the aorta: a prospective study of echocardiographic-angiographic correlations. Circulation, 56: 762, 1977.

Scovil, J., et al.: Echocardiographic studies of abnormalities associated with coarctation of the aorta. Circulation, 53: 953, 1976.

Weyman, A., et al.: Cross-sectional echocardiographic detection of aortic obstruction 2. Coarctation of the aorta. Circulation, 57: 498, 1978.

Wing, J., et al.: Serial echocardiographic profiles in infants and children with coarctation of the aorta. Am. J. Cardiol., 41: 1270, 1978.

Hypertension

Davignon, A., et al.: Hemodynamic studies of labile essential hypertension in adolescents. In Juvenile Hypertension. Edited by L. Levine. New York, Raven Press, 1976.

Dunn, F., et al.: Pathophysiologic assessment of hypertensive heart disease with echocardiography. Am. J. Cardiol., *39*: 789, 1977.

Geva, B., et al.: Determination of left ventricular wall thickening in patients with chronic systemic hypertension. Correlation of electrocardiography and echocardiography. Chest, *76*: 557, 1979.

Goldring, D., et al.: Blood pressure in a high school population. II. Clinical profile of the juvenile hypertensive. J. Pediatr., *95*: 298, 1979.

Guazzi, M., et al.: Cardiac load and function in hypertension. Ultrasonic and hemodynamic study. Am. J. Cardiol., *44*: 1007, 1979.

Karliner, J., et al.: Left ventricular performance in patients with left ventricular hypertrophy caused by systemic arterial hypertension. Br. Heart J., *39*: 1239, 1977.

Olivari, M., et al.: Pulmonary hemodynamics and right ventricular function in hypertension. Circulation, *57*: 1185, 1978.

Richardson, P., et al.: Relationship between hypertension and angina pectoris. Br. J. Clin. Pharmacol., [Suppl.], *7*: 249, 1979.

Ross, A., et al.: Echocardiographic and clinical correlations in systemic hypertension. J. Clin. Ultrasound, *6*: 95, 1978.

Safar, M., et al.: Echocardiographic dimensions in borderline and sustained hypertension. Am. J. Cardiol., *44*: 930, 1979.

Salcedo, E., et al.: Left ventricular mass and wall thickness in hypertension. Comparison of M-mode and two-dimensional echocardiography in two experimental models. Am. J. Cardiol., *44*: 936, 1979.

Savage, D., et al.: Echocardiographic assessment of cardiac anatomy and function in hypertensive subjects. Circulation, *59*: 623, 1979.

Sullivan, J., et al.: Short-term therapy of severe hypertension. Hemodynamic correlates of the antihypertensive response in man. Arch. Intern. Med., *139*: 1233, 1979.

Yamori, Y., et al.: Cardiac hypertrophy in early hypertension. Am. J. Cardiol., *44*: 964, 1979.

Subvalvular Aortic Stenosis

Berger, M., et al.: Unsuspected hypertrophic subaortic stenosis in the elderly diagnosed by echocardiography. J. Am. Geriatr. Soc., *27*: 178, 1979.

Berry, T., et al.: Echocardiographic assessment of discrete subaortic stenosis in childhood. Am. J. Cardiol., *43*: 957, 1979.

Chandraratna, P., et al.: Pre- and postoperative echocardiographic features of discrete subaortic stenosis. Cardiology, *61*: 181, 1976.

Davis, R., et al.: Echocardiographic manifestations of discrete subaortic stenosis. Am. J. Cardiol., *33*: 277, 1974.

Doi, Y., et al.: M-mode echocardiography in hypertrophic cardiomyopathy: diagnostic criteria and prediction of obstruction. Am. J. Cardiol., *45*: 6, 1980.

Fortuin, N.: Echocardiogram of the month: hypertrophic cardiomyopathy. Med. Times, *108*: 50, 1980.

Gilbert, B., et al.: Hypertrophic cardiomyopathy: subclassification by M-mode echocardiography. Am. J. Cardiol., *45*: 861, 1980.

Harrison, E., et al.: Coexisting right and left hypertrophic subvalvular stenosis and fixed left ventricular outflow obstruction due to aortic valve stenosis. Am. J. Cardiol., *40*: 133, 1977.

Hess, P., et al.: Echocardiographic features of combined membranous subaortic stenosis and acquired calcific aortic valvulopathy. Am. Heart J., *94*: 249, 1977.

Hirose, K., et al.: A point-score system for the differential diagnosis between idiopathic cardiomyopathy and ischemic heart disease. Jpn. Circ. J., *44*: 137, 1980.

Isshiki, T., et al.: Cross-sectional echocardiography of the short axis views of the left ventricle in hypertrophic cardiomyopathy. Jpn. Heart J., *21*: 297, 1980.

Johnson, G., et al.: Echocardiographic evaluation of fixed left ventricular outlet obstruction in children: pre- and postoperative assessment of ventricular systolic pressures. Circulation, *56*: 299, 1977.

Johnson, M., et al.: Echocardiography of the aortic valve in non-rheumatic left ventricular outflow tract lesions. Radiology, *112*: 677, 1974.

Kelly, D., et al.: Discrete subaortic stenosis. Circulation, *46*: 309, 1972.

Krajcer, Z., et al.: Septal myomectomy and mitral valve replacement for idiopathic hypertrophic subaortic stenosis. An echocardiographic and hemodynamic study. Circulation, 62: 158, 1980.

Kronzon, I., et al.: Fixed membranous subaortic stenosis. Chest, 67: 473, 1975.

Krueger, S., et al.: Echocardiographic features of combined hypertrophic and membranous subvalvular aortic stenosis: a case report. J. Clin. Ultrasound, 4:31, 1976.

Krueger, S., et al.: Echocardiography in discrete subaortic stenosis. Circulation, 59: 506, 1979.

Lundström, N.: Echocardiography in the diagnosis of subaortic stenosis. Acta Med. Scand. (Suppl.), 627: 192, 1979.

Mariani, M., et al.: Validity and limitations of echocardiography for the diagnosis of discrete subaortic stenosis associated with marked left ventricular muscular hypertrophy. J. Nucl, Med. Allied Sci., 23: 109, 1979.

Maron, B., et al.: Nongenetically transmitted disproportional ventricular septal thickening associated with left ventricular outflow obstruction. Br. Heart J., 41: 345, 1979.

Maron, B., et al.: Hypertrophic cardiomyopathy. Recent observations regarding the specificity of three hallmarks of the disease: asymmetric septal hypertrophy, septal disorganization and systolic anterior motion of the anterior mitral leaflet. Am. J. Cardiol., 45: 141, 1980.

Martin, R., et al.: Idiopathic hypertrophic subaortic stenosis viewed by wide-angle phased-array echocardiography. Circulation, 59: 1206, 1979.

Morrow, A., et al.: Left ventricular myotomy and myectomy in patients with obstructive hypertrophic cardiomyopathy and previous cardiac arrest. Am. J. Cardiol., 46: 313, 1980.

Popp, R., et al.: Echocardiographic findings in discrete subvalvular aortic stenosis. Circulation, 49: 226, 1974.

Roelandt, J., et al.: Long-segment (tunnel) subaortic stenosis. Chest, 72: 222, 1977.

Ross, J., et al.: Nonobstructive and obstructive hypertrophic cardiomyopathies. West. J. Med., 130: 325, 1979.

Sung, C., et al.: Discrete subaortic stenosis in adults. Am. J. Cardiol., 42: 283, 1978.

TenCate, F., et al.: Progression to left ventricular dilatation in patients with hypertrophic obstructive cardiomyopathy. Am. Heart J., 97: 762, 1979.

TenCate, F., et al.: Fixed subaortic stenosis. Value of echocardiography for diagnosis and differentiation between various types. Br. Heart J., 41: 159, 1979.

Thompson, R., et al.: Hypertrophic cardiomyopathy after aortic valve replacement. Am. J. Cardiol. 45: 33, 1980.

Wei, J., et al.: The heterogeneity of hypertrophic cardiomyopathy: an autopsy and one-dimensional echocardiographic study. Am. J. Cardiol., 45: 24, 1980.

Weyman, A., et al.: Cross-sectional echocardiography in evaluating patients with discrete subaortic stenosis. Am. J. Cardiol., 37: 358, 1976.

Supravalvular Aortic Stenosis

Ali, N., et al.: Echocardiographic diagnosis of supravalvular aortic stenosis. South. Med., J., 70: 759, 1977.

Bolen, J., et al.: Echocardiographic features of supravalvular aortic stenosis. Circulation, 52: 817, 1975.

Mori, Y., et al.: Echocardiographic and angiocardiographic features of supravalvular aortic stenosis in children. Jpn. Circ. J., 43: 137, 1979.

Nasrallah, A., et al.: Supravalvular aortic stenosis: echocardiographic features. Br. Heart J., 37: 662, 1975.

Shaub, M., et al.: Echocardiographic diagnosis of supravalvular aortic stenosis. A case report. J. Clin. Ultrasound, 3: 143, 1975.

Usher, B., et al.: Echocardiographic detection of supravalvular aortic stenosis. Circulation, 49: 1257, 1974.

Weyman, A., et al.: Cross-sectional echocardiographic characterization of aortic obstruction. 1. Supravalvular aortic stenosis and aortic hypoplasia. Circulation, 57: 491, 1978.

LEFT VENTRICULAR VOLUME OVERLOAD

Aortic Regurgitation

Abdulla, A., et al.: Limitations of echocardiography in the assessment of left ventricular size and function in aortic regurgitation. Circulation, 61: 148, 1980.

Ando, J., et al.: Congenital aortic regurgitation observed in a thalidomide-deformed child. Jpn. Heart J., 19: 823, 1978.

Borer, J., et al.: Left ventricular function at rest and during exercise after aortic valve replacement in patients with aortic regurgitation. Am. J. Cardiol., 44: 1297, 1979.

Danford, H., et al.: Echocardiographic evaluation of the hemodynamic effects of chronic aortic insufficiency with observations on left ventricular performance. Circulation, 48: 253, 1973.

Gaasch, W., et al.: Echocardiographic examination in aortic regurgitation. Chest, 70: 771, 1976.

Gaasch, W., et al.: Chronic aortic regurgitation: the effect of aortic valve replacement on left ventricular volume, mass and function. Circulation, 58: 825, 1978.

Gray, K., et al.: Echocardiographic assessment of severity of aortic regurgitation. Br. Heart J., 37: 691, 1975.

Honig, H., et al.: Severe aortic regurgitation secondary to idiopathic aortitis. Am. J. Med., 63: 623, 1977.

Johnson, A., et al.: Assessment of left ventricular function in severe aortic regurgitation. Circulation, 54: 975, 1976.

Laskey, W., et al.: Assessment of left ventricular function in aortic insufficiency using echocardiography, gated scintigraphy and contrast angiography. Clin. Nucl. Med., 4: 279, 1979.

McDonald, I.: Echocardiographic assessment of left ventricular function in aortic valve disease. Circulation, 53: 860, 1976.

Mehta, J., et al.: Aortic regurgitation associated with ventricular septal defect. Echocardiographic and hemodynamic observations. Chest, 71: 784, 1977.

Morganroth, J., et al.: Acute severe aortic regurgitation. Pathophysiology, clinical recognition and management. Ann. Intern. Med., 87: 223, 1977.

Paoloni, H., et al.: The role of echocardiography in the assessment of chronic aortic regurgitation. Aust. N.Z. J. Med., 7: 491, 1977.

Reid, G., et al.: Aortic insufficiency in association with juvenile ankylosing spondylitis. J. Pediatr., 95: 78, 1979.

Rowland, T.: Traumatic aortic insufficiency in children: case report and review of the literature. Pediatrics, 60: 893, 1977.

Schieken, R., et al.: Effect of aortic valvular regurgitation upon the impedance cardiogram. Br. Heart J., 40: 958, 1978.

Schuler, G., et al.: Serial noninvasive assessment of left ventricular hypertrophy and function after surgical correction of aortic regurgitation. Am. J. Cardiol., 44: 585, 1979.

Shimada, T., et al.: Acute aortic regurgitation with congestive heart failure due to bacterial endocarditis: diagnosed by echocardiogram and treated successfully by surgery (case report). Jpn. Circ. J., 43: 59, 1979.

Tanaka, H., et al.: Echocardiographic findings in patients with aortitis syndrome. Angiology, 30: 620, 1979.

Tremblay, G.: Echocardiography. IV. Aortic insufficiency. Union Med. Can., 106: 891, 1977.

Venco, A., et al.: Noninvasive assessment of left ventricular function after correction of severe aortic regurgitation. Br. Heart J., 38: 1324, 1976.

Mitral Regurgitation

Ahmad, S., et al.: The echocardiographic diagnosis of rupture of a papillary muscle. Chest, 73: 232, 1978.

Antman, E., et al.: Demonstration of the mechanism by which mitral regurgitation mimics aortic stenosis. Am. J. Cardiol., 42: 1044, 1978.

Burgess, J., et al.: Echocardiographic findings in different types of mitral regurgitation. Circulation, 48: 97, 1973.

Gould, L., et al.: Severe mitral regurgitation with a normal-sized left atrium. Angiology, 29: 174, 1978.

Humphries, W., et al.: Echocardiographic equivalents of flail mitral leaflets. Am. J. Cardiol., *40*: 802, 1977.

Kim, H., et al.: An attempt to correlate the mitral valve echogram with the hemodynamics of patients with pure mitral insufficiency. Jpn. Circ. J., *37*: 403, 1973.

Levisman, J.: Echocardiographic diagnosis of mitral regurgitation in congestive cardiomyopathy. Am. Heart J., *93*: 33, 1977.

Meyer, J., et al.: Systolic mitral flutter, an echocardiographic clue to the diagnosis of ruptured chordae tendineae. Am. Heart J., *93*: 3, 1977.

Millward, D., et al.: Echocardiographic studies of the mitral valve in patients with congestive cardiomyopathy and mitral regurgitation. Am. Heart J., *85*: 413, 1973.

Mintz, G., et al.: Two-dimensional echocardiographic evaluation of patients with mitral insufficiency. Am. J. Cardiol., *44*: 670, 1979.

Morcerf, F., et al.: Echocardiographic determination of the etiology of severe mitral regurgitation. Clev. Clin. Q., *43*: 163, 1976.

Ogawa, S., et al.: Flail mitral valve in rheumatic heart disease. Chest, *71*: 88, 1978.

Pathak, L.: Diagnostic ultrasound in mitral regurgitation. Indian Heart J., *29*: 192, 1977.

Patton, R., et al.: The posterior left atrial echocardiogram of mitral regurgitation. Circulation, *57*: 1134, 1978.

Rashid, A., et al.: Papillary muscle rupture following nonpenetrating chest trauma: report of a case with hemodynamic and serial echocardiographic findings and successful surgical treatment. Heart Lung, *7*: 647, 1978.

Sweatman, T., et al.: Echocardiographic diagnosis of ruptured chordae tendineae. Am. J. Cardiol., *26*: 661, 1970.

Sweatman, T., et al.: Echocardiographic diagnosis of mitral regurgitation due to ruptured chordae tendineae. Circulation, *46*: 580, 1972.

Sze, K., et al.: Systolic flutter of the mitral valve. Am. Heart J., *96*: 157, 1978.

Wanderman, K., et al.: Left ventricular performance in mitral regurgitation assessed with systolic time intervals and echocardiography. Am. J. Cardiol., *38*: 831, 1976.

Wann, L., et al.: Cross-sectional echocardiographic detection of rheumatic mitral regurgitation. Am. J. Cardiol., *41*: 1258, 1978.

Winters, W., et al.: Abnormal mitral valve motion as demonstrated by the ultrasound technique in apparent pure mitral insufficiency. Am. Heart J., *77*: 196, 1969.

Patent Ductus Arteriosus

Alpert, B., et al.: Plasma indomethacin levels in pre-term newborns with symptomatic patent ductus arteriosus: clinical and echocardiographic assessments of response. Adv. Prostaglandin Thromboxane Res., *7*: 883, 1980.

Baylen, B., et al.: The critically ill premature infant with patent ductus arteriosus and pulmonary disease: an echocardiographic assessment. J. Pediatr., *86*: 423, 1975.

Baylen, B., et al.: Left ventricular performance in the critically ill premature infant with patent ductus arteriosus and pulmonary disease. Circulation, *55*: 182, 1977.

Björkhem, G., et al.: Influence of continuous positive airways pressure treatment on ductus arteriosus shunt assessed by echocardiography. Arch. Dis. Child., *52*: 659, 1977.

Clarke, D., et al.: Patent ductus arteriosus ligation and respiratory distress syndrome in premature infants. Ann. Thorac. Surg., *22*: 138, 1976.

Friedman, W., et al.: The patent ductus arteriosus. Clin. Perinatol., *5*: 411, 1978.

Goldberg, S., et al.: Echocardiographic detection and management of patent ductus arteriosus in neonates with respiratory distress syndrome: a two-and-one-half-year prospective study. J. Clin. Ultrasound, *5*: 161, 1977.

Hall, G., et al.: Premature infants with patent ductus arteriosus and respiratory distress; selection for ductal ligation. Ann. Thorac. Surg., *22*: 146, 1976.

Harinck, E., et al.: Anatomical correction of transposition of great arteries with persistent ductus arteriosus. One year after operation. Br. Heart J., *43*: 95, 1980.

Higgins, C., et al.: Patent ductus arteriosus in preterm infants with idiopathic respiratory distress syndrome. Radiographic and echocardiographic evaluation. Radiology, *124*: 189, 1977.

Hirschklau, M., et al.: Echocardiographic diagnosis: pitfalls in the premature infant with a large patent ductus arteriosus. J. Pediatr., *92*: 474, 1978.

Laird, W., et al.: Echocardiography of premature infants with pulmonary disease: a noninvasive method for detecting large ductal left-to-right shunts. Radiology, *122*: 455, 1977.

McGrath, R., et al.: The silent ductus arteriosus. J. Pediatr., *93*, 110, 1978.

Purohit, D., et al.: Effects of assisted ventilation of echocardiographic findings in two infants with patent ductus arteriosus. J. Thorac. Cardiovasc. Surg., *72*: 294, 1976.

Sahn, D., et al.: Real-time cross-sectional echocardiographic imaging and measurement of the patent ductus arteriosus in infants and children. Circulation, *58*: 343, 1978.

Williams, W., et al.: The ductus debate: ligation in prematurity? Ann. Thorac. Surg., *22*: 151, 1976.

Ventricular Septal Defect

Ahmad, M., et al.: Assessment of left-to-right shunt and left ventricular function in isolated ventricular septal defect. Br. Heart J., *41*: 147, 1979.

Aziz, K., et al.: Echocardiographic features of supracristal ventricular septal defect with prolapsed aortic valve leaflet. Am. J. Cardiol., *43*: 854, 1979.

Brandt, B., et al.: Ventricular septal defect following myocardial infarction. Ann. Thorac. Surg., *27*: 580, 1979.

Fuhrman, B., et al.: Predictive value of the echocardiographic left atrial dimension in isolated ventricular septal defect. J. Clin. Ultrasound, *8*: 347, 1980.

Hibi, N., et al.: Cross-sectional and M-mode echocardiographic study on ventricular septal defect. Jpn. Heart J., *20*: 127, 1979.

King, D., et al.: Visualization of ventricular septal defects by cardiac ultrasonography. Circulation, *48*: 1215, 1973.

Lewis, A., et al.: Echocardiographic assessment of left-to-right shunt volume in children with ventricular septal defect. Circulation, *54*: 78, 1976.

Mehta, S., et al.: Echocardiographic estimation of ventricular hypoplasia in complete atrioventricular canal. Circulation, *59*: 888, 1979.

Riggs, T., et al.: Ventricular septal defect in infancy: a combined vectorgraphic and echocardiographic study. Circulation, *59*: 385, 1979.

Sahn, D., et al.: Echocardiographic detection of large left-to-right shunts and cardiomyopathies in infants and children. Am. J. Cardiol., *38*: 73, 1976.

Scanlan, J., et al.: Visualization of ventricular septal rupture utilizing wide-angle two-dimensional echocardiography. Mayo Clin. Proc., *54*: 381, 1979.

Stone, F., et al.: Ventricular septal defect, solitary aortic trunk, and ductal origins of pulmonary arteries. Am. Heart J., *92*: 506, 1976.

Wilson, R., et al.: The echocardiographic appearance of a partially disrupted ventricular septal defect repair. J. Clin. Ultrasound, *4*: 41, 1976.

RIGHT VENTRICULAR PRESSURE OVERLOAD

Allen, H., et al.: Echocardiographic profiles of the long-term cardiac changes in cystic fibrosis. Chest, *75*: 428, 1979.

Alpert, J., et al.: Left ventricular function in massive pulmonary embolism. Chest, *71*: 108, 1977.

Bell, R.: Ultrasound study of the heart in primary pulmonary hypertension. J. Tenn. Med. Assoc., *71*: 364, 1978.

Bracchi, G., et al.: Relations between echocardiography of the pulmonary valve and the hemodynamics of chronic cor pulmonale. Bronchopneumologie, *27*: 131, 1977.

Chipps, B., et al.: Noninvasive evaluation of ventricular function in cystic fibrosis. J. Pediatr., *95*: 379, 1979.

Covarrubias, E., et al.: Echocardiography and pulmonary embolism. Ann. Intern. Med., *87*: 720, 1977.

Eslami, B., et al.: Paradoxical septal motion in a patient with pulmonic stenosis. Chest, 67: 244, 1975.

Flanagan, W., et al.: Echocardiographic correlate of pre-systolic pulmonary ejection sound in congenital valvular pulmonic stenosis. Am. Heart J., 94: 633, 1977.

Goodman, D., et al.: Echocardiographic features of primary pulmonary hypertension. Am. J. Cardiol., 33: 438, 1974.

Gordon, R., et al.: Obstruction of the right ventricular outflow tract due to metastatic hypernephroma. Vasc. Surg., 7: 213, 1973.

Halliday, H., et al.: Respiratory distress syndrome: echocardiographic assessment of cardiovascular function and pulmonary vascular resistance. Pediatrics, 60: 444, 1977.

Harrison, E., et al.: Coexisting right and left hypertrophic subvalvular stenosis and fixed left ventricular outflow obstruction due to aortic valve stenosis. Am. J. Cardiol., 40: 133, 1977.

Hirschfeld, S., et al.: The echocardiographic assessment of pulmonary artery pressure and pulmonary vascular resistance. Circulation, 52: 642, 1975.

Hirschfeld, S., et al.: Echocardiographic abnormalities in patients with cystic fibrosis. Chest, 75: 351, 1979.

Kline, L., et al.: Noninvasive assessment of left ventricular performance in patients with chronic obstructive pulmonary disease. Chest, 72: 558, 1977.

Krayenbuehl, H., et al.: Left ventricular function in chronic pulmonary hypertension. Am. J. Cardiol., 41: 1150, 1978.

Mehl, S., et al.: Combined tricuspid and pulmonic stenosis. Clinical, echocardiographic, hemodynamic, surgical and pathological features. J. Thorac. Cardiovasc. Surg., 74: 55, 1977.

Meyer, R.: Persistence of fetal circulation syndrome: an echocardiographic study. J. Pediatr., 91: 626, 1977.

Nanda, N., et al.: Evaluation of pulmonary hypertension by echocardiography. J. Clin. Ultrasound, 1: 255, 1973.

Nussbaum, E., et al.: Echocardiographic changes in children with pulmonary hypertension secondary to upper airway obstruction. J. Pediatr., 93: 931, 1978.

Oberhänsli, I., et al.: Echocardiographic study of right and left ventricular dimension and left ventricular function in patients with tetralogy of Fallot before and after surgery. Br. Heart J., 41: 40, 1979.

Rosenthal, A., et al.: Echocardiographic assessment of cor pulmonale in cystic fibrosis. Pediatr. Clin. North Am., 23: 327, 1976.

Ryssing, E.: Assessment of cor pulmonale in cystic fibrosis by echocardiography. Acta Paediatr. Scand., 66: 753, 1977.

Steckley, R., et al.: Acute right ventricular overload: an echocardiographic clue to pulmonary thromboembolism. Johns Hopkins Med. J., 143: 122, 1978.

Unger, K., et al.: Evaluation of left ventricular performance in acutely ill patients with chronic obstructive lung disease. Chest, 68: 135, 1975.

Weyman, A., et al.: Echocardiographic patterns of pulmonic valve motion in pulmonic stenosis. Am. J. Cardiol., 34: 644, 1974.

Weyman, A., et al.: Echocardiographic patterns of pulmonary valve motion with pulmonary hypertension. Circulation, 50: 905, 1974.

Weyman, A., et al.: Echocardiographic differentiation of infundibular from valvular pulmonary stenosis. Am. J. Cardiol., 36: 21, 1975.

Weyman, A., et al.: Cross-sectional echocardiographic visualization of the stenotic pulmonary valve. Circulation, 56: 769, 1977.

Winer, H., et al.: Echocardiographic findings in severe paradoxical pulse due to pulmonary embolization. Am. J. Cardiol., 40: 808, 1977.

Yoshida, Y., et al.: Echocardiographic evaluation of pulmonary hypertension by oxygen inhalation method. Tohoku J. Exp. Med., 127: 199, 1979.

RIGHT VENTRICULAR VOLUME OVERLOAD

Atrial Septal Defect

Beppu, S., et al.: Diagnosis of endocardial cushion defect with cross-sectional and M-mode scanning echocardiography. Differentiation from secundum atrial septal defect. Br. Heart J., 38: 911, 1976.

DaCosta, J., et al.: Results following closure of ostium secundum atrial septal defects. J. Cardiovasc. Surg., *19*: 567, 1978.

deLeon, A.: Atrial septal defect in the adult. Curr. Probl. Cardiol., *1*: 2, 1976.

DeMaria, A., et al.: Apparent reduction of aortic and left heart chamber size in atrial septal defect. Am. J. Cardiol., *42*: 545, 1978.

Diamond, M., et al.: Echocardiographic features of atrial septal defect. Circulation, *43*: 129, 1971.

Dillon, J., et al.: Cross-sectional echocardiographic examination of the interatrial septum. Circulation, *55*: 115, 1977.

Eshaghpour, E., et al.: Echocardiography in endocardial cushion defects: a preoperative and postoperative study. Chest, *68*: 172, 1975.

Forman, H., et al.: Lutembacher's syndrome: recognition by echocardiography. J. Clin. Ultrasound, *7*: 53, 1979.

Guimar-aes, L.: Atrial septal defect—echocardiographic assessment before and after surgical repair. Acta Med. Port., *1*: 457, 1980.

Hagan, A., et al.: Ultrasound evaluation of systolic anterior septal motion in patients with and without right ventricular volume overload. Circulation, *50*: 248, 1974.

Hagler, D., et al.: Real-time wide-angle sector echocardiography: atrioventricular canal defects. Circulation, *59*: 140, 1979.

Kamigaki, M., et al.: Echocardiographic analysis of mitral valve motion in atrial septal defect. Am. J. Cardiol., *30*: 343, 1972.

Komatsu, Y., et al.: Echocardiographic analysis of intracardiac anatomy in endocardial cushion defect. Am. Heart J., *91*: 210, 1976.

Lieppe, W., et al.: Two-dimensional echocardiographic findings in atrial septal defect. Circulation, *56*: 447, 1977.

McCann, W., et al.: The echocardiogram in right ventricular volume overload. J.A.M.A., *221*: 1243, 1972.

Mueller, T., et al.: Comparison of interventricular septal motion studied by ventriculography and echocardiography in patients with atrial septal defect. Br. Heart J., *40*: 984, 1978.

Pearlman, A., et al.: Abnormal right ventricular size and ventricular septal motion after atrial septal defect closure: etiology and functional significance. Am. J. Cardiol., *41*: 295, 1978.

Popio, K., et al.: Abnormalities of left ventricular function and geometry in adults with an atrial septal defect: ventriculographic hemodynamic and echocardiographic studies. Am. J. Cardiol., *36*: 302, 1975.

Quash, J., et al.: Echocardiography in Lutembacher's syndrome. Chest, *72*: 676, 1977.

Radtke, W., et al.: Atrial septal defect: echocardiographic observations. Studies in 120 patients. Ann. Intern. Med., *84*: 246, 1976.

Schapira, J., et al.: Single and two-dimensional echocardiographic features of the interatrial septum in normal subjects and patients with an atrial septal defect. Am. J. Cardiol., *43*: 816, 1979.

Spanos, P., et al.: Repair of atrioventricular canal associated with membranous subaortic stenosis. Mayo Clin. Proc., *52*: 121, 1977.

Tajik, A., et al.: Echocardiogram in atrial septal defect. Chest, *62*: 213, 1972.

Tajik, A., et al.: Normal ventricular septal motion in atrial septal defect. Mayo Clin. Proc., *47*: 635, 1972.

Tajik, A., et al.: Echocardiogram in atrial septal defect with small left to right shunt. Chest, *63*: 95, 1973.

Wanderman, K., et al.: Left ventricular performance in patients with atrial septal defect: evaluation with noninvasive methods. Am. J. Cardiol., *41*: 487, 1978.

Williams, R., et al.: Echocardiographic features of endocardial cushion defects. Circulation, *49*: 418, 1974.

Yoshikawa, J., et al.: Echocardiographic diagnosis of endocardial cushion defects. Jpn. Heart J., *16*: 1, 1975.

Total Anomalous Pulmonary Venous Return

Aziz, K., et al.: Echocardiographic features of total anomalous pulmonary venous drainage into the coronary sinus. Am. J. Cardiol., *42*: 108, 1978.

Bass, J., et al.: Echocardiographic differentiation of partial and complete atrioventricular canal. Circulation, *57*: 1144, 1978.

Mortera, C., et al.: Infra-diaphragmatic total anomalous pulmonary venous connection to portal vein. Diagnostic implications of echocardiography. Br. Heart J., *39*: 645, 1977.

Orsmond, G., et al.: Echocardiographic features of total anomalous pulmonary venous connection to the coronary sinus. Am. J. Cardiol., *41*: 597, 1978.

Paquet, M., et al.: Echocardiographic features of total anomalous pulmonary venous connection. Circulation, *51*: 599, 1975.

Sahn, D., et al.: Cross-sectional echocardiographic diagnosis of the sites of total anomalous pulmonary venous drainage. Circulation, *60*: 1317, 1979.

Shah, K., et al.: Echocardiography in total anomalous pulmonary venous return. Indian Heart J., *30*: 168, 1978.

Wilson, R., et al.: Echocardiographic findings in total anomalous pulmonary venous return (TAPVR) to the coronary sinus. Chin. Med. J. (Engl.), *92*: 703, 1979.

RIGHT AND LEFT VENTRICULAR VOLUME OVERLOAD

Identity with Contrast Echo

Allen, H., et al.: New serial contrast technique for assessment of left-to-right shunting patent ductus arteriosus in the neonate. Am. J. Cardiol., *41*: 288, 1978.

Brenner, J., et al.: Contrast echocardiographic findings in an infant with right coronary artery to right ventricular fistula. Am. J. Roentgenol., *130*: 983, 1978.

Danilowicz, D., et al.: Use of contrast echocardiography in the diagnosis of partial anomalous pulmonary venous connection. Am. J. Cardiol., *43*: 248, 1979.

Duff, D., et al.: The use of saline or blood for ultrasonic detection of a right-to-left intracardiac shunt in the early postoperative patient. Am. Heart J., *94*: 402, 1977.

Fraker, T., et al.: Detection and exclusion of interatrial shunts by two-dimensional echocardiography and peripheral venous injection. Circulation, *59*: 379, 1979.

Hermandez, A., et al.: Diagnosis of pulmonary arteriovenous fistula by contrast echocardiography. J. Pediatr., *93*: 258, 1978.

Kerber, R., et al.: Use of an ultrasonic contrast method in the diagnosis of valvular regurgitation and intracardiac shunts. Am. J. Cardiol., *34*: 722, 1974.

Kronik, G., et al.: Contrast M-mode echocardiography in diagnosis of atrial septal defect in acyanotic patients. Circulation, *59*: 372, 1979.

Mortera, C., et al.: Diagnosis of ventriculo-arterial discordance (transposition of the great arteries) by contrast echocardiography. Br. Heart J., *39*: 844, 1977.

Pieroni, D., et al.: The sensitivity of contrast echocardiography in detecting intracardiac shunts. Cathet. Cardiovasc. Diagn., 5: 19, 1979.

Pritchard, D., et al.: Peripheral arteriovenous fistula. Detection by contrast echocardiography. Mayo Clin. Proc., *52*: 186, 1977.

Sahn, D., et al.: The utility of contrast echocardiographic techniques in the care of critically ill infants with cardiac and pulmonary disease. Circulation, *56*: 959, 1977.

Serruys, P., et al.: Intracardiac right-to-left shunts demonstrated by two-dimensional echocardiography after peripheral vein injection. Br. Heart J., *42*: 429, 1979.

Serwer, G., et al.: Use of contrast echocardiography for evaluation of right ventricular hemodynamics in the presence of ventricular septal defects. Circulation, *58*: 327, 1978.

Seward, J., et al.: Echocardiographic contrast studies: initial experience. Mayo Clin. Proc., *50*: 163, 1975.

Seward, J., et al.: Peripheral venous contrast echocardiography. Am. J. Cardiol., *39*: 202, 1977.

Shub, C., et al.: Detecting intrapulmonary right-to-left shunt with contrast echocardiography. Observations in a patient with diffuse pulmonary arteriovenous fistulas. Mayo Clin. Proc., *51*: 81, 1976.

Tajik, A., et al.: Contrast echocardiography. Cardiovasc. Clin., 9: 317, 1978.

Valdes-Cruz, L., et al.: Echocardiographic detection of intracardiac right to left shunts following peripheral vein injections. Circulation, 54: 558, 1976.

Valdes-Cruz, L., et al.: Recognition of residual post-operative shunts by contrast echocardiographic techniques. Circulation, 55: 148, 1977.

Weyman, A., et al.: Negative contrast echocardiography: a new method for detecting left to right shunts. Circulation, 59: 498, 1979.

Williams, R., et al.: Echocardiographic evaluation of valvar and shunt lesions in children. Prog. Cardiovasc. Dis., 20: 423, 1978.

5

Pericardial and
Extrapericardial Disease

Pericardial effusion is an accumulation of fluid between the epicardium (visceral pericardium) and the fibroserous pericardial sac. Some clinical findings and symptoms of pericardial disease include chest pain, shortness of breath, pericardial friction rub, fever, and an enlarged or enlarging cardiac silhouette on a chest roentgenogram. Echocardiographic requisitions do not always catalog a patient's clinical findings, nor do they indicate the need for careful examination of the pericardium. Instead, the patient's primary diagnosis may be indicated on the requisition or hospital chart,[1] and the physician expects an evaluation of the pericardium in conjunction with cardiac chamber dimensions and ventricular function.

RECORDING TECHNIQUE

The M-mode echocardiographic techniques used to detect pericardial fluid are similar to those used to record routine left ventricular studies. The only difference is the use of maximum signal attenuation to isolate the pericardium-lung interface. Under normal circumstances, the pericardium and epicardium show little or no separation from each other, since there is little fluid in the pericardial sac. Normal pericardial thickness does not exceed 4 mm (Fig. 5–1).

Small, loculated effusions along the inferoposterior aspect of the left ventricle are found with short-axis, two-dimensional echocardiography (Fig. 5–2). These small effusions are often undetected with M-mode echocardiography, since medial angulation of the transducer is discouraged during evaluation of the left ventricle. Estimated quantities of pericardial effusion are not accurate with M-mode echocardiography. Long-axis, two-dimensional echocardiography is more suitable to show the distribution of fluid along the anterior and posterior cardiac borders and at the apex (Fig. 5–3). When two-dimensional echocardiographic capabilities are not available, scans from the posterior papillary muscle to the left atrium often show accurate distribution of fluid along the posterior cardiac border (see Fig. 5–12).

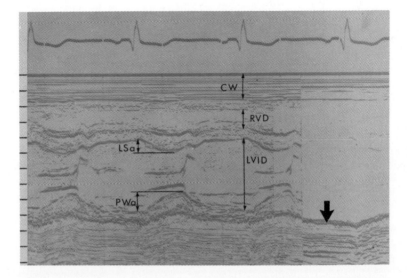

Fig. 5–1. A normal, 16-year-old male. In this routine echocardio-gram of the right and left ventricles and their respective wall motions and dimensions, the echoes reflected from cardiac tissue were damped to isolate the pericardial-lung interface (bold arrow). The right and left ventricular dimensions were measured coincident with the electrocardiographic "R." It is now conventional to obtain diastolic measurements coincident with the onset of ventricular depolarization or "Q." CW, chest wall; LSa, systolic septal amplitude; PWa, posterior wall amplitude during systole; RVD, right ventricular dimension; LVID, left ventricular dimension.

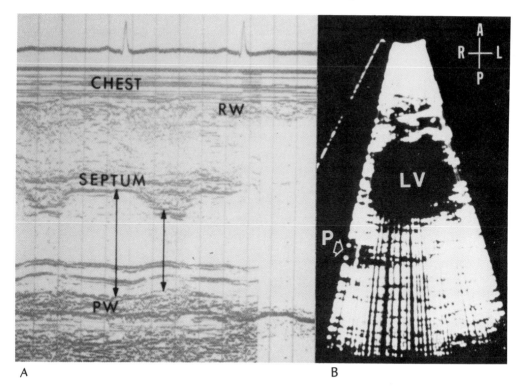

Fig. 5–2. A 44-year-old male patient with coronary artery disease. *A,* Pericardial effusion was not evident on the M-mode echocardiogram. *B,* In this single frame from a short-axis, two-dimensional echocardiogram of the mid-left ventricle, there was a small accumulation of pericardial fluid (P) along the inferoposterior border of the ventricle. RW, right ventricular wall; PW, posterior wall of left ventricle; LV, short-axis plane through left ventricle below the free edges of the mitral valve and above the papillary muscles.

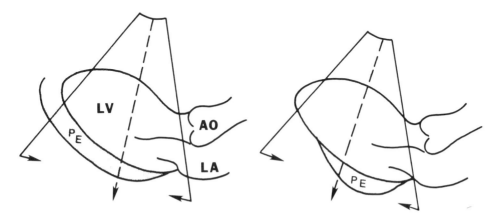

Fig. 5–3. Diagrams showing the superiority of long-axis, two-dimensional echocardiography to evaluate the distribution of pericardial effusion behind the posterior left ventricular wall. The area sampled with M-mode echocardiography (dotted line) erroneously suggests equal quantities of effusion distributed behind each heart. PE, pericardial effusion; LV, left ventricle; AO, aorta; LA, left atrium.

PERICARDIAL DISEASE

Synchronously moving, but separated, epicardium and pericardium may represent either parietal pericardial thickening or small, fibrinous exudates with adhesion (Fig. 5–4). Differentiation between a thickened parietal pericardium and a thickened epicardium is easier when larger quantities of free fluid separate these structures from each other (Fig. 5–5). Apical, two-dimensional echocardiography (see Fig. 4–12) is useful for information about fluid distribution and adhesive strands along the cardiac apex and the lateral left ventricular wall (Figs. 5–5 to 5–8). Fresh blood, effusions of a malignant origin, and serosanguineous effusions are nearly homogeneous fluids and are poorly echo-reflective. Fibrinous effusions and purulent pericarditis produce nonhomogeneous exudates that are often more echo-reflective than the ventricular muscle.

The clinical significance of echographic evidence for pericardial thickening or effusion cannot be determined from the isolated echogram. Insignificant pericardial effusions have evolved into larger quantities of fluid or cardiac tamponade

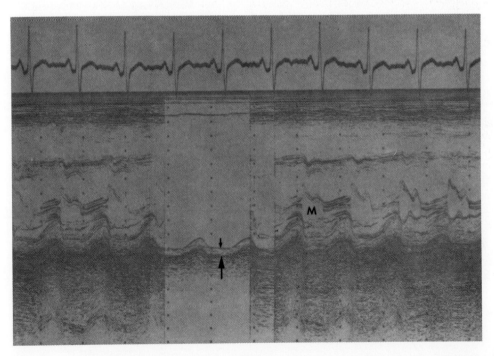

Fig. 5–4. A 30-year-old male patient eight days after the removal of two mediastinal abscesses secondary to dental abscess. There was echocardiographic evidence of a thickened pericardium when reflected signals were attenuated (arrows). At the time of operation, the pericardium was thickened, with inflammation of the pericardial surface. Little pericardial effusion was present at the time of operation. Pericardial aspiration and window were not done. (See Fig. 5–16.) M, mitral leaflet motion.

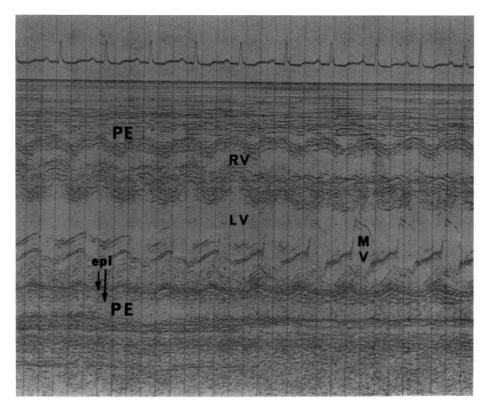

Fig. 5–5. A 58-year-old male patient with chronic renal failure, amyloidosis, anemia, and hypertension. The echocardiogram showed pericardial effusion anterior and posterior to the heart. The increased echo-reflectiveness from the pericardium and the epicardium suggested thickening of these structures. Progressive constrictive pericarditis required surgical intervention. (See Figs. 5–6 to 5–8.) PE, pericardial effusion; epi, epicardium; RV, right ventricle: LV, left ventricle; MV, mitral valve. (Tracing recorded by Julie Arthur, Medical College of Ohio, Toledo, Ohio.)

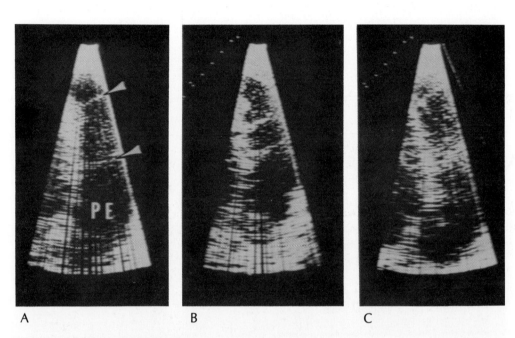

A   B   C

Fig. 5–6.   Still-frames from apical, two-dimensional echocardiograms recorded from the patient in Figure 5–5. *A,* (March 26) A large quantity of pericardial effusion (PE) with adhesive strands (arrowheads) separated the lateral left ventricular wall from the pericardium. *B,* (April 3) The quantity of pericardial effusion decreased following aspiration of 200 ml sanguineous fluid. Adhesions were more echo-reflective. *C,* (April 10) Individual adhesive strands were poorly differentiated. More echo-reflective material appeared in the effusion. The patient developed cardiac tamponade each time hemodialysis was attempted and was referred to a surgeon for pericardiectomy. (See Figs. 5–7 and 5–8). (Illustration *A* similar to Chang, S., and Chang, J.: Cross-sectional echocardiography and progressive constrictive pericarditis. *In* Recent Advances in Ultrasound Diagnosis. Vol. II. Edited by A. Kurjak. (International Congress Series, No. 498. Proceedings of International Symposium on "Recent Advances in Ultrasound Diagnosis," 1979.) Amsterdam, Excerpta Medica, 1980.)

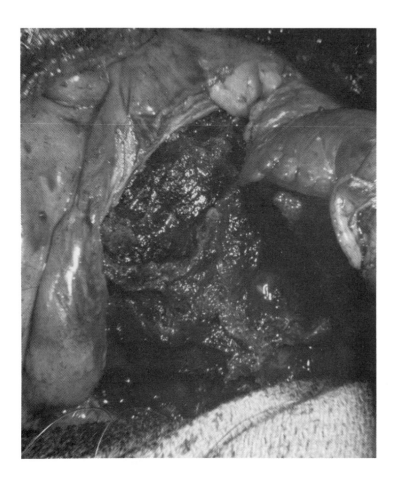

Fig. 5–7. Same patient as in Figures 5–5 and 5–6. The *in vivo* appearance of the heart's surface when the pericardium was opened. The parietal pericardium was thickened and was adherent to underlying structures enclosing a large quantity of sanguineous fluid. The surface of the heart was encased with grumous material.

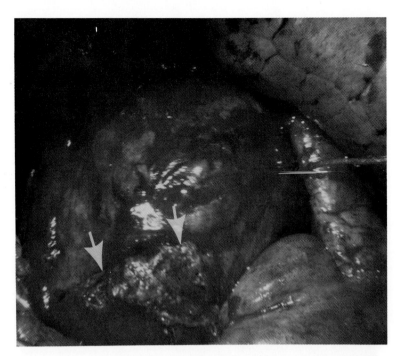

Fig. 5–8. The appearance of a thick, tough epicardium after removal of the grumous material shown in Figure 5–7. The arrows indicate the initial site of the exploratory incision to expose the underlying cardiac myocardium.

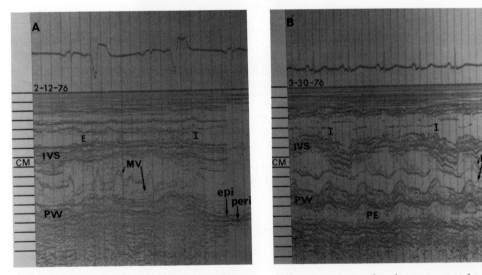

Fig. 5–9. A 51-year-old male. *A,* One day following a quadruple coronary bypass operation. There was a slight separation between the epicardium (epi) and the pericardium (peri); both structures moved in unison compatible with adhesion. *B,* The same patient, 19 days after the operation, showed moderate pericardial effusion, congestive heart failure, and subacute cardiac tamponade. The septum was markedly displaced with inspiration (I). The patient was referred for cardiac catheterization and the following pressures were obtained: mean right atrial, 26 mm Hg; right ventricle, 74/32 mm Hg; pulmonary artery, 74/36 mm Hg; mean pulmonary wedge, 32 mm Hg; left ventricle, 150/30 mm Hg. E, expiration; MV, mitral leaflet motion; PW, posterior left ventricular wall; IVS, interventricular septum.

(Fig. 5–9). Whereas an echocardiogram can support the clinical diagnosis of tamponade, no single echocardiographic feature is pathognomonic for this condition. Clinical correlation is always necessary.

Moderate and Large Pericardial Effusions

Increasing separation between the epicardium and the pericardium results when fluid accumulation is continuous. Except when loculated (Figs. 5–2 and 5–10), most effusions are distributed evenly around the heart and allow it to move freely within the surrounding volume of fluid (Figs. 5–11 and 5–12). Mitral valve motion frequently resembles that seen with mitral valve prolapse. This prolapse movement occurs when the heart is completely unrestrained by the pericardium (see Fig. 7–50).

The patient shown in Figure 5–13 appeared to have a "swinging heart," all ventricular structures moving synchronously with systole. Closer inspection showed a predominantly posterior pericardial effusion with little fluid accumulation along the anterior cardiac border. Two-dimensional echocardiography was not available to evaluate fluid distribution elsewhere around the heart. Dyskinetic septal movement was secondary to an associated right ventricular volume overload.

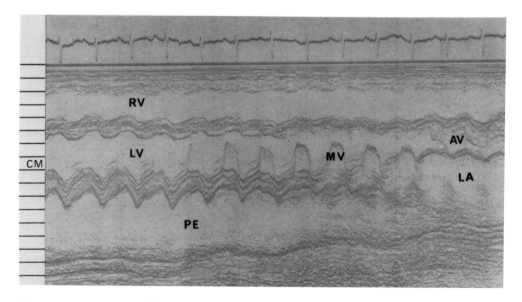

Fig. 5–10. A 20-year-old female patient with thalassemia major, anemia, and congestive heart failure. The tracing was recorded from a sitting, dyspneic patient 16 days after aspiration of 1020 ml sanguineous fluid. Pericardial fluid had re-accumulated and was loculated behind the heart. Another pericardiocentesis was unsuccessful. PE, pericardial effusion; RV, right ventricle; LV, left ventricle; MV, mitral valve motion; AV, aortic valve motion; LA, left atrium.

(Text continues on page 158.)

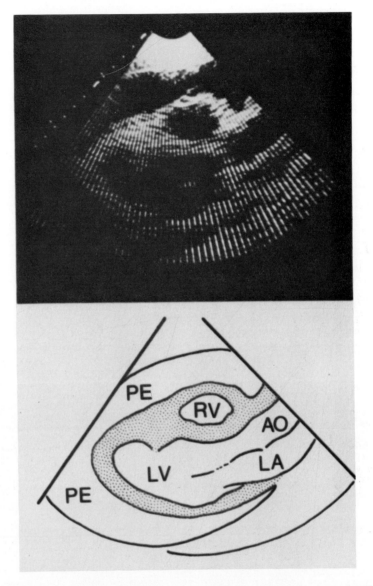

Fig. 5–11. A 47-year-old female patient with liver carcinoma and pericardial involvement. A still-frame and its diagram from a long-axis, two-dimensional echocardiogram show a massive quantity of pericardial effusion (PE) evenly distributed around the heart. The heart moved freely in the fluid without evidence of adhesion. Pericardiocentesis yielded 900 ml thin, cloudy, dark red fluid. Pathologists reported the presence of atypical reactive mesothelial cells, but no neoplastic cells. The patient was referred to a surgeon for a pericardial window. At the time of operation, 500 ml fluid were aspirated. RV, right ventricle; LV, left ventricle; AO, aorta; LA, left atrium.

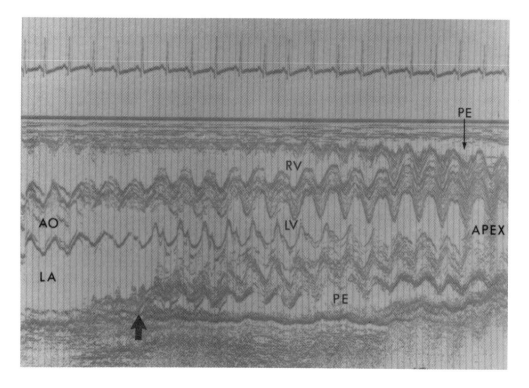

Fig. 5–12. A 37-year-old female patient with chronic renal failure. A compressed scan from the aorta toward the apex disclosed pericardial effusion along the anterior and posterior cardiac borders. The quantity of effusion was less near the atrioventricular junction (bold arrow). AO, aorta; LA, left atrium; RV, right ventricle; LV, left ventricle; PE, pericardial effusion.

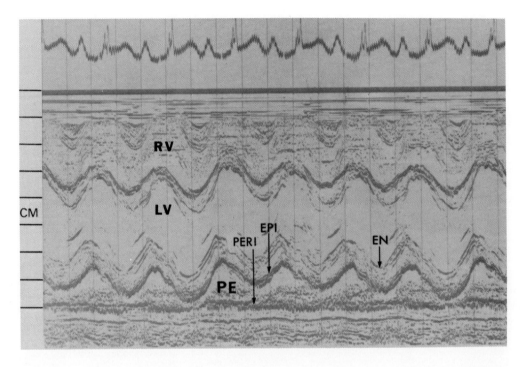

Fig. 5–13. A four-year-old female patient with a small atrial septal defect, Qp:Qs, 1.5:1 ratio. The right and left ventricular wall motion was synchronous. A large quantity of posterior pericardial effusion and minimal anterior effusion were recorded at approximately 45 mm/sec with 200-msec time line intervals. Abnormal septal motion was due, in part, to the presence of pericardial effusion and to right ventricular volume overload. PE, pericardial effusion; EPI, epicardium; EN, endocardial surface of posterior left ventricular wall; PERI, pericardium; RV, right ventricle; LV, left ventricle.

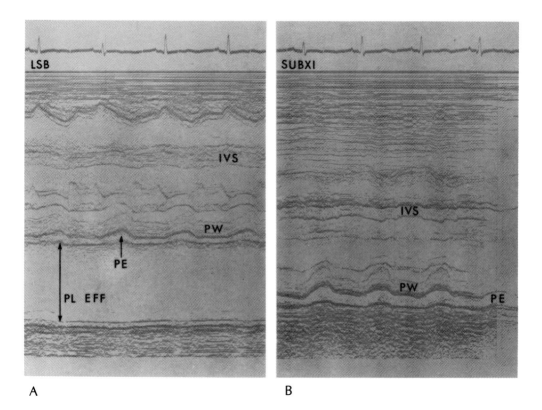

A   B

Fig. 5–14. A 70-year-old male patient with congestive heart failure. *A,* The echocardiogram recorded at the left parasternum (LSB) showed pericardial effusion (PE) and a large
quantity of pleural effusion (PL EFF). *B,* When the transducer was repositioned at the
subcostal examination site, the sound beam was parallel to the lung surface and only the
pericardial effusion was evident. IVS, interventricular septum; PW, posterior left ventricular wall.

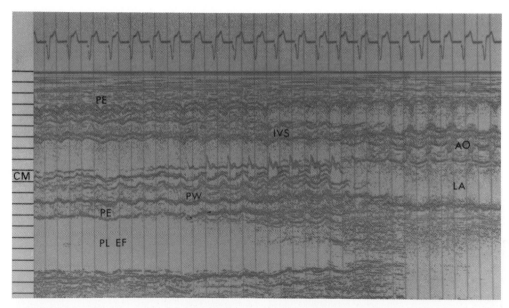

Fig. 5–15. A 67-year-old female patient with congestive heart failure. The compressed scan from the ventricle to the aorta was recorded two days after pericardiocentesis for effusion secondary to pacemaker insertion. A large, left pleural effusion was also present. PE, pericardial effusion; PL EF, pleural effusion; PW, posterior left ventricular wall; IVS, interventricular septum; AO, aorta; LA, left atrium.

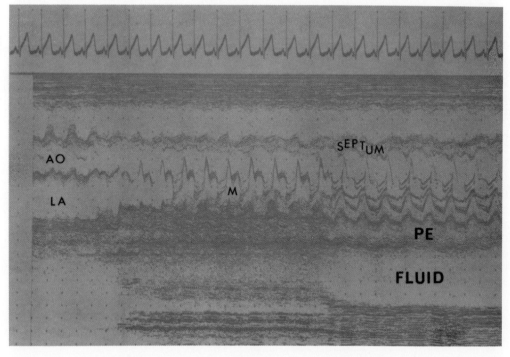

Fig. 5–16. A tracing from the patient in Figure 5–4. The compressed scan from the aorta to the left ventricle showed the relationship between pericardial and extrapericardial exudates. Pericardial effusion was removed by pericardiocentesis. The pleural cavity was explored at the time of operation, and an egg-shaped abscess, 6 cm in diameter, containing 400 ml of pus (fluid) was disclosed. AO, aorta; LA, left atrium; M, mitral valve motion; PE, pericardial effusion.

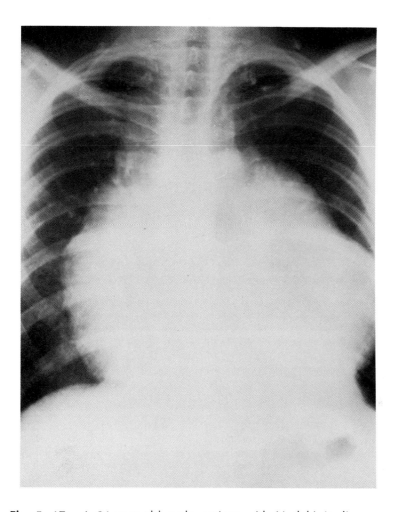

Fig. 5–17. A 21-year-old male patient with Hodgkin's disease. There was massive enlargement of cardiac silhouette. Radiologists were uncertain whether the enlargement was due to pericardial effusion or to mediastinal fluid. (See Fig. 5–18.) (Courtesy of Salvatore Biasi, M.D., National Institute for Study and Cure of Cancer, Milan, Italy.)

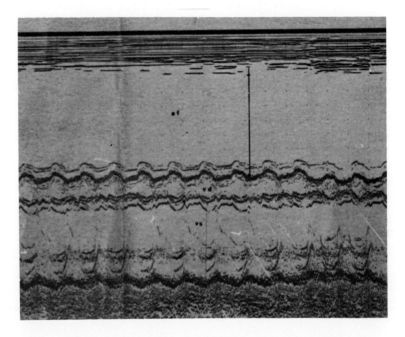

Fig. 5–18. An echocardiogram recorded on the patient whose chest roentgenogram appears in Figure 5–17. There was a large, echo-free (ef) space between the chest wall and the right ventricular wall, thought to represent mediastinal fluid. Two hundred milliliters of clear fluid were aspirated. (See Fig. 5–19.) vd, right ventricle; vs, left ventricle. (Courtesy of Salvatore Biasi, M.D., National Institute for Study and Cure of Cancer, Milan, Italy.)

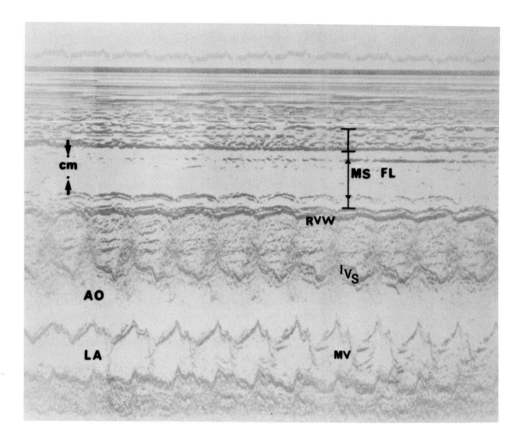

Fig. 5–19. An echocardiogram from the patient in Figures 5–17 and 5–18 following pericardiocentesis. The increased amplification of echoes reflected near the chest wall showed the presence of soft tissue not previously seen in Figure 5–18. The clear space anterior to the right ventricular wall (RVW) showed residual mediastinal fluid (MS FL). After one month of chemotherapy, the patient died. At necropsy, the mediastinal space was filled with neoplasm. The pericardium, epicardium, and myocardium were totally infiltrated. Both atria were undamaged. There was no pericardial effusion. AO, aorta; LA, left atrium; IVS, interventricular septum; MV, mitral leaflet motion. (Courtesy of Salvatore Biasi, M.D., National Institute for Study and Cure of Cancer, Milan, Italy.)

EXTRACARDIAC EFFUSIONS

It is unusual for a large pericardial effusion to be loculated along the anterior or posterior cardiac borders. In these cases, the exudates could be due to extracardiac fluid, as found with pleural effusion (Figs. 5–14 and 5–15), cysts (Fig. 5–16), or tumors (Figs. 5–17 to 5–19).

REFERENCE

1. Fowler, N.: The recognition and management of pericardial disease and its complications. *In* The Heart. 4th Ed. Edited by J.W. Hurst, R. B. Logue, R. Schlant, and N. Wenger. New York, McGraw-Hill, 1978, p. 1640.

BIBLIOGRAPHY

CONSTRICTIVE PERICARDITIS

Candell-Riera, J., et al.: Echocardiographic features of the interventricular septum in chronic constrictive pericarditis. Circulation, 57: 1154, 1978.

Cohen, M., et al.: Constrictive pericarditis: early and late complication of cardiac surgery. Am. J. Cardiol., 43: 657, 1979.

D'Cruz, I., et al.: Echocardiographic diagnosis of partial pericardial constriction of the left ventricle. Radiology, 127: 755, 1978.

Eklayam, U., et al.: Echocardiographic findings in constrictive pericarditis. A case report. Isr. J. Med. Sci., 12: 1308, 1976.

Foote, W., et al.: False-positive echocardiographic diagnosis of pericardial effusion. Result of tumor encasement of the heart simulating constrictive pericarditis. Chest, 71: 546, 1977.

Gibson, T., et al.: An echocardiographic study of the interventricular septum in constrictive pericarditis. Br. Heart J., 38: 738, 1976.

Hancock, E.: Constrictive pericarditis. Clinical clues to diagnosis. J.A.M.A., 232: 176, 1975.

Lewis, J., et al.: Echocardiography: pericardial thickening and constrictive pericarditis. Am. J. Cardiol., 42: 383, 1978.

Pool, P., et al.: Echocardiographic manifestation of constrictive pericarditis. Abnormal septal motion. Chest, 68: 684, 1975.

Schloss, M., et al.: Cystic thymoma simulating constrictive pericarditis. The role of echocardiography in the differential diagnosis. J. Thorac. Cardiovasc. Surg., 70: 143, 1975.

Schnittger, I., et al.: Echocardiography: pericardial thickening and constrictive pericarditis. Am. J. Cardiol., 42: 388, 1978.

Shabetai, R.: Cardiac tamponade and constrictive pericarditis diagnosis. I. J. Maine Med. Assoc., 63: 123, 1972.

Shah, K., et al.: Apexcardiography and echocardiography in constrictive pericarditis. Indian Heart J., 30: 328, 1978.

Voelkel, A., et al.: Echocardiographic features of constrictive pericarditis. Circulation, 58: 871, 1978.

Wise, D., et al.: Constrictive pericarditis. Cardiovasc. Clin., 7: 197, 1976.

CARDIAC TAMPONADE

Antman, E., et al.: Low-pressure cardiac tamponade. Ann. Intern. Med., 91: 403, 1979.

Bulkley, B., et al.: Clinical pathologic conference. Purulent pericarditis with asymmetric cardiac tamponade: a cause of death months after coronary artery bypass surgery. Am. Heart J., 93: 776, 1977.

Burggraf, G., et al.: Effects of dextran infusion on left ventricular volume and pressure in man. Cathet. Cardiovasc. Diagn., 4: 383, 1978.

Cos'io, F., et al.: Abnormal septal motion in cardiac tamponade with pulse paradoxus. Echocardiographic and hemodynamic observations. Chest, 71: 787, 1977.

D'Cruz, I., et al.: Diagnosis of cardiac tamponade by echocardiography. Circulation, 52: 460, 1975.

Dosios, T., et al.: Cardiac tamponade complicating percutaneous catheterization of subclavian vein. Surgery, 78: 261, 1975.

Fernando, H., et al.: Late cardiac tamponade following open-heart surgery: detection by echocardiography. Ann. Thorac. Surg., 24: 174, 1977.

Foote, W., et al.: False-positive echocardiographic diagnosis of pericardial effusion. Result of tumor encasement of the heart simulating constrictive pericarditis. Chest, 71: 546, 1977.

Fowler, N.: Physiology of cardiac tamponade and pulsus paradoxus. I: mechanism of pulsus paradoxus in cardiac tamponade. Mod. Concepts Cardiovasc. Dis., 47: 109, 1978.

Fowler, N., et al.: The paradox of the paradoxical pulse. Trans. Am. Clin. Climatol. Assoc., 90: 27, 1979.

Hancock, E.: Cardiac tamponade. Med. Clin. North Am., 63: 223, 1979.

Hardesty, R., et al.: Delayed postoperative cardiac tamponade: diagnosis and management. Ann. Thorac. Surg., 26: 155, 1978.

Hassani, S., et al.: Ultrasonography of cardiac tamponade. N.Y. State J. Med., 78: 1385, 1978.

Hochberg, M., et al.: Delayed cardiac tamponade associated with prophylactic anticoagulation in patients undergoing coronary bypass grafting. Early diagnosis with two-dimensional echocardiography. J. Thorac. Cardiovasc. Surg., 75: 777, 1978.

Kuhn, L.: Acute and chronic cardiac tamponade. Cardiovasc. Clin., 7: 177, 1976.

Jacobs, W., et al.: Cardiomegaly and paradoxical pulse. Arch. Intern. Med., 138: 1125, 1978.

Jones, M., et al.: Late isolated left ventricular tamponade. Clinical, hemodynamic, and echocardiographic manifestations of a previously unreported postoperative complication. J. Thorac. Cardiovasc. Surg., 77: 142, 1979.

Martins, J., et al.: Can cardiac tamponade be diagnosed by echocardiography? Experimental studies. Circulation, 60: 737, 1979.

Nathan, M., et al.: Unusual echocardiographic findings in pericardial tamponade. Am. Heart J., 98: 225, 1979.

Orzan, F., et al.: Atypical late cardiac tamponade after mitral valve replacement: case presentation with hemodynamic and echocardiographic observations. Cathet. Cardiovasc. Diagn., 3: 297, 1977.

Pearl, W., and Spicer, M.: Cardiac tamponade. South. Med. J., 73: 1091, 1980.

Pories, W., et al.: Cardiac tamponade. Surg. Clin. North Am., 55: 573, 1975.

Schiller, N., et al.: Right ventricular compression as a sign of cardiac tamponade: an analysis of echocardiographic ventricular dimensions and their clinical implications. Circulation, 56: 774, 1977.

Settle, H., et al.: Echocardiographic study of cardiac tamponade. Circulation, 56: 951, 1977.

Slater, E.: Cardiac tamponade and peripheral eosinophilia in a patient receiving cromolyn sodium. Chest, 73: 878, 1978.

Stein, L., et al.: Recognition and management of pericardial tamponade. J.A.M.A., 225: 503, 1973.

Sweetwood, H.: Cardiac tamponade when dyspnea spells sudden death. Registered Nurse, 43: 35, 1980.

Winer, H., et al.: Absence of paradoxical pulse in patients with cardiac tamponade and atrial septal defects. Am. J. Cardiol., 44: 378, 1979.

PERICARDIAL DISEASE

Allen, J., et al.: The role of serial echocardiography in the evaluation and differential diagnosis of pericardial disease. Am. Heart J., 93: 560, 1977.

Bowie, P., et al.: Malignant thymoma in a nine-year-old boy presenting with pleuropericardial effusion. J. Thorac. Cardiovasc. Surg., 77: 777, 1979.

Brigden, W.: The pericardium. Acute pericarditis. Br. J. Hosp. Med., 21: 7, 1979.

Brown, A.: Pericardial disease. Practitioner, 224: 249, 1980.

Burch, G.: Acute viral pericarditis. Cardiovasc. Clin., 7: 149, 1976.

Burney, D., et al.: Rheumatoid pericarditis. Clinical significance and operative management. J. Thorac. Cardiovasc. Surg., 77: 511, 1979.

Chandraratna, P., et al.: Echocardiographic contrast studies during pericardiocentesis. Ann. Intern. Med., 87: 199, 1977.

Charnilas, Y., et al.: Isolated idiopathic chylopericardium. J. Thorac. Cardiovasc. Surg., 73: 719, 1977.

Chowdhury, J., et al.: Disseminated coccidioidomycosis with pericarditis. Successful treatment with amphotericin B. Chest, 71: 533, 1977.

Dunn, M., et al.: Clinical aspects of acute pericarditis. Cardiovasc. Clin., 7: 131, 1976.

Eslami, B., et al.: The echocardiogram after pericardectomy. Jpn. Heart J., 20: 1, 1979.

Felner, J., et al.: Echocardiographic identification of a pericardial cyst. Chest, 68: 386, 1976.

Horowitz, M., et al.: Echocardiographic diagnosis of pericardial disease. Am. Heart J., 94: 420, 1979.

Kotler, M., et al.: The inflamed heart: pericarditis in the elderly. Geriatrics, 35: 63, 1980.

Kumar, S., et al.: Pericarditis in renal disease. Prog. Cardiovasc. Dis., 22: 357, 1980.

Kundu, C., et al.: Pericardial effusion complicating psittacosis infection. Br. Heart J., 42: 603, 1979.

Lacey, C., et al.: Primary liposarcoma of the pericardium. Thorax, 34: 120, 1979.

Lajos, T., et al.: Pericardial decompression. Ann. Thorac. Surg., 19: 47, 1975.

Markiewicz, W.: Echocardiographic detection of pericardial effusion and pericardial thickening in malignant lymphoma. Radiology, 123: 161, 1977.

Martin, R., et al.: Radiation-related pericarditis. Am. J. Cardiol., 35: 216, 1975.

Payvandi, M., et al.: Echocardiography in congenital and acquired absence of the pericardium: an echocardiographic mimic of right ventricular volume overload. Circulation, 53: 86, 1976.

Ross, P., et al.: A case of isolated primary chylopericardium. Br. Heart J., 41: 508, 1979.

Schiller, N.: Echocardiography in pericardial disease. Med. Clin. North Am., 64: 253, 1980.

Shanley, J., et al.: Chronic pericarditis due to a streptomyces species. Am. J. Clin. Pathol., 72: 107, 1979.

Teichholz, L.: Echocardiographic evaluation of pericardial diseases. Prog. Cardiovasc. Dis., 21: 133, 1978.

Tierney, R.: Pericardial disease in children. Paediatrician, 7: 52, 1978.

Unverferth, D., et al.: The differential diagnosis of paracardiac lesions: pericardial cysts. Cathet. Cardiovasc. Diagn., 5: 31, 1979.

PERICARDIAL EFFUSION

General

Abe, H.: Rotational excursion of heart in massive pericardial effusion studied by phased array echocardiography. Br. Heart J., 41: 513, 1979.

Alimurung, B., et al.: Echocardiography in the diagnosis of idiopathic hypertrophic subaortic stenosis coexisting with pericardial effusion. Chest, 76: 187, 1979.

Berger, M., et al.: Pericardial effusion diagnosed by echocardiographic findings in 171 patients. Chest, 74: 174, 1978.

Casarella, W., et al.: Pitfalls in the ultrasonic diagnosis of pericardial effusion. Am. J. Roentgenol., 110: 760, 1970.

Chiaramida, S., et al.: Echocardiographic identification of intrapericardial fibrous strands in acute pericarditis with pericardial effusion. Chest, 77: 85, 1980.

Cobbe, S.: Pericardial effusions. Br. J. Hosp. Med., 23: 250, 1980.

D'Cruz, I., et al.: Potential pitfalls in quantification of pericardial effusions by echocardiography. Br. Heart J., 39: 529, 1977.

Elkayam, U., et al.: Pericardial effusion and mitral valve involvement in systemic lupus erythematosus. Ann. Rheum. Dis., 36: 349, 1977.

Ellis, K., et al.: Pericarditis and pericardial effusion. Radiologic and echocardiographic diagnosis. Radiol. Clin. North Am., 11: 393, 1973.

Farooki, Z., et al.: Hemophilus influenzae pericarditis associated with meningitis. Clin. Pediatr., *13*: 609, 1974.

Feigenbaum, H.: Echocardiographic diagnosis of pericardial effusion. Am. J. Cardiol., *26*: 475, 1970.

Firestein, G., et al.: Left ventricular function in presence of small pericardial effusion. Echocardiography study. Br. Heart J., *43*: 382, 1980.

Foote, W., et al.: False-positive echocardiographic diagnosis of pericardial effusion. Result of tumor encasement of the heart simulating constrictive pericarditis. Chest, *71*: 546, 1977.

Fortuin, N.: The enlarged heart. Pericardial effusion. Med. Times, *108*: 75, 1980.

Friedman, M., et al.: Two-dimensional echocardiography and B-mode ultrasonography for the diagnosis of loculated pericardial effusion. Circulation, *60*: 1644, 1979.

Garbor, G., et al.: Electrical and mechanical alteration in pericardial effusion. Chest, *59*: 341, 1971.

Glaser, J.: Echocardiographic diagnosis of septic pericarditis in infancy. J. Pediatr., *83*: 697, 1973.

Goldberg, B., et al.: Ultrasonically guided pericardiocentesis. Am. J. Cardiol., *31*: 490, 1973.

Gould, L., et al.: Pericardial effusion as an early complication of acute myocardial infarction. Am. Fam. Physician, *19*: 107, 1979.

Greene, D., et al.: Unusual echocardiographic manifestation of pericardial effusion. Am. J. Cardiol., *39*: 112, 1977.

Hagler, D.: Echocardiographic interpretation of pericardial effusion. J. Pediatr., *86*: 645, 1975.

Haider, R., et al.: Congenital pericardio-peritoneal communication with herniation of omentum into the pericardium. A rare cause of cardiomegaly. Br. Heart J., *35*: 981, 1973.

Hamilton, C., et al.: Chronic pericardial effusion and autoimmune antibodies: a case report. Nebr. Med. J., *59*: 351, 1974.

Hassani, S., et al.: Demonstration of pericardial effusion by real-time ultrasonography. J. Natl. Med. Assoc., *70*: 645, 1978.

Hernandez-Lopez, E., et al.: Simultaneous electrical and mechanical alternans in pericardial effusion. Echocardiographic documentation. Arch. Intern. Med., *140*: 840, 1980.

Horowitz, M., et al.: Sensitivity and specificity of echocardiographic diagnosis of pericardial effusion. Circulation, *50*: 239, 1974.

Jacobs, W., et al.: Echocardiographic interpretation of pericardial effusion. Arch. Intern. Med., *138*: 622, 1978.

Kerber, R., et al.: Echocardiographic evaluation of pericardial effusion in myxedema. Incident and biochemical and clinical correlations. Circulation, *52*: 823, 1975.

Krueger, S., et al.: Echocardiographic detection of pericardial effusion. Nebr. Med. J., *60*: 203, 1975.

Laird, W., et al.: The frequency of pericardial effusions in bacterial meningitis. Pediatrics, *63*: 764, 1979.

Lemire, F., et al.: Further echocardiographic observations in pericardial effusion. Mayo Clin. Proc., *51*: 13, 1976.

Lin, T., et al.: Pericardial angiosarcoma simulating pericardial effusion by echocardiography. Chest, *73*: 881, 1978.

Manyari, D., et al.: Detection of pericardial effusion by chest roentgenography versus echocardiography. Can. Med. Assoc. J., *119*: 445, 1978.

Markiewicz, W., et al.: Pericardial rub in pericardial effusion: lack of correlation with amount of fluid. Chest, *77*: 643, 1980.

Martin, R., et al.: Localization of pericardial effusion with wide angle phased array echocardiography. Am. J. Cardiol., *42*: 904, 1978.

Martin, R., et al.: Intrapericardial abnormalities in patients with pericardial effusion. Findings by two-dimensional echocardiography. Circulation, *61*: 568, 1980.

Parashar, S.: Echocardiographic study of pericardial effusion. Indian Heart J., *31*: 98, 1979.

Pedersen, J.: Multitransducer scanning in pericardial effusion. Diagnosis and aid in puncture. J. Clin. Ultrasound, *2*: 224, 1974.

Prakash, R., et al.: Echocardiographic pseudo-idiopathic hypertrophic subaortic stenosis in a patient with pericardial effusion. J. Clin. Ultrasound, 5: 350, 1977.

Prakash, R., et al.: Reliability of echocardiography in quantitating pericardial effusion: a prospective study. J. Clin. Ultrasound, 5: 398, 1977.

Riba, A., et al.: Unsuspected substantial pericardial effusions detected by echocardiography. J.A.M.A., 236: 2623, 1976.

Rinkenberger, R., et al.: Mechanism of electrical alternans in patients with pericardial effusion. Cathet. Cardiovasc. Diagn., 4: 63, 1978.

Sakamoto, T., et al.: Unusual diastolic heart beat in pericardial effusion. Jpn. Heart J., 13: 379, 1972.

Salem, B., et al.: Electrocardiographic pseudo-infarction pattern: appearance with a large posterior pericardial effusion after cardiac surgery. Am. J. Cardiol., 42: 681, 1978.

Salem, B., et al.: Echocardiographic swinging heart motion in loculated anterior pericardial effusion. South. Med. J., 72: 999, 1979.

Sbarbaro, J., et al.: Pericardial effusion and electrical alternans: echocardiographic assessment. Postgrad. Med., 63: 105, 1978.

Shah, P., et al.: Echocardiography in the diagnosis of pericardial effusion. Cardiovasc. Clin., 7: 125, 1976.

Skolnick, M., et al.: Ultrasonic detection of pericardial effusions adjacent to the right atrium during routine examination of the upper abdomen. Clin. Radiol., 30: 295, 1979.

Tajik, A.: Echocardiography in pericardial effusion. Am. J. Med., 63: 29, 1977.

Tehranzadeh, J., et al.: The differential density sign of pericardial effusion. Radiology, 133: 23, 1979.

Vignola, P., et al.: Correlation of echocardiographic and clinical findings in patients with pericardial effusion. Am. J. Cardiol., 37: 701, 1976.

Walinsky, P.: Pitfalls in the diagnosis of pericardial effusion. Cardiovasc. Clin., 9: 111, 1978.

Warren, B., et al.: Echocardiographic observation of ventricular volume changes and swinging septal position in massive pericardial effusion. J. Clin. Ultrasound, 3: 282, 1975.

Weisse, A.: Loculated pericardial effusion in acute pericarditis: diagnosis by combined echocardiographic and radioisotopic techniques. Chest, 76: 113, 1979.

Zoneraich, S., et al.: New, poorly recognized echocardiographic findings. Occurrence in patients with pericardial effusion. J.A.M.A., 236: 1954, 1976.

Renal

Ali-Regiaba, S., et al.: Treatment of uraemic pericarditis by anterior pericardectomy. Lancet, 2: 12, 1974.

Goldstein, D., et al.: Clinically silent pericardial effusions in patients on long-term hemodialysis. Pericardial effusions in hemodialysis. Chest, 72: 744, 1977.

Horton, J., et al.: Natural history of asymptomatic pericardial effusions in patients on maintenance hemodialysis. Proc. Clin. Dial. Transplant Forum, 7: 76, 1977.

Kleiman, J., et al.: Pericardial effusions in patients with end-stage renal disease. Br. Heart J., 40: 190, 1978.

Silverberg, S., et al.: Pericarditis in patients undergoing long-term hemodialysis and peritoneal dialysis. Incident, complications and management. Am. J. Med., 63: 874, 1977.

Winney, R., et al.: Echocardiography in uraemic pericarditis with effusion. Nephron, 18: 201, 1977.

Wray, T., et al.: Uremic pericarditis: A prospective echocardiographic and clinical study. Clin. Nephrol., 6: 295, 1976.

Wright, F.: The diagnosis of free and loculated pericardial effusions during hemodialysis by diagnostic radiology, isotope scintiscanning and ultrasound. Br. J. Clin. Pract., 26: 143, 1972.

Yoshida, K., et al.: Uremic pericardial effusion: detection and evaluation of uremic pericardial effusion by echocardiography. Clin. Nephrol., 13: 260, 1980.

Zarate, A., et al.: Pericardial effusion associated with minoxidil therapy in dialyzed patients. Int. J. Artif. Organs, 3: 15, 1980.

Simulated Pericardial Effusion

Canedo, M., et al.: Echocardiographic features of cardiac compression by a thymoma simulating cardiac tamponade and obstruction of the superior vena cava. Br. Heart J., 39: 1038, 1977.

Chandraratna, P., et al.: Echocardiographic evaluation of extracardiac masses. Br. Heart J., 40: 741, 1978.

Child, J., et al.: Echocardiographic differentiation of mediastinal tumors from primary cardiac disease. Chest, 67: 108, 1975.

Cohen, J., et al.: Echocardiographic features of a calcified pericardial tumor. J. Med. Soc. N.J., 77: 587, 1980.

Farooki, Z., et al.: Echocardiographic features in a case of intrapericardial teratoma. J. Clin. Ultrasound, 6: 108, 1978.

Felner, J., et al.: Echocardiographic identification of a pericardial cyst. Chest, 68: 386, 1975.

Gottdiener, J., et al.: Posterior cardiac displacement by anterior mediastinal tumor. Chest, 77: 784, 1980.

Gupta, V., et al.: Amoebic liver abscess ruptured into pericardium. Indian Heart J., 32: 113, 1980.

Koch, P., et al.: Displacement of the heart by a giant mediastinal cyst. Am. J. Cardiol., 40: 445, 1977.

Lin, T., et al.: Pericardial angiosarcoma simulating pericardial effusion by echocardiography. Chest, 73: 881, 1978.

Millman, A., et al.: Pericardial tumor or fibrosis mimicking pericardial effusion by echocardiography. Ann. Intern. Med., 86: 434, 1977.

Shah, A., et al.: Echocardiographic features of cardiac compression by mediastinal pancreatic pseudocyst. Chest, 77: 440, 1980.

Snyder, S.: Massive pericardial coelomic cyst. Diagnostic features and unusual presentation. Chest, 71: 100, 1977.

Tingelstad, J., et al.: Conformation of a retrosternal mass by echocardiogram. J. Clin. Ultrasound, 4: 129, 1976.

6

Practical Left Ventricular Function

Because it is noninvasive, M-mode echocardiography has been an attractive method by which to evaluate left ventricular pumping performance. The primary limitation of this method lies in the smallness of those areas of left ventricular muscle in which motion may be monitored from one or more intercostal spaces (Fig. 6–1). These muscle segments may be near or remote from each other.

Correct transducer placement is not ideal on patients who are too sick to maneuver into different examination positions, or who have had recent thoracic operations or other open-wound chest trauma. Some patients with emphysema or chronic obstructive lung disease have such small "precordial windows" that echographic records obtained along the para-sternum are unsuitable for evaluation of left ventricular function (Fig. 6–2). Although one may use the subcostal approach to record more cardiac wall and valvular movement, the tracings may also be inadequate for full analysis of ventricular function or definition of a specific disease process (Fig. 6–3). The most exquisite measurement methods cannot compensate for incomplete or carelessly performed tracings. It is better to have no data than to derive erroneous function calculations from records of poor quality.

VENTRICULAR PERFORMANCE BY M-MODE ECHOCARDIOGRAPHY

I favor five variables for routine M-mode echographic evaluation of left ventricular performance. These are left ventricular dimension and wall thickness at the end of diastole, minor axis shortening,[1] relative velocity of contraction,[2] and echographic systolic time intervals.[3] These variables are routinely reported on each patient whenever possible (see Appendix, "Echocardiography Consultation Request"). On *rare* occasions, I estimate an ejection fraction from the mitral-septal separation,[4] the stroke volume through the mitral valve,[5] and the velocity of circumferential fiber shortening.[6] I prefer not to estimate ventricular volume, except for investigative monitoring of acute pharmacologic changes. Each patient

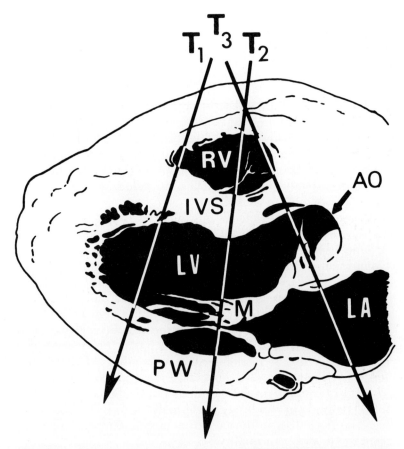

Fig. 6–1. The standard pathway of ultrasound through the right and left ventricles (T$_2$). To examine cardiac structures nearer to the apex or the aorta, the transducer must be angled toward these structures or moved to another intercostal space (T$_1$, T$_3$). RV, right ventricle; IVS, interventricular septum; LV, left ventricle; M, anterior mitral leaflet; PW, posterior left ventricular wall; AO, aorta; LA, left atrium. (Adapted from: McAlpine, W.: Heart and Coronary Arteries, New York, Springer-Verlag, 1975.)

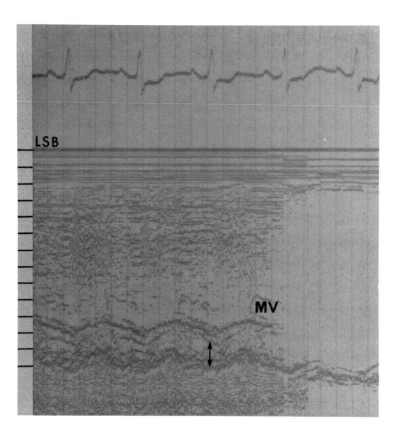

Fig. 6–2. A 70-year-old female patient with idiopathic hyper-trophic subaortic stenosis. The tracing recorded along the left parasternum was technically unsuitable to measure septal thickness or left ventricular dimension (see Fig. 6–3). At cardiac catheteriza-tion, the patient demonstrated a 150-mm Hg subaortic pressure gradient with amyl nitrite inhalation. MV, mitral valve motion; arrow, posterior left ventricular wall thickness.

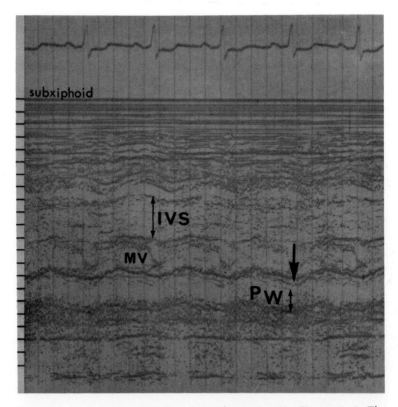

Fig. 6–3. A subcostal tracing from the patient in Figure 6–2. The left ventricular cavity was unusually small secondary to extraordinary myocardial thickening. Systolic septal motion was dyskinetic, and left ventricular fractional shortening was not calculated. IVS, interventricular septum; MV, mitral valve motion; PW, posterior left ventricular wall; bold arrow, slightly thickened or calcified mitral annulus.

serves as his own control, without comparison to other patients.

1. Left Ventricular Wall Thickness (see Chap. 2, "Measurements")

2. Diastolic and Systolic Left Ventricular Dimensions (see Chap. 2, "Measurements")

3. Systolic Time Intervals (see Chap. 2, "Systolic Time Intervals")

4. Minor Axis Shortening[1]

Equation: $\%FS = \dfrac{D - S}{D} \times 100$

Normal (adult): 24 – 42%

% FS = minor axis, or fractional, shortening

D = diastolic left ventricular dimension (Fig. 6–4)

S = systolic left ventricular dimension (Fig. 6–4)

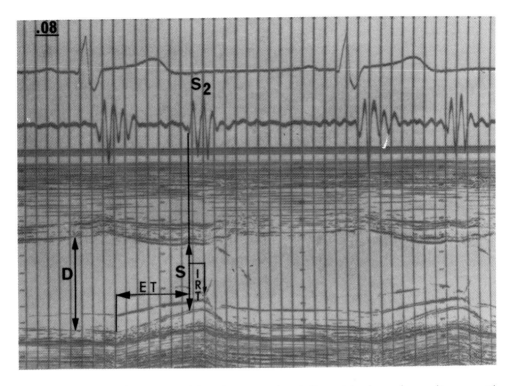

Fig. 6–4. A normal 15-year-old male; a routine left ventricular echocardiogram. The patient was in the left lateral decubitus position with a 20° elevation of the head and thorax. Paper recording speed was approximately 100 mm/sec. Time lines were 40 msec apart. S_2, second heart sound; D, diastolic left ventricular dimension; ET, ejection time; S, systolic left ventricular dimension; IRT, isovolumic relaxation time, measured from the onset of the second heart sound to the mitral valve D-point, expressed in milliseconds.

The percentage of minor axis shortening is a ratio between the diastolic and the systolic left ventricular dimension during the same cardiac cycle. This ratio is influenced by the position of the transducer and of the patient (Figs. 6–5 and 6–6; Table 6–1). It is also affected by cardiac rhythm, ingestion of medication, alcohol and food, surgical procedures, emotional status, associated disease, and measuring techniques. Patients with uniform ventricular contraction exhibit similar values of minor axis shortening at different examination sites (Fig. 6–7).[7,8] Patients with coronary artery disease frequently exhibit focal contraction abnormalities that result in diverse values of minor axis shortening. Since evidence of diminished function can be obtained through poor examination techniques or in technically difficult situations, echocardiographic descriptions of left ventricular function must be carefully correlated with other clinical information. Used in conjunction with other data, minor axis shortening is useful to follow a patient's *trend* toward functional improvement or deterioration (Figs. 6–8 and 6–9).

(Text continues on page 182.)

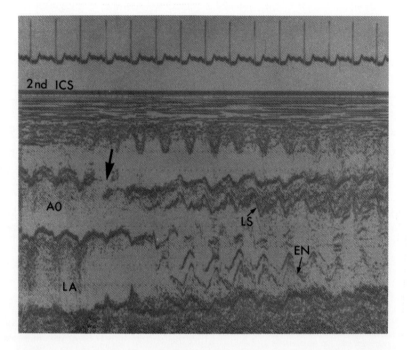

Fig. 6–5. A 48-year-old female patient with a high cardiac output state and systemic hypertension; mild mitral valve prolapse and minimal mitral regurgitation were demonstrated at cardiac catheterization. Mitral valve prolapse was not accentuated by isoproterenol (Isuprel). Large arrow, an artifact mimicking discontinuity between the anterior aortic wall and the membranous septum. This phenomenon is common in adult patients when the transducer is positioned in closer proximity to the great vessels than to the base of the left ventricle. AO, aorta; LA, left atrium; LS, left side of interventricular septum; EN, endocardial surface of posterior left ventricular wall.

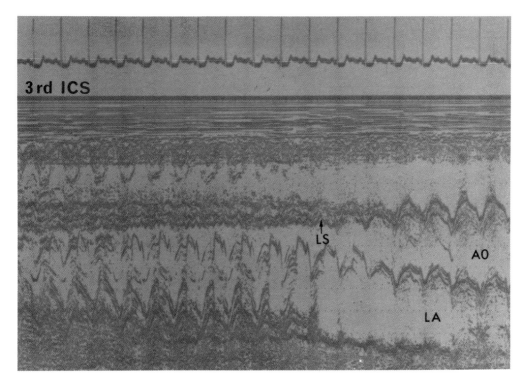

Fig. 6-6. A recording from the patient shown in Figure 6–5. With the transducer relocated from the second to the third intercostal space, the sound beam was no longer perpendicular to the plane of septal motion. The septum appeared erroneously hypokinetic. Aortic-septal continuity was intact. LS, left side of septum; AO, aorta; LA, left atrium.

Table 6–1.
Effect of the Position of Patient and Transducer Upon Percentage of Minor Axis Shortening in 22 Persons Without Cardiovascular Disease

Patient	Age (yr)	% Minor axis shortening position of patient		
		Supine (%)	Left lateral (%)	Subxiphoid (%)
A	57	30	34	42
B	62	37	34	38
C	40	36	34	38
D	41	31	33	35
E	45	26	29	33
F	56	48	46	42
G	48	26	36	30
H	41	29	30	36
I	41	32	34	33
J	58	23	25	31
K	44	26	40	42
L	56	30	41	37
M	41	37	33	37
N	50	35	41	44
O	48	38	46	42
P	50	25	30	25
Q	45	31	27	33
R	51	40	32	45
S	55	40	30	36
T	42	30	32	30
U	60	37	36	37
V	58	41	41	36
Mean	50	33	35	36
Range	(40–62)	(23–48)	(25–46)	(25–45)

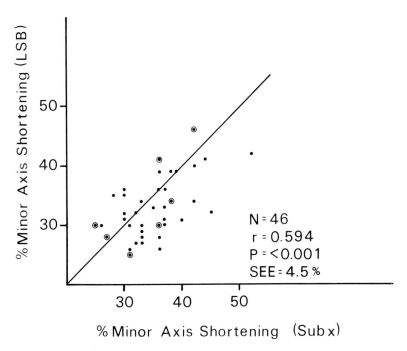

Fig. 6–7. Comparison of left ventricular fractional shortening obtained at left parasternum (LSB) and subxiphoid (Subx) in 46 individuals without evidence of cardiovascular disease. Ages ranged from 40 to 65 years. ⊙ = two patients having identical data; N, number of patients; r, correlation coefficient; P, probability; SEE, standard error of estimate.

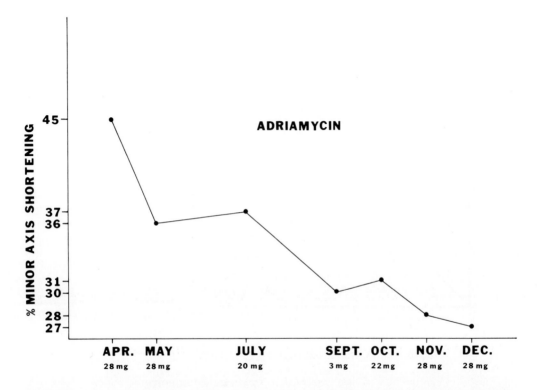

Fig. 6–8. A two-year-old female patient with acute monomyelocytic leukemia of the bone marrow. The child died four months following withdrawal from adriamycin in December. Prior to the initiation of chemotherapy and before each monthly administration of medication, an echocardiogram was obtained to evaluate the status of the left ventricular fractional shortening. With the exception of stable periods in May to July and September to October, there was progressive deterioration of the left ventricular function.

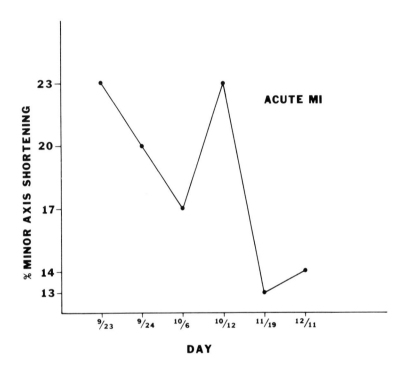

Fig. 6–9. A 63-year-old male patient with an acute anterior
myocardial infarction. The patient received propranolol (Inderal)
and anticoagulants until 10/6, when Inderal was discontinued. The
remainder of the patient's hospital course was uneventful. An
echocardiogram, obtained a week following hospital discharge,
showed significant deterioration of left ventricular function. The
patient's activity level at home was nearly equivalent to bedrest,
although he denied any symptoms and insisted that he could do any
activity he wished.

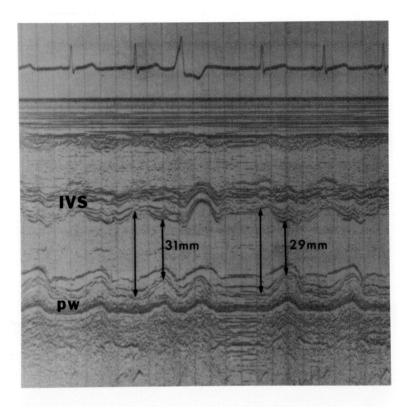

Fig. 6–10. A normal 42-year-old female. The septum moved paradoxically in response to abnormal depolarization. Following a compensatory pause, the septum and the posterior left ventricular wall exhibited slightly more inward movement during systole than was evident before the premature ventricular contraction. IVS, interventricular septum; pw, posterior left ventricular wall.

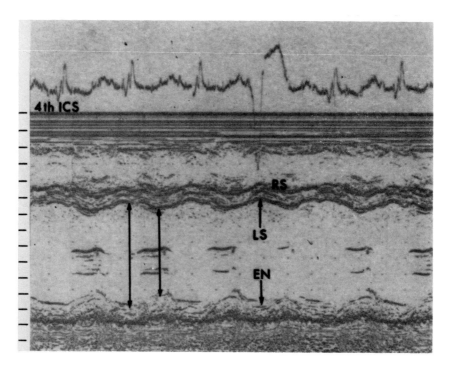

Fig. 6–11. A 70-year-old male patient with coronary artery disease. The right ventricular wall, the septum, and the posterior left ventricular wall failed to show a significant accentuation of wall motion following the extrasystolic beat. RS, right side of septum; LS, left side of septum; EN, endocardial surface of posterior left ventricular wall. (From Chang, S.: The representative septum. Med. Ultrasound, 0(8): 7, 1976.)

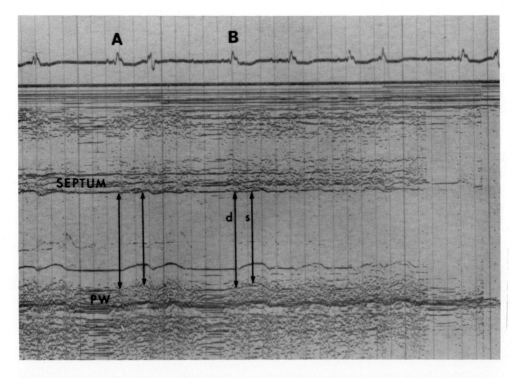

Fig. 6–12. A 65-year-old male patient with ischemic cardiomyopathy. The septum was unresponsive during and following premature ventricular contraction. PW, posterior left ventricular wall; d, diastolic left ventricular dimension; s, systolic left ventricular dimension.

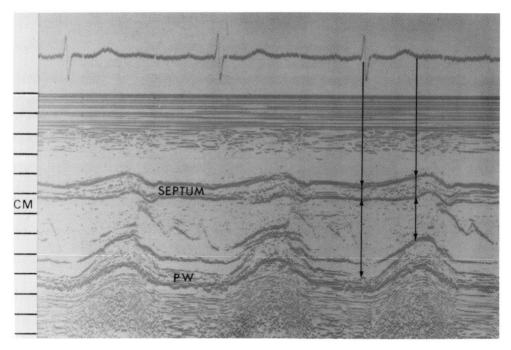

Fig. 6–13. A 40-year-old female patient with a surgical absence of the pericardium. The septal movement was akinetic throughout systole, but it did exhibit some systolic myocardial thickening. Posterior left ventricular wall motion (PW) contributed most to fractional shortening.

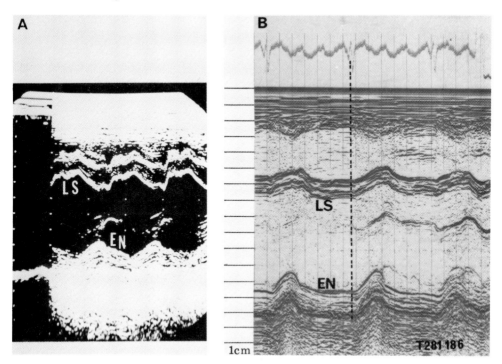

Fig. 6–14. A 50-year-old male patient with severe aortic regurgitation. *A,* A preoperative left ventricular echogram displayed exaggerated septal movement. *B,* The postoperative paradoxical septal motion persisted six years after aortic valve replacement. LS, left septal-blood interface; EN, endocardial-blood interface of posterior left ventricular wall. (From: Feigenbaum, H.: Echocardiography, 2nd Ed. Philadelphia, Lea & Febiger, 1976.)

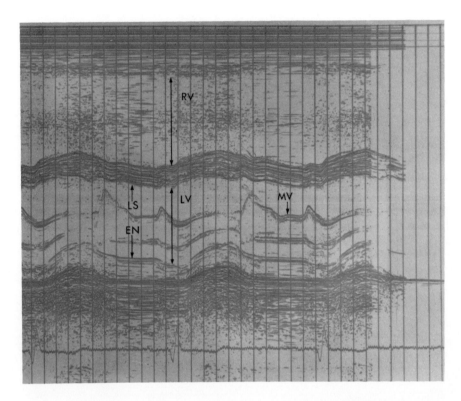

Fig. 6–15. A 60-year-old male patient with a large atrial septal defect and three-vessel coronary artery disease. Fractional shortening was not calculated because paradoxical septal motion causes an underestimation of the ventricular performance. The following data were obtained at catheterization: right atrium, 4 mm Hg (mean); right ventricle, 34/6 mm Hg; pulmonary artery, 34/14 mm Hg; left ventricle, 140/8 mm Hg; left ventricular end-diastolic pressure rose to 16 mm Hg following left ventriculogram; aorta, 140/76 mm Hg; ejection fraction, 53%. There was a large left-to-right shunt at the atrial level. The QpQs ratio could not be calculated, owing to inaccurate blood sample data. RV, right ventricle; LV, left ventricle; LS, left septum; EN, endocardial surface of posterior left ventricular wall; MV, mitral valve motion.

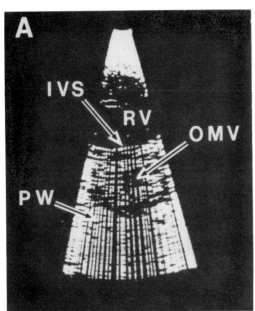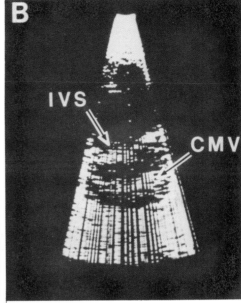

Fig. 6–16. A 59-year-old female patient with an atrial septal defect, QpQs ratio, 3:1, and a history of rheumatic fever. Still-frames from a short-axis, two-dimensional echocardiogram show an enlarged right ventricle and some flattening of the anterior septum. *A*, The mitral valve was unusually echo-reflective, consistent with tissue thickening or calcification. *B*, The systolic shape of the left ventricle was distorted from its expected round symmetry. This was caused by leftward displacement of the septum. The following data were obtained at catheterization: right atrium, 2 mm Hg (mean); right ventricle, 43/0 mm Hg; pulmonary artery, 21/10 mm Hg; left atrium, 10 mm Hg (mean); left ventricle, 132/5 mm Hg; aorta, 112/62 mm Hg. The coronary arteries were normal. There was some scalloping and calcification of the mitral leaflets without mitral regurgitation. The patient was referred to a surgeon for repair of a large secundum atrial septal defect and a smaller patent foramen ovale. The mitral valve, as viewed through the atrial defect, was unremarkable. IVS, interventricular septum; RV, right ventricle; PW, posterior left ventricular wall; OMV, open mitral valve; CMV, closed mitral valve.

Premature ventricular contractions provide a bonus variable for left ventricular performance.[9] The normal ventricular myocardium shows increased minor axis shortening following an extrasystolic beat (Fig. 6–10). The impaired myocardium fails to demonstrate significant systolic enhancement of wall excursion or systolic thickening (Figs. 6–11 and 6–12).

Intrathoracic surgical procedures significantly influence septal movement in the adult (Figs. 6–13 and 6–14), as does right ventricular volume overload (Figs. 6–15 and 6–16). Minor axis shortening should not be calculated in these situations.

5. Relative Velocity of Contraction (RVC)[2]

$$\text{Equation: (a),} \quad \text{Vcf} = \frac{D - S}{D(ET + IRT)}$$

$$(\text{normal} = 1.18 \pm 0.20 \text{ sec}^{-1})$$

$$\text{(b),} \quad \text{RVC} = \frac{\text{Vcf}}{(0.014)\,(\text{HR}) + 0.14}$$

$$(\text{normal} = 1.03 \pm 0.09 \text{ dia/sec})$$

Vcf = velocity of "circumferential" fiber shortening[6]
  D = diastolic left ventricular dimension (see Fig. 6–4)
  S = systolic left ventricular dimension (see Fig. 6–4)
 ET = ejection time
IRT = isovolumic relaxation time, measured from the onset of the second heart sound to the onset of mitral valve opening (see Fig. 6–4)

The relative velocity of contraction assists in the recognition of the left ventricle's decreased ability to pump blood, but like other equations, it does not identify the cause of the dysfunction.

6. Stroke Volume.

There are three ways by which to calculate stroke volume.

The mitral valve method[5] is:

$$\text{Equation:} \quad \left[\left(\frac{EE}{HR} + PR \right) (100) \right] + \frac{2(DE)}{HR}$$

Normal (adult):   81 ± 17.5 ml
  (range, 40 − 116 ml)

EE = maximum, early diastolic anterior, and posterior mitral leaflet separation, expressed in millimeters (Fig. 6–17)
HR = heart rate
PR = electrocardiographic duration of atrial depolarization, expressed in hundredths of a second (Fig. 6–17)
DE = accelerating anterior mitral leaflet opening, expressed in millimeters per second (Fig. 6–17)

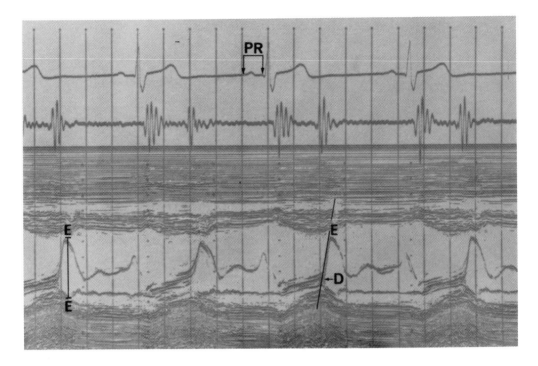

Fig. 6–17. A normal 15-year-old male. Calculation of the estimated stroke volume through the mitral valve requires a maximum separation of the anterior and posterior mitral leaflets (EE) and a continuous record of leaflet motion from the onset of the mitral valve opening (D) to its maximum point of excursion (E). The electrocardiographic PR interval must be free of electrical interference.

Use of this equation requires a mitral valve echogram showing maximum leaflet separation recorded simultaneously with well-defined electrocardiographic "P" waves. When mitral stenosis or aortic regurgitation is present, estimates of stroke volume are invalid.

The echocardiographic estimation of the ejection fraction may not be accurate when left ventricular diastolic pressure is significantly elevated or when the electrocardiographic PR intervals are prolonged beyond 200 msec.

The cube method[10] is:

$$\text{Equation:} \quad SV = D^3 - S^3$$

SV = stroke volume (ml)
 D = diastolic left ventricular dimension (see Fig. 6–4)
 S = systolic left ventricular dimension (see Fig. 6–4)

This formula assumes a symmetrically shaped left ventricle with uniform contraction. As the heart enlarges, there is decreased correlation between this calculation of left ventricular volume and cardiac output as measured by the thermodilution or Fick methods.[11]

The Fortuin method[12] is:

$$\text{Equation:} \quad \text{EDV} = (59)(D) - 153$$
$$\text{ESV} = (47)(S) - 120$$
$$\text{SV} = \text{EDV} - \text{ESV}$$

EDV = end-diastolic volume
   D = diastolic left ventricular dimension (see Fig. 6–4)
ESV = end-systolic volume
    S = systolic left ventricular dimension (see Fig. 6–4)
  SV = stroke volume (ml)

This equation has generally been applied to the enlarged heart. Although it has shown good correlation with Fick's measurements of cardiac output, it also tends to overestimate stroke volume.

7. Mitral-Septal Separation[4]

EPSS ≤ 5 mm = angiographic ejection fraction > 55%

(I have found that if the EPSS is equal to or less than 8 mm, the angiographic ejection fraction equaled or exceeded 55%, as shown in Figure 6–19.)

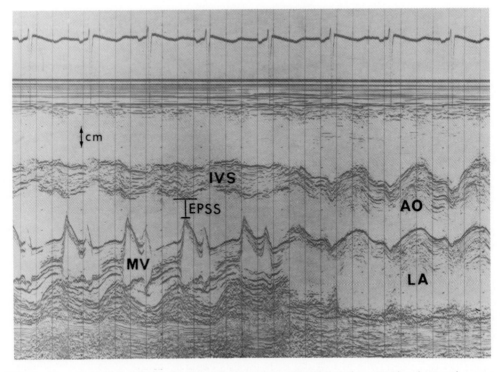

Fig. 6–18. A 29-year-old male illicit drug user. A scan from the mitral valve to the aorta identified maximum mitral leaflet separation. Mitral-septal separation (EPSS) was measured perpendicularly from the most open position of the anterior mitral leaflet to the most posterior position of the septum within the same cardiac cycle. MV, mitral valve motion; IVS, interventricular septum; AO, aorta; LA, left atrium.

EPSS = millimeters of separation between the maximum, early open mitral valve and the most posterior displacement of the septum within the same cardiac cycle (Fig. 6–18)

The appropriate site at which to measure M-mode echographic mitral-septal separation is located by scanning inferiorly from the aorta toward the mitral valve until both mitral leaflets demonstrate maximum separation at or just below the atrioventricular junction. One should measure the perpendicular distance between the mitral valve's E-point and the maximum posterior displacement of the septum within the same cardiac cycle (Fig. 6–18). These echographic estimations of

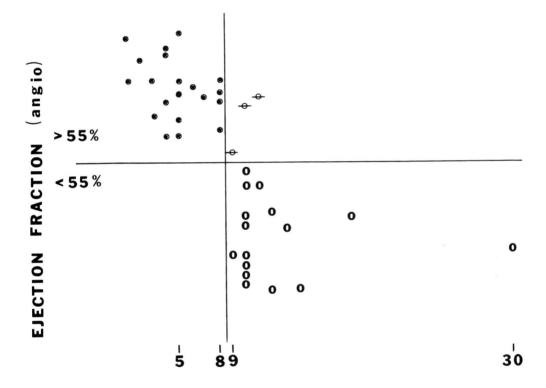

MITRAL – SEPTAL SEPARATION (mm)

Fig. 6–19. A comparison of the echographic mitral-septal separation estimate of left ventricular ejection fraction and the ejection fraction estimated from the left ventriculogram in 39 patients with coronary artery disease. The upper left quadrant shows angiographic ejection fractions exceeding 55% when mitral-septal separation was ≤ 8.5 mm. The majority of patients with mitral-septal separation ≥ 9 mm demonstrated a decreased ejection fraction by angiography (lower right quadrant). The upper right quadrant shows three patients with normal angiographic ejection fractions and mitral-septal separation ≥ 9 mm. These three patients had dilated left ventricular outflow tracts secondary to obstruction of the left anterior descending coronary artery. This resulted in an underestimation of the echographic ejection fraction.

ejection fractions have compared well with ejection fractions obtained at cardiac catheterization (Fig. 6–19). There are limitations to this measurement, however. Overestimation of the left ventricular ejection fraction occurs in patients having apical and lateral wall contraction abnormalities or paradoxical septal movement. Patients with anteroseptal contraction abnormalities, left bundle branch block, mitral stenosis, and aortic regurgitation have an increased distance between the septum and the open mitral valve that leads to the underestimation of the left ventricular ejection fraction.

8. Mean Velocity of Circumferential Fiber Shortening (Vcf)[6]

$$\text{Equation:} \qquad \text{Vcf} = \frac{D - S}{(D)\,(ET)}$$

Normal (adult): $1.29 \pm 0.23 \text{ sec}^{-1}$

D = diastolic left ventricular dimension (see Fig. 6–4)
S = systolic left ventricular dimension (see Fig. 6–4)
ET = ejection time

The ejection time and the ventricular dimensions must be measured from areas with identical electrocardiographic R–R intervals to minimize the effect of changing heart rate. The rate of shortening (Vcf) is useful to detect patients who require an abnormally long time to achieve normal end-systolic dimensions. Unfortunately, the rate of shortening is heart-rate dependent. For this reason, I prefer to use the equation for "relative velocity of contraction" to detect subtle myocardial dysfunction.

EVALUATION OF LEFT VENTRICULAR PERFORMANCE WITH TWO-DIMENSIONAL ECHOCARDIOGRAPHY

Diagnostic acuity has been enhanced with the addition of two-dimensional echocardiography to the noninvasive arsenal. Many different planes of examination allow the assessment of large areas of regional wall movement and establish spatial relationships between the cardiac chambers and great vessels. Euphoric initial experiences with two-dimensional echocardiography might lead one to think that the examination techniques are simple. In fact, identification of cardiac anatomic structures and movement requires as much technical skill as it does in M-mode echocardiography.

Problems with adult examination are almost exclusively due to lung interference or chest deformity. Adult subcostal studies are feasible only with equipment capable of depth compression equal to or greater than 20 cm. Technical problems of instrumentation, transducer placement, and anatomic identification during an examination are compounded when examining wiggly infants. The neonatal heart is minuscule, as compared with that of an adult, with heart rates ranging from 100 to 200 beats per min. Noisy, mechanically oscillating transducers frighten infants and young children and are abrasive to their skin unless suspended in mounds of unstable jelly. There is less room to maneuver large transducers to achieve ideal planes of examination, especially when life-support equipment is in place.

Planes of Examination

Long Axis (see Fig. 8–1)

Long-axis, two-dimensional echocardiography is used at the beginning of an examination to establish the normalcy of the ventricular outflow tract, mitral valve, and proximal aorta. It is also used to localize the base of the left ventricle with respect to the transducer. Septal wall thickness and movement can be ascertained qualitatively from the two-dimensional echogram. I prefer to obtain more quantitative measurements from the M-mode echocardiogram.

Short Axis

One should rotate the adult patient into a partial left lateral decubitus position. Place the transducer along the parasternum, perpendicular to the mitral valve so the sound beam bisects the heart across its minor axis in an imaginary plane between the right flank and the left shoulder (Fig. 6–20). The transducer may be rotated clockwise or counterclockwise and angled superiorly or inferiorly until the left ventricular cavity assumes a symmetrically round appearance, with the mitral leaflets bridging this circumferential shape from right to left.

Short-axis, two-dimensional echocardiography is used to identify overt, focal contraction abnormalities of the medial septum and the inferior and lateral left ventricular walls. Distortion of a ventricular cavity from its expected round shape is the first visual indication of regional dysfunction. One's attention must then be directed to the quality of wall motion exhibited in the distended area to exclude the possibility of an aneurysm or a pseudoaneurysm. An example of an anterolateral ventricular aneurysm is shown in Figure 6–21.

Lateral ventricular wall motion is often difficult to record, owing to lung interference, but it can be achieved if the patient exhales and holds his breath for a short time during recording. Sometimes we rotate the transducer 180° counterclockwise into a "reversed short axis" plane to see the curvature and motion of the lateral ventricular wall. Audio notation of this maneuver is recorded for the benefit of those who review videotapes at a later time.

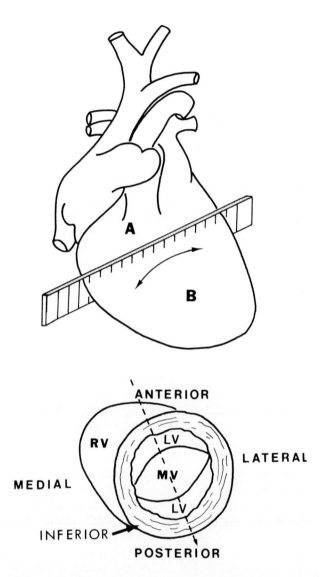

Fig. 6–20. Diagram of basilar ventricular anatomy seen with short-axis, two-dimensional echocardiography. The transducer was positioned along the left parasternum. The sound beam bisected the ventricle in an imaginary plane between the right flank and the left shoulder. This view provides information concerning lateral, medial, and inferior ventricular wall curvature and motion unavailable to the M-mode echographic plane of examination (dotted line).

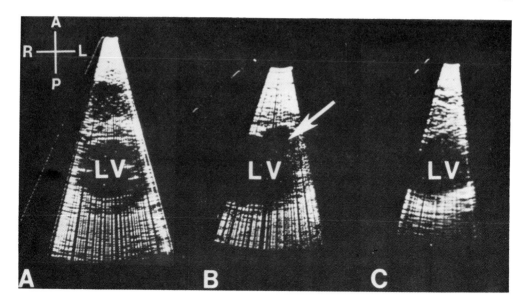

Fig. 6–21. *A,* A normal 49-year-old male. A short-axis, two-dimensional echocardiogram of the left ventricle showed a symmetrically round cavity. *B,* A 57-year-old man with a complete occlusion of the left anterior descending coronary artery distal to the first septal perforator. A short-axis, two-dimension echogram of the left ventricle showed distension and akinesis of the anterolateral wall (arrow). The left ventriculogram showed a large aneurysmal sac in the anterior free wall of the left ventricle. The inferior segment of the aneurysm was irregular, suggesting thrombus. At operation, the aneurysm was broadly based without any discrete neck and contained large quantities of soft, loosely adherent clot. *C,* A postoperative two-dimension echocardiogram showed a small, symmetrically round ventricular cavity. LV, left ventricle; A, anterior; P, posterior; R, right; L, left.

That area of the left ventricle occupied by the papillary muscles is seen with inferior angulation of the sound beam below the mitral valve and chordae tendineae. Occasionally, the transducer must be relocated inferiorly and laterally to obtain the desired position. The papillary muscles extend into the left ventricular cavity at approximately five o'clock and eight o'clock positions and form a dumbbell or mushroom-shaped cavity during systole (Fig. 6–22). With the exception of the papillary muscles, no other organized echoes should be reflected from this area of the ventricle. Large quantities of extraneous echoes protruding into the ventricular cavity are consistent with myxomas or thrombus formation (Fig. 6–23). The differential diagnosis cannot be made with echocardiography.

Occasionally, many echoes fill an enlarged and hypokinetic left ventricular cavity, as seen in Figure 6–24. The echoes persisted even at low signal amplification, but an apical filling defect could not be demonstrated in this patient during cardiac catheterization.

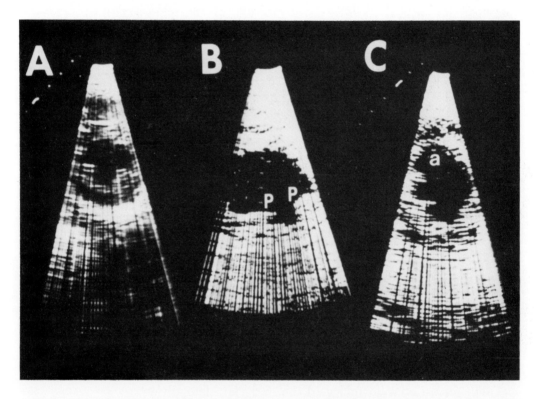

Fig. 6–22. Still frames of parasternal short-axis, two-dimensional echograms at the level of the papillary muscles from: *A,* A normal 23-year-old female patient; *B,* A 62-year-old female patient with coronary artery disease and congestive heart failure; *C,* A 45-year-old male patient with an anteroseptal aneurysm. p, papillary muscle; a, aneurysm.

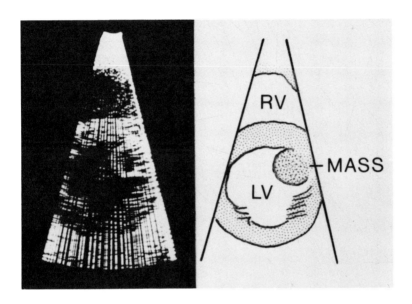

Fig. 6–23. A 58-year-old male patient with diabetes, congestive heart failure, coronary artery disease, and cardiomyopathy. This still-frame and its diagram from a short-axis, two-dimensional echocardiogram show echoes protruding into the anterolateral aspect of the ventricular cavity. These echoes could represent a thrombus or a myxoma. (See Fig. 6–32.) Following a short, uneventful hospital course, the patient was discharged. Dipyridamole (Persantin) and an aspirin-magnesium aluminum hydroxide compound (Ascriptin) were prescribed because of a history of cerebrovascular embolism and the presence of the ventricular mass. RV, right ventricle; LV, left ventricle.

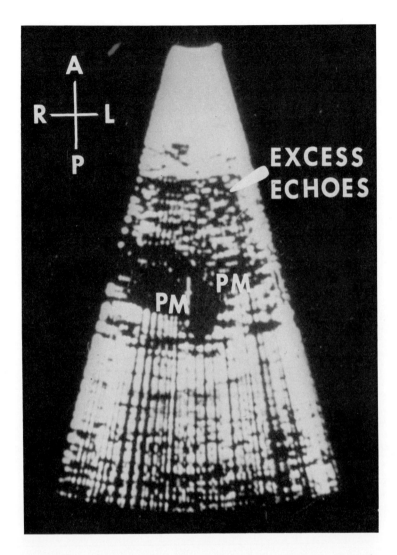

Fig. 6–24. A 40-year-old male patient with coronary artery disease. In this short-axis, two-dimensional echocardiogram at the level of the papillary muscles (PM), apical dilatation displaced the papillary muscles laterally and medially, causing the cavity to appear more round. Excess echoes in the anterior, anteromedial, and lateral aspects of the ventricular cavity suggested the presence of a mural thrombus or an area of nearly stagnated blood. No filling defects were demonstrated on the left ventriculograms, right anterior oblique and lateral projections. There was marked hypokinesis of the anterolateral, apical, and distal inferior ventricular walls. The estimated angiographic ejection fraction was 36%. The patient was not a surgical candidate. A, anterior; P, posterior; R, right; L, left.

Four-Chamber Apical View

One should rotate the patient into a partial or steep left lateral position with elevation of the torso between 20 and 50°. This maneuver brings the cardiac apex closer to the chest wall. The transducer should be positioned on the left ventricular apex (point of maximal impulse) with the ultrasound directed toward the mitral valve or the aorta. The plane of interrogation should be between the right flank and the left shoulder (Fig. 6–25).

Most normal left ventricles are strawberry-shaped, the ventricular base being wider than the narrow, tapered apex. During systole, the septal, apical, and lateral ventricular walls should move uniformly inward. The apical-lateral ventricular segment is the most difficult area to evaluate (Fig. 6–26). This area frequently appears akinetic, even in normal individuals,

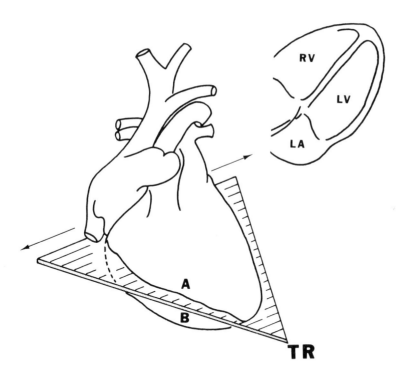

Fig. 6–25. Schematics for two-dimensional examination of the heart from the left ventricular apex (apical four-chamber view). The transducer is located in the vicinity of the "point of maximal impulse" and is directed toward the crux of the heart, where atrial and ventricular septa meet. Sound beams bisect the heart through a long axis from right to left. Inset: the diagram shows section (A) lifted from section (B) to a fully opened position. This is one presentation of the heart on an echograph monitor during examination of the left ventricle. RV, right ventricle; LA, left atrium; LV, left ventricle; TR, transducer.

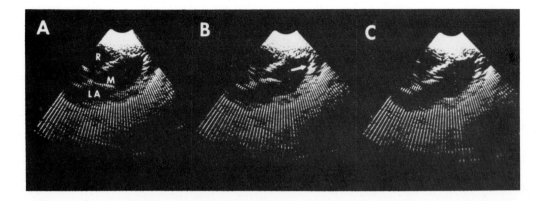

Fig. 6–26. An 18-year-old male patient, normal. The transducer was placed near the right ventricular apex. Although this apical view does not present the maximum longitudinal plane through the left ventricle, it does provide the best plane to evaluate wall motion of the apical-lateral segment (arrow). *A,* End-systole; *B,* Early diastole; *C,* Mitral valve fully open. LA, left atrium; M, mitral valve, R, right ventricle.

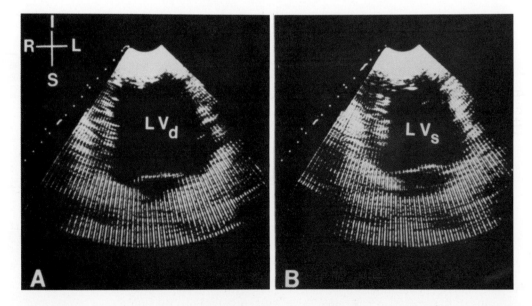

Fig. 6–27. A 40-year-old male patient with chest pain, cardiomegaly, and aortic insufficiency secondary to a markedly dilated aortic root. M-mode echographic fractional shortening was diminished at 21 to 25%. *A* (LV_d), Diastolic apical, long-axis two-dimensional echogram shows left ventricular chamber enlargement. *B* (LV_s), The systolic strawberry shape of the ventricle was preserved secondary to uniform global contraction. I, inferior or apex; S, superior, toward ventricular base; R, right; L, left.

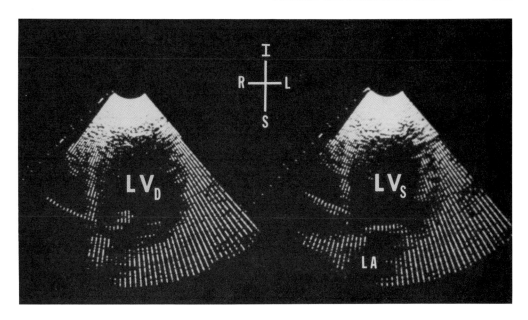

Fig. 6–28. A 54-year-old male patient with congestive heart failure and alcoholic cardiomyopathy. The chest roentgenogram showed a large global heart with evidence of biventricular hypertrophy and pulmonary vascular congestion. The M-mode echogram showed normal left ventricular wall thickness. Generalized dilatation of the left ventricle produced a globular-shaped chamber. There was little change in shape between diastole and systole, owing to generalized hypokinetic wall motion. LV_s, systole; LV_d, diastole; LA, left atrium; I, inferior or apex; S, superior or toward ventricular base; R, right; L, left.

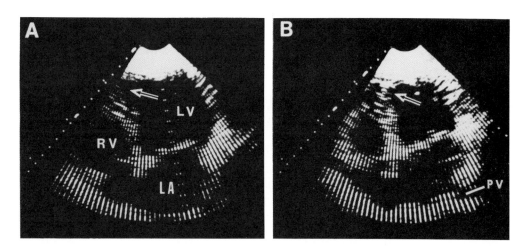

Fig. 6–29. A 24-year-old male illicit drug user with mitral stenosis and regurgitation. Hospital admission followed a car accident secondary to the patient's episode of syncope. *A,* The enlarged left ventricle showed an unusual diastolic distortion of the anteroapical segment (arrow). *B,* Uniform, inward systolic contraction excluded a discrete ventricular aneurysm. Left atrial enlargement was also present. LV, left ventricle; RV, right ventricle; LA, left atrium; PV, pulmonary vein.

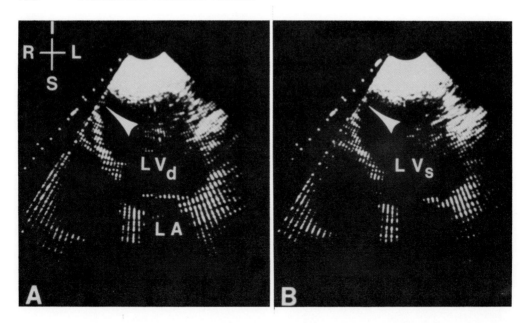

Fig. 6–30. A 65-year-old male patient with congestive heart failure, coronary artery disease and clinical findings of ventricular aneurysm. *A,* A four-chamber apical view showed an enlargement of the left ventricle with distortion of diastolic shape, particularly in anteroapical segment (arrowhead). *B,* During systole, this area expanded outward, consistent with a ventricular aneurysm. The patient died; an autopsy was not obtained. LV_d, diastolic shape of left ventricle; LA, left atrium; LV_s, systolic shape of left ventricle; I, inferior or apex; S, superior or toward ventricular base; R, right; L, left.

and requires extensive manipulation of the transducer or the patient to align the ultrasound correctly with the wall's plane of movement.

The left ventricular strawberry shape is maintained when enlargement of this chamber is uniform (Fig. 6–27). Globular or square-shaped ventricles occur with excessive apical dilatation (Figs. 6–28 and 6–29). Some patients exhibit diastolic distortion of the anteroapical segment, but inward systolic contraction excludes a ventricular aneurysm (Fig. 6–29). Outward systolic distension, with enlargement of this segment, is consistent with a significant ventricular aneurysm (Fig. 6–30).

Examination of the Left Ventricular Inferior Wall

Two-dimensional echocardiographic records of left ventricular inferior wall motion are achieved by rotating the transducer approximately 60 to 90° *counterclockwise* from the four-chamber apical plane of examination (Fig. 6–31). This two-chamber or "simulated left posterior oblique view" is similar to the left posterior oblique view seen during cineangiography. It is also similar to the original long-axis apical view described by Feigenbaum, H., et al., except the trans-

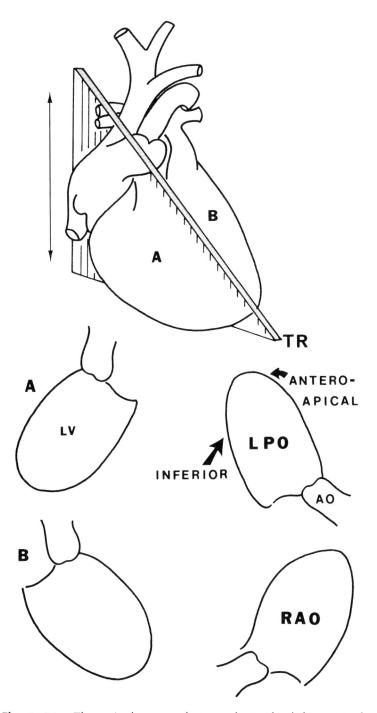

Fig. 6–31. The apical approach to evaluate the left ventricular inferior wall is shown at the top. *A,* The simulated left posterior oblique view obtained by rotating the transducer 60 to 90° counterclockwise from the apical four-chamber position. The presentation on the monitor shows the ventricular apex directed anteriorly and leftward; the mitral valve and aorta are oriented posteriorly and rightward. *B,* The simulated right anterior oblique view obtained by rotating the transducer 60 to 90° clockwise from the four-chamber view. The presentation on the monitor is the mirror-image of the simulated left posterior oblique view (LPO). RAO, right anterior oblique; AO, aorta; LV, left ventricle; TR, transducer.

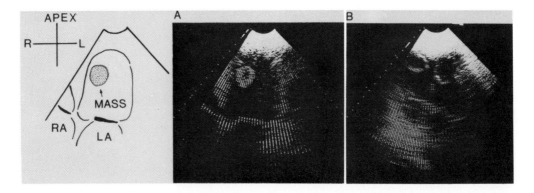

Fig. 6–32. A 58-year-old male patient. (See Fig. 6–23.) *A,* A still-frame and its diagram from an apical two-dimensional echocardiogram show a large, globular mass localized near the left ventricular apex. *B,* The transducer was rotated approximately 90° counterclockwise. This simulated a left posterior oblique plane and disclosed the presence of *two* masses. Both masses were presumed to be organized thrombi, based upon the patient's clinical history. This patient was not a surgical candidate and is presently being followed in an outpatient clinic. No further embolic events have occurred following his hospital discharge.

ducer is on, not over, the apical impulse.[13,14] Generally, movement of the inferior wall can be recorded more easily in this plane than in its counterpart, the "simulated right anterior oblique" view, which requires 60 to 90° *clockwise* rotation of the transducer from the four-chamber apical plane (Fig. 6–31).

Using the two- and four-chamber apical views, two large apical masses were detected (Fig. 6–32). The patient's clinical situation did not warrant surgical removal of these masses. The presumptive cause was thrombi secondary to severe coronary artery disease and akinetic wall motion following an acute myocardial infarction.

REFERENCES

1. McDonald, I., et al.: Analysis of left ventricular wall motion by reflected ultrasound: application to assessment of myocardial function. Circulation, *46:* 14, 1972.
2. Knapp, W.: Relationships between mean velocity of circumferential fiber shortening (Vcf) and heart rate—the diagnostic value of normalization of Vcf to heart rate. J. Clin. Ultrasound, *6:* 10, 1978.
3. Stefadouros, M., et al.: Systolic time intervals by echocardiography. Circulation, *51:* 114, 1975.
4. Massie, B.: Mitral-septal separation: New echocardiographic index of ventricular function. Am. J. Cardiol., *39:* 1008, 1977.
5. Rasmussen, S., et al.: Stroke volume calculated from the mitral valve echogram in patients with and without ventricular dyssynergy. Circulation, *58:* 125, 1978.
6. Cooper, R., et al.: Ultrasound determinations of mean fiber shortening rate in man. Am. J. Cardiol., *29:* 257, 1972.
7. Crawford, M., et al.: Subxiphoid echocardiography: accuracy for assessing left ventricular size and performance. Am. J. Cardiol., *43:* 410, 1979. (Abstr.).

8. Starling, M., et al.: Accuracy of subxiphoid echocardiography for assessing left ventricular size and performance. Circulation, *61*: 367, 1980.

9. Cohn, P., et al.: Noninvasively induced postextrasystolic potentiation of ischemic and infarcted myocardium in patients with coronary artery disease. Am. Heart J., *97*: 187, 1979.

10. Pombo, J., et al.: Left ventricular volumes and ejection fraction by echocardiography. Circulation, *43*: 480, 1971.

11. Alpert, J., et al.: Blood flow measurement: the cardiac output. *In* Cardiac Catheterization and Angiography. Edited by W. Grossman. Philadelphia, Lea & Febiger, 1976, pp. 44, 62.

12. Fortuin, N., et al.: Determinations of left ventricular volumes by ultrasound. Circulation, *44*: 575, 1971.

13. Feigenbaum, H.: Echocardiography. 2nd Ed. Philadelphia, Lea & Febiger, 1976, p. 336.

14. Feigenbaum, H., et al.: Role of echocardiography in patients with coronary artery disease. Am. J. Cardiol., *37*: 775, 1976.

BIBLIOGRAPHY

CORONARY ARTERY DISEASE

Acute

Bates, R., et al.: Cardiac rupture—challenge in diagnosis and management. Am. J. Cardiol., *40*: 429, 1977.

Bergeron, G., et al.: Echocardiographic analysis of mitral valve motion after acute myocardial infarction. Circulation, *51*: 82, 1975.

Chandraratna, P., et al.: Echocardiographic observations on ventricular septal rupture complicating acute myocardial infarction. Circulation, *51*: 506, 1975.

Corya, B., et al.: Echocardiography in acute myocardial infarction. Am. J. Cardiol., *36*: 1, 1975.

DeJoseph, R., et al.: Echocardiographic findings of ventricular septal rupture in acute myocardial infarction. Am. J. Cardiol., *36*: 346, 1975.

Eisenmann, B., et al.: Anatomic, clinical and therapeutic features of acute cardiac rupture. Successful surgical management fourteen hours after myocardial infarction. J. Thorac. Cardiovasc. Surg., *76*: 78, 1978.

Farcot, J., et al.: Two-dimensional echocardiographic visualization of ventricular septal rupture after acute anterior myocardial infarction. Am. J. Cardiol., *45*: 370, 1980.

Hanrath, P., et al.: Relationship between pulmonary artery pressure and echocardiographic mitral valve closure in patients with acute myocardial infarction. *In* Myocardial Failure. Edited by G. Riecker, et al. Berlin, Springer, 1977.

Heger, J., et al.: Cross-sectional echocardiography in acute myocardial infarction: detection and localization of regional left ventricular asynergy. Circulation, *60*: 531, 1979.

Heger, J., et al.: Cross-sectional echocardiographic analysis of the extent of left ventricular asynergy in acute myocardial infarction. Circulation, *61*: 1113, 1980.

Heikkilä, J., et al.: Echoventriculographic detection, localization and quantification of left ventricular asynergy in acute myocardial infarction. A correlative echo and electrocardiographic study. Br. Heart J., *37*: 46, 1975.

Heikkilä, J., et al.: Echoventriculography in acute myocardial infarction. Infarct size and reliability by pathologic anatomic correlations. Clin. Cardiol., *3*: 26, 1980.

Kerber, R., et al.: Effect of intra-aortic balloon counterpulsation on the motion and perfusion of acutely ischemic myocardium: an experimental echocardiographic study. Circulation, *53*: 853, 1976.

Kerber, R., et al.: Effects of acute coronary occlusion on the motion and perfusion of the normal and ischemic interventricular septum. Circulation, *54*: 928, 1976.

Kerber, R., et al.: Echocardiography in experimentally induced myocardial ischemia. Am. J. Med., *63*: 21, 1977.

Kerber, R., et al.: Evaluation of regional myocardial function in ischemic heart disease by echocardiography. Prog. Cardiovasc. Dis., *20*: 441, 1978.

Kerin, N., et al.: Ventricular septal defect complicating acute myocardial infarction. Echocardiographic demonstration confirmed by angiocardiograms and surgery. Chest, 70: 560, 1976.

Kossowsky, W., et al.: Acute myocardial infarction in idiopathic hypertrophic subaortic stenosis. Chest, 64: 529, 1973.

Lew, W., et al.: Assessment of mitral valve E point-septal separation as an index of left ventricular performance in patients with acute previous myocardial infarction. Am. J. Cardiol., 41: 836, 1978.

Nieminen, M., et al.: Echoventriculography in acute myocardial infarction. III: clinical correlations and implication of the noninfarcted myocardium. Am. J. Cardiol., 38: 1, 1976.

Nixon, J., et al.: Serial echocardiography in patients with acute myocardial infarction: its value and prognostic significance. Eur. J. Cardiol., 9: 161, 1979.

Orlando, J., et al.: Correlation of mean pulmonary artery wedge pressure, left atrial dimension and PTF-VI in patients with acute myocardial infarction. Circulation, 55: 750, 1977.

Prakash, R.: Echocardiographic evaluation of cardiac function and drug effects in acute myocardial infarction. J. Am. Geriatr. Soc., 26: 203, 1978.

Prakash, R., et al.: Spontaneous changes in hemodynamics in uncomplicated acute myocardial infarction: a prospective study. Angiology, 28: 677, 1977.

Rackley, C., et al.: Left ventricular function in acute and chronic coronary artery disease. Annu. Rev. Med., 26: 105, 1975.

Stefan, G., et al.: Echocardiographic findings in experimental myocardial infarction of the posterior left ventricular wall. Am. J. Cardiol., 30: 629, 1972.

Stefan, G., et al.: Ventricular septal rupture and mitral regurgitation in a patient with an acute myocardial infarction (clinical conference). Chest, 75: 614, 1979.

Weiner, I., et al.: Prognostic value of echocardiographic evaluation of septal function in acute anteroseptal myocardial infarction. Am. Heart J., 97: 726, 1979.

Wharton, C., et al.: Changes in left ventricular movement after acute myocardial infarction measured by reflected ultrasound. Br. Med. J., 4: 75, 1971.

General

Brandt, B., et al.: Ventricular septal defect following myocardial infarction. Ann. Thorac. Surg., 27: 580, 1979.

Chandraratna, P., et al.: Echocardiographic assessment of left ventricular function in coronary arterial disease. Br. Heart J., 39: 139, 1977.

Cody, R., et al.: M-mode echocardiography in anteroseptal myocardial infarction. Lack of sensitivity. Chest, 77: 781, 1980.

Corya, B., Echocardiography in ischemic heart disease. Am. J. Med., 63: 10, 1977.

Corya, B., et al.: Anterior left ventricular wall echoes in coronary artery disease. Linear scanning with a single element transducer. Am. J. Cardiol., 34: 652, 1974.

Corya, B., et al.: Echocardiographic features of congestive cardiomyopathy compared with normal subjects and patients with coronary artery disease. Circulation, 49: 1153, 1974.

Corya, B., et al.: M-mode echocardiography in evaluating left ventricular function and surgical risk in patients with coronary artery disease. Chest, 72: 181, 1977.

Corya, B., et al.: Systolic thickening and thinning of the septum and posterior wall in patients with coronary artery disease, congestive cardiomyopathy and atrial septal defect. Circulation, 55: 109, 1977.

Dortimer, A., et al.: Distribution of coronary artery disease. Prediction by echocardiography. Circulation, 54: 724, 1976.

Erbel, R., et al.: Regional myocardial function in coronary artery disease at rest and during atrial pacing. Eur. J. Cardiol., 11: 183, 1980.

Feigenbaum, H.: Echocardiography in patients with coronary artery disease. Clev. Clin. Q., 45: 17, 1978.

Feigenbaum, H., et al.: Role of echocardiography in patients with coronary artery disease. Am. J. Cardiol., 37: 775, 1976.

Fogelman, A., et al.: Echocardiographic study of the abnormal motion of the posterior left ventricular wall during angina pectoris. Circulation, *46*: 905, 1972.

Fujii, J., et al.: Detection of the site and extent of the left ventricular asynergy in myocardial infarction by echocardiography and B-scan imaging. Jpn. Heart J., *17*: 630, 1976.

Gaudiani, V., et al.: Alterations in regional contractility following cardiopulmonary bypass with intraoperative ischemia. J. Thorac. Cardiovasc. Surg., *76*: 70, 1978.

Gerson, M., et al.: Noninvasive documentation of Prinzmetal's angina. Am. J. Cardiol., *43*: 329, 1979.

Glasser, S.: Ventricular asynergy. Heart Lung, *6*: 817, 1977.

Goldstein, S., et al.: Changes in left ventricular wall dimension during regional myocardial ischemia. Am. J. Cardiol., *34*: 56, 1974.

Gordon, M., et al.: Interventricular septal motion in patients with proximal and distal left anterior descending coronary artery lesions. Circulation, *55*: 338, 1977.

Gorlin, R.: Evaluation of the patient with coronary heart disease. Major Probl. Intern. Med., *11*: 173, 1976.

Hagameijer, F., et al.: Echocardiography and rupture of the heart. Br. Heart J., *43*: 45, 1980.

Hamer, S., et al.: Masquerading myocardial infarction. Heart Lung, *7*: 334, 1978.

Henning, H., et al.: Left ventricular performance assessed by radionuclide angiocardiography and echocardiography in patients with previous myocardial infarction. Circulation, *52*: 1069, 1975.

Jacobs, J., et al.: Detection of left ventricular asynergy by echocardiography. Circulation, *43*: 263, 1973.

Joffe, C., et al.: Echocardiographic diagnosis of left anterior descending coronary artery disease. Am. J. Cardiol., *40*: 11, 1977.

Johnson, M.: Echocardiographic evaluation of left ventricular size and function and its application in coronary artery disease. Adv. Cardiol., *17*: 105, 1976.

Karliner, J.: Noninvasive evaluation of the patient with suspected coronary artery disease. Curr. Probl. Cardiol., *3*: 1, 1978.

Kerber, R., et al.: Correlation between echocardiographically demonstrated segmental dyskinesis and regional myocardial perfusion. Circulation, *52*: 1097, 1975.

Kleiger, R., et al.: Postmyocardial infarction complications requiring surgery. Arch. Intern. Med., *137*: 1580, 1977.

Kolibash, A., et al.: The relationship between abnormal echocardiographic septal motion and myocardial perfusion in patients with significant obstruction of the left anterior descending artery. Circulation, *56*: 780, 1977.

Kramer, N., et al.: Differentiation of posterior myocardial infarction from right ventricular hypertrophy and normal anterior loop by echocardiography. Circulation, *58*: 1057, 1978.

Lorell, B., et al.: Right ventricular infarction. Clinical diagnosis and differentiation from cardiac tamponade and pericardial constriction. Am. J. Cardiol., *43*: 465, 1979.

Ludbrook, P., et al.: Comparison of ultrasound and cineangiographic measurements of left ventricular performance in patients with and without wall motion abnormalities. Br. Heart J., *35*: 1026, 1973.

Ludbrook, P., et al.: Posterior wall velocity: an unreliable index of total left ventricular performance in patients with coronary artery disease. Am. J. Cardiol., *33*: 475, 1974.

McDonald, I.: Echocardiography in ischaemic heart disease. Med. J. Aust., *1*: 4, 1977.

Maron, B., et al.: Prevalence and characteristics of disproportionate ventricular septal thickening in patients with coronary artery disease. Circulation, *57*: 250, 1978.

Massie, B., et al.: Echocardiography in ischemic heart disease: present status and future prospectives. Am. Heart J., *96*: 543, 1978.

Mimbs, J., et al.: Detection of myocardial infarction in vitro based on altered attenuation of ultrasound. Circ. Res., *41*: 192, 1977.

Mimbs, J., et al.: Changes in ultrasonic attenuation indicative of early myocardial ischemic injury. Am. J. Physiol., 236: 340, 1979.

Morrison, C., et al.: The use of echocardiography in determination of reversible posterior wall asynergy. Am. Heart J., 94: 140, 1977.

Nieminen, M., et al.: Global and regional left ventricular contractility and coronary collaterals in stable ischemic heart disease. Clin. Cardiol., 3: 163, 1980.

Ohuchi, Y., et al.: Real-time, phased-array, cross-sectional echocardiographic evaluation of left ventricular asynergy and quantitation of left ventricular function. A comparison of left ventricular cineangiography. Jpn. Heart J., 21: 1, 1980.

Papadopol, S., et al.: Echocardiography in ischemic heart disease. Med. Interne, 17: 3, 1979.

Rasmussen, S., et al.: Detection of myocardial scar tissue by M-mode echocardiography. Circulation, 57: 230, 1978.

Schwartz, J., et al.: Noninvasive evaluation of left ventricular size and function in patients with coronary artery disease. Isr. Med. J., 71: 543, 1978.

Sharpe, D., et al.: The noninvasive diagnosis of right ventricular infarction. Circulation, 57: 483, 1978.

Shettigar, U., et al.: P wave analysis in ischaemic heart disease. An echocardiographic, haemodynamic, and angiographic assessment. Br. Heart J., 39: 894, 1977.

Swan, H.: Mechanical function of the heart and its alteration during myocardial ischemia and infarction. Specific reference to coronary atherosclerosis. Circulation, 60: 1587, 1979.

Sweet, R., et al.: Relationship between echocardiography, cardiac output, and abnormally contracting segments in patients with ischaemic heart disease. Circulation, 52: 634, 1975.

Teichholz, L.: Echocardiography in coronary artery disease. Cardiovasc. Clin., 9: 139, 1978.

Walsh, R., et al.: Leg arterial insufficiency in patients with significant coronary artery disease. Angiology, 31: 185, 1980.

Wharton, T., et al.: Clinical and angiographic implications of a depressed echocardiographic ejection fraction in coronary artery disease. Cathet. Cardiovasc. Diagn., 3: 259, 1977.

Wilson, C.: Evaluation of coronary heart disease—noninvasive methods. Nebr. Med. J., 65: 167, 1980.

Ventricular Aneurysm

Catherwood, E., et al.: Pseudoaneurysm of the left ventricle complicated by Salmonella typhimurium infection. Recognition by two-dimensional echocardiography. Am. J. Med., 68: 782, 1980.

Catherwood, E., et al.: Two-dimensional echocardiographic recognition of left ventricular pseudoaneurysm. Circulation, 62: 294, 1980.

Chiaramida, S., et al.: Cross-sectional echocardiographic diagnosis of acquired aneurysm of the interventricular septum. J. Clin. Ultrasound, 8: 356, 1980.

Dillon, J., et al.: M-mode echocardiography in the evaluation of patients for aneurysmectomy. Circulation, 53: 657, 1976.

Grube, E., et al.: Non-invasive diagnosis of a false left ventricular aneurysm by echocardiography and pulsed Doppler echocardiography. Br. Heart J., 43: 232, 1980.

Gussenhaven, W., et al.: Echocardiographic pattern in an aneurysm of the membranous interventricular septum. Chest, 77: 541, 1980.

Hansen, G., et al.: Sonographic evaluation of a left ventricular aneurysm presenting as an upper abdominal mass. J. Clin. Ultrasound, 8: 151, 1980.

Katz, R., et al.: Noninvasive diagnosis of left ventricular pseudoaneurysm: role of two-dimensional echocardiography and radionuclide gated pool imaging. Am. J. Cardiol., 44: 372, 1979.

Lewin, R., et al.: Two-dimensional real-time echocardiographic detection of a left ventricular aneurysm associated with mobile pedunculated thrombi. Chest, 77: 704, 1980.

Morcerf, F., et al.: Echocardiographic findings in false aneurysms of the left ventricle. Clev. Clin. Q., 43: 71, 1976.

Mills, P., et al.: Echo-phonocardiographic diagnosis of left ventricular pseudoaneurysm. Chest, 72: 365, 1977.

Ogawa, S., et al.: Delayed peak of the posterior wall. A new echocardiographic index of posterior wall aneurysm. Chest, 73: 382, 1978.

Onik, G., et al.: False left ventricular aneurysm: diagnosis by noninvasive means. J. Nucl. Med., 21: 177, 1980.

Peterson, J., et al.: Echocardiographic recognition of left ventricular aneurysm. Am. Heart J., 83: 244, 1972.

Roelandt, J., et al.: Echocardiographic diagnosis of pseudoaneurysm of the left ventricle. Circulation, 53: 466, 1975.

Sabah, I., et al.: Noninvasive diagnosis of pseudoaneurysm of the left ventricle. Jpn. Heart J., 20: 95, 1979.

Sahn, D., et al.: Echocardiographic recognition of ventricular septal aneurysm: a case report. J. Clin. Ultrasound, 3: 297, 1975.

Saksena, F., et al.: Infective aneurysm of the left ventricle; angiographic and echocardiographic features. Am. Heart J., 96: 385, 1978.

Sears, T., et al.: Left ventricular pseudoaneurysm identified by cross-sectional echocardiography. Ann. Intern. Med., 90: 935, 1979.

Sharratt, G., et al.: Intraoperative left ventricular perforation with false aneurysm formation. Br. Heart J., 38: 1154, 1976.

Silvestre, A., et al.: Septal aneurysm and right ventricular obstruction: a case report. Angiology, 30: 56, 1979.

Snider, A., et al.: Echocardiographic evaluation of ventricular septal aneurysms. Circulation, 59: 920, 1979.

Spindola-Franco, H., et al.: Pseudoaneurysm of the left ventricle. Radiographic and angiocardiographic diagnosis. Radiology, 127: 29, 1978.

Thadani, U., et al.: Submitral annular left ventricular aneurysm—unusual echocardiographic and angiographic features. Cathet. Cardiovasc. Diagn., 4: 163, 1978.

van Mechelen, R., et al.: Noninvasive diagnosis of pseudoaneurysm of left ventricle. Br. Heart J., 40: 812, 1978.

Watson, L., et al.: Left ventricular aneurysm: pre-operative hemodynamics, chamber volume and results of aneurysmectomy. Circulation, 52: 868, 1975.

EVALUATION OF PERFORMANCE

General

Anderson, P., et al.: The force-interval relationship of the left ventricle. Circulation, 60: 334, 1979.

Belenkie, I., et al.: Assessment of left ventricular dimensions and function by echocardiography. Am. J. Cardiol., 31: 755, 1973.

Brinker, J., et al.: Leftward septal displacement during right ventricular loading in man. Circulation, 61: 626, 1980.

Conetta, D., et al.: Effects of transient regional ischemia on left ventricular diastolic function. J. Clin. Ultrasound, 8: 233, 1980.

Clark, R., et al.: Serial echocardiographic evaluation of left ventricular function in valvular disease, including reproducibility guidelines for serial studies. Circulation, 62: 564, 1980.

Fortuin, N., et al.: Evaluation of left ventricular function by echocardiography. Circulation, 46: 26, 1972.

Fortuin, N., et al.: The evaluation of left ventricular function by echocardiography. Am. J. Med., 63: 1, 1977.

Gibson, D., et al.: Stress-strain characteristics of left ventricular myocardium in man. Br. Heart J., 36: 398, 1974.

Gibson, D., et al.: Relation between diastolic left ventricular wall stress and strain in man. Br. Heart J., 36: 1066, 1974.

Grossman, W., et al.: Quantitative assessment of left ventricular diastolic stiffness in man. Circulation, 47: 567, 1973.

Karliner, J.: Clinical reliability of determining left ventricular function by echocardiography. Cardiovasc. Clin., 9: 151, 1978.

Kisslo, J., et al.: Dynamic cardiac imaging using a focused, phased-array ultrasound system. Am. J. Med., 63: 61, 1977.

Lewis, B., et al.: Current concepts of left ventricular relaxation and compliance. Am. Heart J., *99*: 101, 1980.

McDonald, I.: Assessment of myocardial function by echocardiography. Adv. Cardiol., *12*: 221, 1974.

Mason, S., et al.: The use of echocardiography for quantitative evaluation of left ventricular function. Prog. Cardiovasc. Dis., *21*: 119, 1978.

Meller, J., et al.: Noninvasive assessment of left ventricular function. Adv. Intern. Med., *24*: 331, 1979.

Meyer, R.: Echocardiography—application in assessing cardiac performance in clinical care. Anesthesiology, *49*: 71, 1978.

Murray, J., et al.: Echocardiographic determination of left ventricular performance. Ann. Intern. Med., *72*: 777, 1970.

Murray, J., et al.: Echocardiographic determination of left ventricular dimensions, volumes and performance. Am. J. Cardiol., *30*: 252, 1972.

Nimura, Y., et al.: Ultrasoundcardiogram and left ventricular function. Jpn. J. Clin. Med., *32*: 297, 1974.

Parisi, A., et al.: Echocardiography as an index of cardiac performance. Hosp. Pract., *13*: 101, 1978.

Parisi, A., et al.: Echocardiographic evaluation of left ventricular function. Med. Clin. North Am., *64*: 61, 1980.

Popp, R.: Echocardiographic evaluation of left ventricular function. N. Engl. J. Med., *296*: 856, 1977.

Shors, C.: Cardiac function determined by echocardiogram. Crit. Care Med., *3*: 5, 1975.

UCLA Conference (Moderated by K. Shine): noninvasive assessment of myocardial function. Ann. Intern. Med., *92*: 78, 1980.

Indices of Function

Ambrose, J., et al.: The influence of left ventricular late diastolic filling on the A-wave of the left ventricular pressure trace. Circulation, *60*: 510, 1979.

Benzing, G., et al.: Evaluation of left ventricular performance: Circumferential fiber shortening and tension. Circulation, *49*: 925, 1974.

Carr, K., et al.: Measurement of left ventricular ejection fraction by mechanical cross-sectional echocardiography. Circulation, *59*: 1196, 1979.

Chilton, R., et al.: Echocardiographic systolic time intervals. Left ventricular performance in coronary artery disease. Arch. Intern. Med., *140*: 240, 1980.

Cooper, R., et al.: Ultrasound determinations of mean fiber shortening rate in man. Am. J. Cardiol., *29*: 257, 1972.

Cooper, R., et al.: Comparison of ultrasound and cineangiographic measurements of the mean rate of circumferential shortening in man. Circulation, *46*: 914, 1972.

Crawford, M., et al.: Accuracy and reproducibility of new M-mode echocardiographic recommendations for measuring left ventricular dimensions. Circulation, *61*: 137, 1980.

Folland, E., et al.: Noninvasive evaluation of left ventricular function: the ejection fraction. Compr. Ther., *5*: 47, 1979.

Gibson, D., et al.: Assessment of disordered left ventricular contraction from simultaneous measurements of left ventricular pressure and dimension. Br. Heart J., *35*: 862, 1973.

Jugdutt, B., et al.: Noninvasive assessment of left ventricular function from the mitral valve echogram. Relation of final anterior mitral leaflet closing velocity to peak dp/dt and aortic velocity. Circulation, *58*: 861, 1978.

Karliner, J., et al.: Mean velocity of fiber shortening; a simplified measure of left ventricular myocardial contractility. Circulation, *44*: 323, 1971.

Karliner, J., et al.: Factors influencing the ejection fraction and the mean rate of circumferential fiber shortening during atrial fibrillation in man. Cardiovasc. Res., *8*: 18, 1974.

Karliner, J., et al.: Usefulness and limitations of assessment of internal shortening velocity by ultrasound in man. Chest, *68*: 361, 1975.

Kessler, K.: Ejection fraction derived by M-mode echocardiography. A table and comments. Cathet. Cardiovasc. Diagn., *5*: 295, 1979.

Knapp, W.: Relationships between mean velocity of circumferential fiber shortening (Vcf) and heart rate—the diagnostic value of a normalization of Vcf to heart rate. J. Clin. Ultrasound, *6*: 10, 1978.

Ludbrook, P., et al.: Comparison of ultrasound and cineangiographic measurements of left ventricular performance in patients with and without wall motion abnormalities. Br. Heart J., 35: 1026, 1973.

McDonald, I., et al.: Analysis of left ventricular wall motion by reflected ultrasound. Application to assessment of myocardial function. Circulation, 46: 14, 1972.

Massie, B., et al.: Mitral-septal separation: new echocardiographic index of left ventricular function. Am. J. Cardiol., 39: 1008, 1977.

Moynihan, P., et al.: A system for quantitative evaluation of left ventricular function with two-dimensional ultrasonography. Med. Instrum., 14: 111, 1980.

Nakamura, Y., et al.: The changes in pattern of myocardial shortening by reduction of regional coronary blood flow. Jpn. Heart J., 21: 225, 1980.

Paraskos, J., et al.: A noninvasive technique for the determination of circumferential fiber shortening in man. Circ. Res., 29: 610, 1971.

Quinones, M., et al.: Echocardiographic assessment of left ventricular function: with special reference to normalized velocities. Circulation, 50: 42, 1974.

Quinones, M., et al.: Echocardiographic determination of left ventricular stress-velocity relations in man: with reference to the effects of loading and contractility. Circulation, 51: 689, 1975.

Quinones, M., et al.: Influence of acute changes in pre-load, afterload, contractile state and heart rate of ejection and isovolumic indices of myocardial contractility in man. Circulation, 53: 293, 1976.

Quinones, M., et al.: Percentage of shortening of the echocardiographic left ventricular dimension. Its use in determining ejection fraction and stroke volume. Chest, 74: 59, 1978.

Quinones, M., et al.: Noninvasive quantification of left ventricular wall stress. Validation of method and application to assessment of chronic pressure overload. Am. J. Cardiol., 45: 782, 1980.

Rankin, L., et al.: Alterations in preload and ejection phase indices of left ventricular performance. Circulation, 51: 910, 1975.

Ratshin, R., et al.: Determination of left ventricular preload and afterload by quantitative echocardiography in man. Circ. Res., 34: 711, 1974.

Sasayama, S., et al.: Echocardiographic approach for the clinical assessment of left ventricular function:—the analysis of end-systolic pressure (wall stress)—diameter relation and force-velocity relation of ejecting ventricle. Jpn. Circ. J., 43: 357, 1979.

Sobrino, J., et al.: Left ventricular cavity obliteration: hemodynamic behavior of the postextrasystolic beat. Am. Heart J., 99: 319, 1980.

Wilson, J., et al.: Echocardiographic indices of left ventricular function: a comparison. Chest, 76: 441, 1979.

Isovolumic Time Intervals

Antani, J., et al.: Ejection phase indexes by invasive and noninvasive methods: an apexcardiographic, echocardiographic and ventriculographic correlative study. Am. J. Cardiol., 43: 239, 1979.

Araoye, M., et al.: Isovolumic relaxation time in normal subjects and patients with cardiac disease: comparison of determinations made with echocardiographic techniques and apexcardiography. Angiology, 29: 7, 1978.

Bourlen, F., et al.: Relation between isovolumic relaxation period of left ventricle and pulmonary artery pressure in d-transposition of the great arteries. Br. Heart J., 43: 226, 1980.

Doran, J., et al.: Detection of abnormal left ventricular wall movement during isovolumic contraction and early relaxation. Comparison of echo- and angiocardiography. Br. Heart J., 40: 367, 1978.

Gibson, D., et al.: Regional abnormalities of left ventricular wall movement during isovolumic relaxation in patients with ischemic heart disease. Eur. J. Cardiol., 7: 251, 1978.

Hanrath, P., et al.: Left ventricular relaxation and filling pattern in different forms of left ventricular hypertrophy: an echocardiographic study. Am. J. Cardiol., 45: 15, 1980.

Hirschfeld, S., et al.: The isovolumic contraction time of the left ventricle. Circulation, 54: 751, 1976.

Ito, M., et al.: Isometric contraction and relaxation times of right and left ventricles in normal subjects and in patients with right ventricular overloading measured with bidirectional echocardiography. Jpn. Heart J., *19*: 193, 1978.

Lewis, B., et al.: Isovolumic relaxation period in man. Am. Heart J., *100*: 490, 1980.

Peterson, K., et al.: Comparison of isovolumic and ejection phase indices of myocardial performance in man. Circulation, *49*: 1088, 1974.

Upton, M., et al.: Echocardiographic assessment of abnormal left ventricular relaxation in man. Br. Heart J., *38*: 1001, 1976.

Ziady, G., et al.: The use of echocardiography to measure isometric contraction time. Am. Heart J., *89*: 200, 1975.

Normal

Brenner, J., et al.: Effect of phasic respiration on left ventricular dimension and performance in a normal population. Circulation, *57*: 122, 1978.

DeMaria, A., et al.: Systematic correlation of cardiac chamber size and ventricular performance determined with echocardiography and alterations in heart rate in normal persons. Am. J. Cardiol., *43*: 1, 1979.

Gerstenbligh, G., et al.: Echocardiographic assessment of a normal adult aging population. Circulation, *56*: 273, 1977.

Hirschfeifer, J., et al.: Influence of acute alterations in heart rate and systemic arterial pressure on echocardiographic measures of left ventricular performance in normal human subjects. Circulation, *52*: 835, 1975.

Katz, R., et al.: Effects of a natural volume overload state (pregnancy) on left ventricular performance in normal human subjects. Circulation, *58*: 434, 1978.

Kessler, K., et al.: Left ventricular size and function in women receiving oral contraceptives. Obstet. Gynecol., *55*: 211, 1980.

Marsh, J., et al.: Left ventricular end-systolic pressure-dimension and stress-length relations in normal human subjects. Am. J. Cardiol., *44*: 1311, 1979.

Rubler, S., et al.: Cardiac size and performance during pregnancy estimated with echocardiography. Am. J. Cardiol., *40*: 534, 1977.

Specific Disease, Symptom, Procedure

Abdulla, A., et al.: Limitations of echocardiography in the assessment of left ventricular size and function in aortic regurgitation. Circulation, *61*: 148, 1980.

Acquatella, H., et al.: Left ventricular function in terminal uremia. A hemodynamic and echocardiographic study. Nephron, *22*: 160, 1978.

Ahmad, M., et al.: Left ventricular function during lower body negative pressure. Aviat. Space Environ. Med., *48*: 512, 1977.

Benotti, J., et al.: Clinical profile of restrictive cardiomyopathy. Circulation, *61*: 1206, 1980.

Boden, W., et al.: Elevated ejection fractions in patients with anginal syndrome and normal coronary arteriograms. Cathet. Cardiovasc. Diagn., *4*: 249, 1978.

Borer, J., et al.: Echocardiographic observations in patients with systemic infiltrative disease involving the heart. Am. J. Cardiol., *39*: 184, 1977.

Bradford, J., et al.: Left ventricular lipoma: echocardiographic and angiographic features. South. Med. J., *73*: 663, 1980.

Cohen, M., et al.: Echocardiographic assessment of left ventricular function in patients with chronic uremia. Clin. Nephrol., *12*: 156, 1979.

Come, P.: Echocardiography in diagnosis and management of cardiovascular disease. Study of the left ventricle and pericardium and recognition of intracardiac mass lesions. Compr. Ther., *6*: 56, 1980.

Come, P., et al.: Echocardiographic diagnosis of left ventricular thrombi. Am. Heart J., *100*: 523, 1980.

Corya., B., et al.: Echocardiographic findings after acute carbon monoxide poisoning. Br. Heart J., *38*: 712, 1976.

Covarrubias, E., et al.: Left ventricular function in sickle cell anemia: a noninvasive evaluation. South. Med. J., *73*: 342, 1980.

Cunha, C., et al.: Pre-operative M-mode echocardiography as a predictor of surgical results in chronic aortic insufficiency. J. Thorac. Cardiovasc. Surg., 79: 256, 1980.

Danilowicz, D., et al.: Echocardiography in Duchenne muscular dystrophy. Muscle Nerve, 3: 298, 1980.

D'Cruz, I., et al.: Echocardiographic detection of cardiac involvement in patients with chronic renal failure. Arch. Intern. Med., 138: 720, 1978.

Elkayam, U., et al.: Echocardiographic findings in cardiogenic shock due to right ventricular myocardial infarction. Cathet. Cardiovasc. Diagn., 5: 289, 1979.

Farah, M., et al.: Echocardiographic evaluation of left ventricular function in Duchenne's muscular dystrophy. Am. J. Med., 69: 248, 1980.

Farcot, J., et al.: Two-dimensional echocardiographic visualization of ventricular septal rupture after acute anterior myocardial infarction. Am. J. Cardiol., 45: 370, 1980.

Gottdiener, J., et al.: Effects of self-induced starvation on cardiac size and function in anorexia nervosa. Circulation, 58: 425, 1978.

Gomes, J., et al.: Inotropic effect of post-stimulation potentiation in man: an echocardiographic study. Am. J. Cardiol., 43: 745, 1979.

Guazzi, M., et al.: Echocardiographic and hemodynamic correlates in Prinzmetal angina pectoris: a case report. Angiology, 30: 708, 1979.

Henry, W., et al.: Observations on the optimum time for operative intervention for aortic regurgitation. I. Evaluation of the results of aortic valve replacement in symptomatic patients. Circulation, 61: 471, 1980.

Henry, W., et al.: Observations on the optimum time for operative intervention for aortic regurgitation. II. Serial echocardiographic evaluation of asymptomatic patients. Circulation, 61: 484, 1980.

Heymsfield, S., et al.: Cardiac abnormalities in cachectic patients before and during nutritional repletion. Am. Heart J., 95: 584, 1978.

Hilton, C., et al.: Inadequate cardioplegic protection with obstructed coronary arteries. Ann. Thorac. Surg., 28: 323, 1979.

Ito, Y.: On some points of the congestive heart failure. Jpn. Circ. J., 42: 1201, 1978.

Karjalainen, J., et al.: Influenza Al myocarditis in conscripts. Acta Med. Scand., 207: 27, 1980.

Kramer, L., et al.: Cardiac dysfunction in a patient with familial hypokalemic periodic paralysis. Chest, 75: 189, 1979.

Kubac, G., et al.: Malignant granular cell myoblastoma with metastatic cardiac involvement; case report and echocardiogram. Am. Heart J., 100: 227, 1980.

Leon, M., et al.: Detection of early cardiac dysfunction in patients with severe beta-thalassemia and chronic iron overload. N. Engl. J. Med., 301: 1143, 1979.

Lewis, B., et al.: Left ventricular function in chronic renal failure. Br. Heart J., 38: 1229, 1976.

Lewis, B., et al.: Left ventricular function in B-thalassemia and the effect of multiple transfusions. Am. Heart J., 96: 636, 1978.

Lewis, B., et al.: Echocardiographic left ventricular function in thyrotoxicosis. Am. Heart J., 97: 460, 1979.

Lewis, B., et al.: Left ventricular function in liver cirrhosis: an echocardiographic study. Isr. J. Med. Sci., 16: 489, 1980.

McDonald, I.: Echocardiographic assessment of left ventricular function in aortic valve disease. Circulation, 53: 860, 1976.

McDonald, I.: Echocardiographic assessment of left ventricular function in mitral valve disease. Circulation, 53: 865, 1976.

MacDonald, W., et al.: Echocardiographic assessment of cardiac structure and function in patients with rheumatoid arthritis. Am. J. Med., 63: 890, 1977.

Naqvi, N., et al.: Diagnosis of left ventricular thrombus by two-dimensional echocardiography. Eur. J. Cardiol., 11: 235, 1980.

O'Rourke, R., et al.: Timing of valve replacement in patients with chronic aortic regurgitation. Circulation, 61: 493, 1980.

Parisi, A., et al.: Echocardiographic evaluation of the Valsalva maneuver in healthy subjects and patients with and without heart failure. Circulation, 54: 921, 1976.

Riley, S., et al.: Echocardiographic assessment of cardiac performance in patients with arteriovenous fistulas. Surg. Gynecol. Obstet., *146*: 203, 1978.

Stewart, J., et al.: Malapposition of the mitral valve: A two-dimensional echocardiographic sign of left ventricular dysfunction. Radiology, *130*: 399, 1979.

Sutton, M., et al.: Angina in idiopathic hypertrophic subaortic stenosis. A clinical correlate of regional left ventricular dysfunction. A video metric and echocardiographic study. Circulation, *61*: 561, 1980.

Venco, A., et al.: Noninvasive assessment of left ventricular function in myotonic muscular dystrophy. Br. Heart J., *40*: 1262, 1978.

von Bibra, H., et al.: The effects of arteriovenous shunts on cardiac function in renal dialysis patients —an echocardiographic evaluation. Clin. Nephrol., *9*: 205, 1978.

Weiss, S., et al.: Cardiac involvement in progressive systemic sclerosis (P.S.S.)—an echocardiographic study. Z. Rheumatol., *39*: 190, 1980.

Wilson, J., et al.: Noninvasive assessment of load reduction in patients with asymptomatic aortic regurgitation. Am. J. Med., *68*: 664, 1980.

EXERCISE

Alpert, B., et al.: Hemodynamic responses to supine exercise in children with left-sided cardiac disease. Am. J. Cardiol., *45*: 1025, 1980.

Allen, H., et al.: A quantitative echocardiographic study of champion childhood swimmers. Circulation, 55: 142, 1977.

Amon, K., et al.: Upright exercise echocardiography. J. Clin. Ultrasound, 7: 373, 1979.

Bennett, D., et al.: Echocardiographic left ventricular dimensions in the supine and upright positions and on upright exercise in normal subjects (proceedings). J. Physiol., *275*: 77, 1978.

Cahill, N., et al.: A pilot study on left ventricular dimensions and wall stress before and after submaximal exercise. Br. J. Sports Med., *13*: 122, 1979.

Crawford, M., et al.: Echocardiographic evaluation of left ventricular size and performance during handgrip and supine and upright bicycle exercise. Circulation, 59: 1188, 1979.

DeMaria, A., et al.: Alterations in ventricular mass and performance induced by exercise training in man evaluated by echocardiography. Circulation, 57: 237, 1978.

Ehsani, A., et al.: Rapid changes in left ventricular dimensions and mass in response to physical conditioning and deconditioning. Am. J. Cardiol., *42*: 52, 1978.

Falsetti, H.: Invasive and noninvasive evaluation of exercise in humans. Med. Sci. Sports, 9: 262, 1977.

Fortuin, N., et al.: Studies by echocardiography of regional and global cardiac function during exercise. Trans. Am. Clin. Climatol. Assoc., *90*: 174, 1979.

Galbo, H., et al.: Cardiac function during rest and supine cycling examined with a new noninvasive technique. J. Appl. Physiol., *36*: 113, 1974.

Gilbert, C., et al.: Echocardiographic study of cardiac dimensions and function in the endurance-trained athlete. Am. J. Cardiol., *40*: 528, 1977.

Goldstein, R., et al.: Effect of glyceryl trinitrate on echocardiographic left ventricular dimensions during exercise in the upright position. Br. Heart J., *42*: 245, 1979.

Hiasa, Y., et al.: Echocardiographic and phonocardiographic evaluation of the changes of the P-terminal force in V_1 by the exercise. Tokushima J. Exp. Med., *25*: 135, 1978.

Horwitz, L., et al.: Role of the Frank-Starling mechanism in exercise. Circ. Res., *31*: 868, 1972.

Ikäheimo, M., et al.: Noninvasive evaluation of the athletic heart: sprinters versus endurance runners. Am. J. Cardiol., *44*: 24, 1979.

Ishise, S.: Hemodynamic and left ventricular volumic alteration in response to isometric handgrip exercise. Jpn. Circ. J., *42*: 411, 1978.

Koro, T., et al.: Cardiovascular function test by lowgrade submaximal exercise. Jpn. Circ. J., *43*: 183, 1979.

Lamont, L.: Echocardiographic findings in athletes: a review. Am. Correct. Ther. J., *34*: 46, 1980.

Laird, W., et al.: Cardiovascular response to isometric exercise in normal adolescents. Circulation, 59: 651, 1979.

Longhurst, J., et al.: Echocardiographic left ventricular masses in distance runners and weight lifters. J. Appl. Physiol., 48: 154. 1980.

Mason, S., et al.: Exercise echocardiography: detection of wall motion abnormalities during ischemia. Circulation, 59: 50, 1979.

Morganroth, J., et al.: The athlete's heart syndrome: a new perspective. Ann. N.Y. Acad. Sci., 301: 931, 1977.

Nishimura, T., et al.: Echocardiographic evaluation of long-term effects of exercise on left ventricular hypertrophy and function in professional bicyclists. Circulation, 61: 832, 1980.

Parker, B., et al.: The noninvasive cardiac evaluation of long distance runners. Chest, 73: 376, 1978.

Paulsen, W., et al.: Ventricular response to isometric and isotonic exercise: echocardiographic assessment. Br. Heart J., 42: 521, 1979.

Redwood, D., et al.: Design and function of a mechanical assembly for recording echocardiograms during upright exercise. Cardiovasc. Res., 9: 145, 1975.

Roeske, W., et al.: Noninvasive evaluation of ventricular hypertrophy in professional athletes. Circulation, 53: 286, 1976.

Rost, R., et al.: A comparative echocardiographic examination of the hearts of highly trained athletes and untrained persons. J. Sports Med. Phys. Fitness, 15: 305, 1975.

Smithen, C., et al.: Independent effects of heart rate and exercise on left ventricular wall movement measured by reflected ultrasound. Am. J. Cardiol., 30: 43, 1972.

Stefadouros, M., et al.: Noninvasive study of effect of isometric exercise on left ventricular performance in normal man. Br. Heart J., 36: 988, 1974.

Stein, R., et al.: Continuous ventricular dimensions in man during supine exercise and recovery. An echocardiographic study. Am. J. Cardiol., 41: 655, 1978.

Stein, R., et al.: The cardiac response to exercise training: echocardiographic analysis at rest and during exercise. Am. J. Cardiol., 46: 219, 1980.

Sugishita, Y., et al.: Dynamic exercise echocardiography. Circulation, 60: 743, 1979.

Sugishita, Y., et al.: Exercise and echocardiography—dynamic exercise echo-cardiography. Jpn. Circ. J., 43: 205, 1979.

Underwood, R., et al.: Noninvasive analysis of cardiac function of elite distance runners—echocardiography, vectorcardiography and cardiac intervals. Ann. N.Y. Acad. Sci., 301: 297, 1977.

Wann, L., et al.: Exercise cross-sectional echocardiography in ischemic heart disease. Circulation, 60: 1300, 1979.

Weiss, J., et al.: Evidence of Frank-Starling effect in man during severe semisupine exercise. Circulation, 59: 655, 1979.

Zeldis, S., et al.: Cardiac hypertrophy in response to dynamic conditioning in female athletes. J. Appl. Physiol., 44: 849, 1978.

Zoneraich, S., et al.: Assessment of cardiac function in marathon runners by graphic noninvasive techniques. Ann. N.Y. Acad. Sci., 301: 900, 1977.

Zoneraich, S., et al.: Evaluating the endurance athlete's heart: a noninvasive graphic study. Angiology, 30: 223, 1979.

PEDIATRIC

Björkhem, G.: Echocardiographic assessment of left ventricular function. Investigation of infants, children and teenagers without heart disease. Eur. J. Cardiol., 6: 83, 1977.

Björkhem, G., et al.: Echocardiographic studies of children operated on for congenital heart disease: evaluation during the first postoperative year. Eur. J. Cardiol., 11: 33, 1980.

Ghafour, A., et al.: Echocardiographic evaluation of left ventricular function in children with congestive cardiomyopathy. Am. J. Cardiol., 44: 1332, 1979.

Gutgesell, H., et al.: Evaluation of left ventricular size and function by echocardiography: results in normal children. Circulation, 56: 457, 1977.

Henry, W., et al.: Echocardiographic measurements in normal subjects: growth-related changes that occur between infancy and early adulthood. Circulation, 57: 278, 1978.

Kaye H., et al.: Validity of echocardiographic estimates of left ventricular size and performance in infants and children. Br. Heart J., 37: 371, 1975.

Levitsky, S., et al.: Anomalous left coronary artery in the infant: recovery of ventricular function following early direct aortic implantation. J. Thorac. Cardiovasc. Surg., 79: 598, 1980.

Meyer, R.: Echocardiography—application in assessing cardiac performance in clinical care. Anesthesiology, 49: 71, 1978.

Rees, A., et al.: Left ventricular performance in children with homozygous sickle cell anemia. Br. Heart J., 40: 690, 1978.

Riggs, T., et al.: Neonatal circulatory changes: an echocardiographic study. Pediatrics, 59: 338, 1977.

Riggs, T., et al.: The pediatric spectrum of dynamic left ventricular obstruction. Am. Heart J., 99: 301, 1980.

Sahn, D., et al.: Echocardiographic assessment of left ventricular performance in normal newborns. Circulation, 49: 232, 1974.

St. John Sutton, M., et al.: Cardiac function in the normal newborn: additional information by computer analysis of the M-mode echocardiogram. Circulation, 57: 1198, 1978.

St. John Sutton, M., et al.: Assessment of left ventricular function in secundum atrial septal defect by computer analysis of the M-mode echocardiogram. Circulation, 60: 1082, 1979.

Yabek, S., et al.: Echocardiographic determination of left atrial volumes in children with congenital heart disease. Circulation, 53: 268, 1976.

OPERATIVE AND POSTOPERATIVE

Becker, R., et al.: Myocardial protection during coronary surgery; controlled comparison of hypothermic hyperkalemic cardioplegic arrest to intermittent aortic arrest. N.Y. State J. Med., 79: 2043, 1979.

Borow, K., et al.: End-systolic volume as a predictor of postoperative left ventricular performance in volume overload from valvular regurgitation. Am. J. Med., 68: 655, 1980.

Burggraf, G., et al.: Echocardiographic studies of left ventricular wall motion and dimensions after valvular heart surgery. Am. J. Cardiol., 35: 473, 1975.

Chang, J., et al.: Evaluation of cardiac function during neurosurgical procedure in the sitting position. Surg. Forum, 28: 467, 1977.

Favaloro, R.: Direct myocardial revascularization: a 10 year journey. Myths and realities. Louis F. Bishop lecture. Am. J. Cardiol., 43: 109, 1979.

Gaudiani, V., et al.: Continuous epicardial echocardiographic monitoring of left ventricular function in the postoperative period. Surg. Forum, 28: 248, 1977.

Guadiani, V., et al.: Continuous epicardial echocardiographic assessment of postoperative left ventricular function. J. Thorac. Cardiovasc. Surg., 76: 64, 1978.

Hagl, S., et al.: Acute effects of aortocoronary bypass surgery on left ventricular function and regional myocardial mechanics: a clinical study. Ann. Thorac. Surg., 26: 548, 1978.

Hill, R., et al.: Perioperative assessment of segmental left ventricular function in man. Effects of nitroprusside after bypass operations. Arch. Surg., 115: 609, 1980.

Kavey, R., et al.: Perioperative echocardiographic evaluation of cardiovascular function: assessment of changing hemodynamic state. Circulation, 62: 773, 1980.

McNamara, D.: Primary care of the patient following heart surgery. Med. Times, 106: 65, 1978.

Matsumoto, M., et al.: Application of transesophageal echocardiography to continuous intraoperative monitoring of left ventricular performance. Am. J. Cardiol., 46: 95, 1980.

Righetti, A., et al.: Interventricular septal motion and left ventricular function after coronary bypass surgery. Evaluation with echocardiography and radionuclide angiography. Am. J. Cardiol., 39: 372, 1977.

Righetti, A., et al.: Echocardiographic and roentgenographic determination of left ventricular size after coronary arterial bypass graft surgery. Chest, 72: 455, 1977.

Spotnitz, H., et al.: Effects of open heart surgery on end-diastolic pressure-diameter relations of the human left ventricle. Circulation, 59: 662, 1979.

Strom, J., et al.: Effects of hypothermic hyperkalemic cardioplegic arrest on ventricular performance during cardiac surgery. N.Y. State J. Med., 78: 2210, 1978.

Vignola, P., et al.: Abnormal interventricular septal motion following cardiac surgery: clinical, surgical, echocardiographic and radionuclide correlates. Am. Heart J., 97: 27, 1979.

RESPONSE TO DRUGS, ALCOHOL

Abrams, J.: Long-acting nitroglycerin preparations do work. An assessment by noninvasive techniques. *In* Noninvasive Cardiovascular Diagnosis. Edited by E.B. Diethrich. Baltimore, University Park Press, 1978.

Amsterdam, E., et al.: Sustained salutary effects of oral controlled-release nitroglycerin on ventricular function in congestive heart failure. Clin. Cardiol., 2: 19, 1979.

Andy, J., et al.: Cardiovascular effects of dibutamine in severe congestive heart failure. Am. Heart J., 94: 175, 1977.

Arce-Gomez, E., et al.: Ejection fraction determined through echocardiography in anginal patients treated with pentaeritritol. Curr. Ther. Res., 21: 177, 1977.

Askanas, A., et al.: The heart in chronic alcoholism: a noninvasive study. Am. Heart J., 99: 9, 1980.

Autenrieth, G., et al.: Echocardiographic evaluation of myocardial performance during infusion of angiotensin and hand-grip exercise. *In* Myocardial Failure. Edited by G. Riecker, et al. Berlin, Springer, 1977.

Barash, P., et al.: Ventricular function in children during halothane anesthesia. Anesthesiology, 49: 79, 1978.

Bax, N., et al.: Cardiac effects of disopyramide and lignocaine assessed by echocardiography (proceedings). Br. J. Clin. Pharmacol., 8: 398, 1979.

Bett, J., et al.: Echocardiographic comparison of haemodynamic effects of metoprolol and propranolol. Br. Heart J., 43: 541, 1980.

Biancaniello, T., et al.: Doxorubicin cardiotoxicity in children. J. Pediatr., 97: 45, 1980.

Björkhem, G., et al.: Echocardiographic assessment of left ventricular function during the injection of adriamycin. Acta Paediatr. Scand., 66: 595, 1977.

Bloom, K., et al.: Echocardiography in adriamycin cardiotoxicity. Cancer, 41: 1265, 1978.

Burggraf, G., et al.: Left ventricular volume changes after amyl nitrite and nitroglycerin in man as measured by ultrasound. Circulation, 44: 136, 1974.

Burggraf, G., et al.: Effects of dextran infusion on left ventricular volume and pressure in man. Cathet. Cardiovasc. Diagn., 4: 383, 1978.

Carliner, N., et al.: Quinidine therapy in hospitalized patients with ventricular arrhythmias. Am. Heart J., 98: 708, 1979.

Chandraratna, P., et al.: Effects of acebutolol and propranolol on left ventricular performance assessed by echocardiography. Clin. Pharmacol. Ther., 27: 460, 1980.

Child, J., et al.: Cardiac effects of acute ethanol ingestion unmasked by autonomic blockade. Circulation, 59: 120, 1979.

Chlebus, H.: Role of non-invasive methods in clinical evaluation of drugs in ischaemic heart disease. Bibl. Cardiol., 35: 167, 1976.

Colucci, W., et al.: Long-term therapy of heart failure with prazosin: a randomized double blind trial. Am. J. Cardiol., 45: 337, 1980.

Crawford, M., et al.: Favorable effects of oral maintenance digoxin therapy on left ventricular performance in normal subjects; echocardiographic study. Am. J. Cardiol., 38: 843, 1976.

Crawford, M., et al.: Effects of oral propranolol on left ventricular sizes and performance during exercise and acute pressure loading. Circulation, 61: 549, 1980.

Delgado, C., et al.: Acute effects of low doses of alcohol on left ventricular function measured by echocardiography. Circulation, 51: 535, 1975.

DeMaria, A., et al.: Effects of nitroglycerin in left ventricular cavity size and cardiac performance determined by ultrasound in man. Am. J. Med., 57: 754, 1974.

Dillon, J.: Evaluation of drug therapy in heart disease employing echocardiography. *In* Assessment of Pharmaco-Dynamic Effects in Human Pharmacology. Edited by H. Dengler. Stuttgart, Schattauer, 1975.

Dumovic, P., et al.: Effect of therapeutic dosage of lithium on the heart. Br. J. Clin. Pharmacol., 9: 599, 1980.

Edwards, D., et al.: Radiographic and echocardiographic evaluation of newborns treated with indomethacin for patent ductus arteriosus. Am. J. Roentgenol., *131*: 1009, 1978.

Ewy, G., et al.: Detection of adriamycin cardiotoxicity by echocardiography. Ariz. Med., 35: 402, 1978.

Ewy. G., et al.: Noninvasive cardiac evaluation of patients receiving adriamycin. Cancer Treat. Rep., 62: 915, 1978.

Frishman, W., et al.: Noninvasive assessment of clinical response to oral propranolol therapy. Am. J. Cardiol., 35: 635, 1975.

Gash, A., et al.: Effects of smoking marihuana on left ventricular performance and plasma norepinephrine: studies in normal man. Ann. Intern. Med., 89: 448, 1978.

Gibson, D.: Use of M-mode echocardiography in clinical pharmacology. Br. J. Clin. Pharmacol., 7: 443, 1979.

Gomes, J., et al.: The effect of isosorbide dinitrate on left ventricular size, wall stress and left ventricular function in chronic refractory heart failure. Am. J. Med., 65: 794, 1978.

Gottdiener, J.: Noninvasive assessment of cardiac dysfunction in the cancer patient. Cancer Treat. Rep., 62: 949, 1978.

Hanrath, P., et al.: Effect of verapamil on left ventricular isovolumic relaxation time and regional left ventricular filling in hypertrophic cardiomyopathy. Am. J. Cardiol., 45: 1258, 1980.

Hardarson, T., et al.: Prolonged salutary effects of isosorbide dinitrate and nitroglycerin ointment on regional left ventricular function. Am. J. Cardiol., 40: 90, 1977.

Heikkilä, J., et al.: Rapid monitoring of regional myocardial ischaemia with echocardiography and ST segment shifts in man. Modification of "infarct size" and hemodynamics by dopamine and beta blockade. Acta Med. Scand. (Suppl.), 623: 71, 1978.

Henderson, I., et al.: Serial studies of cardiac function in patients receiving adriamycin. Cancer Treat. Rep., 62: 923, 1978.

Hirota, Y., et al.: Dynamic echoventriculography. Noninvasive assessment of effects of nitroglycerin, phenylephrine, isoproterenol, and propranolol on the human cardiovascular system. Jpn. Heart J., *19*: 719, 1978.

Hofstetter, R., et al.: Effect of digoxin on left ventricular contractility in newborns and infants estimated by echocardiography. Eur. J. Cardiol., 9: 1, 1979.

Kerber, R., et al.: Effect of acute ischemia, nitroglycerin and nitroprusside on regional myocardial thickening, stress and perfusion. Experimental echocardiographic studies. Circulation, 60: 121, 1979.

Kerin, N., et al.: Evaluation of phentolamine as a provocative test for idiopathic hypertrophic subaortic stenosis. Am. Heart J., 97: 204, 1979.

Klugar, J., et al.: The clinical pharmacology and antiarrhythmic efficacy of acetylprocainamide in patients with arrhythmias. Am. J. Cardiol., 45: 1250, 1980.

Komer, R., et al.: Effects of nitroglycerin on echocardiographic measurements of left ventricular wall thickness and regional myocardial performance during acute coronary ischemia. Circulation, 59: 926, 1979.

Kraunz, R., et al.: Ultrasound measurements of ventricular wall motion following administration of vasoactive drugs. Am. J. Cardiol., 27: 464, 1971.

Leier, C., et al.: The cardiovascular effects of the continuous infusion of dobutamine in patients with severe cardiac failure. Circulation, 56: 468, 1977.

LeJemtel, T., et al.: Amrinone: a new non-glycosidic, non-adrenergic cardiotonic agent effective in the treatment of intractable myocardial failure in man. Circulation, 59: 1098, 1979.

Lewis, A., et al.: Echocardiographic assessment of anthracycline cardiotoxicity in children. Med. Pediatr. Oncol., 5: 167, 1978.

Lindenfeld, J., et al.: Adrenergic responsiveness after abrupt propranolol withdrawal in normal subjects and in patients with angina pectoris. Circulation, 62: 704, 1980.

Maclean, D.: Noninvasive assessment of the effects of drugs on acute myocardial infarct size in man. Br. J. Clin. Pharmacol., 7: 537, 1979.

Martin, M., et al.: Acebutolol in hypertension—double blind trial against placebo. Br. J. Clin. Pharmacol., 6: 351, 1978.

Martin, M., et al.: Echocardiography in cardiovascular drug assessment. Br. Heart J., 41: 536, 1979.

Meltzer, R., et al.: Two-dimensional echocardiographic quantification of infarct size alteration by pharmacologic agents. Am. J. Cardiol., 44: 257, 1979.

Moyer, J., et al.: Echocardiographic assessment of the effect of an antihypertensive regimen on left ventricular performance. Am. J. Cardiol., 43: 594, 1979.

Ochs, H., et al.: Intravenous quinidine: pharmacokinetic properties and effects on left ventricular performance in humans. Am. Heart J., 99: 468, 1980.

Packer, M., et al.: Importance of left ventricular chamber size in determining the response to hydralazine in severe chronic heart failure. N. Engl. J. Med., 303: 250, 1980.

Prakash, R.: Echocardiographic evaluation of cardiac function and drug effects in acute myocardial infarction. J. Am. Geriatr. Soc., 26: 203, 1978.

Ramos, A., et al.: Echocardiographic evaluation of adriamycin cardiotoxicity in children. Cancer Treat. Rep., 60: 1281, 1976.

Rathod, R., et al.: Echocardiographic assessment of ventricular performance following induction with two anesthetics. Anesthesiology, 49: 86, 1978.

Reeves, W., et al.: Echocardiography in chronic alcoholics following prolonged periods of abstinence. Am. Heart J., 95: 578, 1978.

Rubler, S., et al.: Noninvasive estimation of myocardial performance in patients with diabetes. Effect of alcohol administration. Diabetes, 27: 127, 1978.

Ryan, W., et al.: Effects of tocainide on left ventricular performance at rest and during acute alterations in heart rate and systemic arterial pressure. Br. Heart J., 41: 175, 1979.

Schinz, A., et al.: Time sequence of direct vascular and inotropic effects following intravenous administration of digoxin in normal man. Int. J. Clin. Pharmacol. Biopharm., 15: 189, 1977.

Shubrooks, S., et al.: Left ventricular wall motion response to intravenous propranolol. Circulation, 52: 124, 1975.

Tashkin, D., et al.: Short-term effects of smoked marihuana on left ventricular function in man. Chest, 72: 20, 1977.

Timmis, G., et al.: The relative resistance of normal young women to ethanol-induced myocardial depression. Angiology, 30: 733, 1979.

Weber, K., et al.: Long-term vasodilator therapy with trimazosin in chronic cardiac failure. N. Engl. J. Med., 303: 242, 1980.

VOLUME

Alpert, B., et al.: The comparison between noninvasive and invasive methods of stroke volume determination in children. Am. Heart J., 98: 763, 1979.

Ambrose, J., et al.: The ventricular "A" wave: a new echocardiographic index of late diastolic filling of the left ventricle. Am. Heart J., 96: 615, 1978.

Bennett, D., et al.: Test of reliability of echocardiographic estimation of left ventricular dimensions and volumes. Br. Heart J., 38: 1133, 1976.

Bhatt, D., et al.: Accuracy of echocardiography in assessing left ventricular dimensions and volume. Circulation, 57: 699, 1978.

Branzi, A., et al.: Ultrasound determination of left ventricular position for volume angiography. Chest, 62: 29, 1972.

Fagrell, B., et al.: Noninvasive beat-to-beat analysis of stroke volume and digital pulse volume in patients with complete heart block and artificial pacing. Acta Med. Scand., 205: 185, 1979.

Folland, E., et al.: Assessment of left ventricular ejection fraction and volumes by real-time, two-dimensional echocardiography. A comparison of cineangiographic and radionuclide techniques. Circulation, 60: 760, 1979.

Fortuin, N., et al.: Determinations of left ventricular volumes by ultrasound. Circulation, 44: 575, 1971.

Furukawa, K., et al.: The study of the third heart sound in relation to the left ventricular filling and wall movement by echocardiography. Jpn. Heart J., 18: 611, 1977.

Gibson, D.: Measurement of left ventricular volumes in man by echocardiography—comparison with biplane angiographs. Br. Heart J., 33: 614, 1971.

Gibson, D., et al.: Measurement of instantaneous left ventricular dimension and filling rate in man using echocardiography. Br. Heart J., 35: 1141, 1973.

Grossman, W., et al.: Left ventricular stiffness associated with chronic pressure and volume overloads in man. Circ. Res., 35: 793, 1974.

Jacobs, W., et al.: Echocardiographic aortic ejection area as a reflection of left ventricular stroke volume. J. Clin. Ultrasound, 7: 369, 1979.

Layton, C., et al.: Assessment of left ventricular filling and compliance using an ultrasound technique. Br. Heart J., 35: 559, 1973.

Linhart, J., et al.: Left ventricular volume measurement by echocardiography: fact or fiction? Am. J. Cardiol., 36: 114, 1975.

Machii, K., et al.: Echocardiographic left ventricular volume determination by direct measurements of the major and minor axes. Jpn. Circ. J., 41: 501, 1977.

MacKay, R.: Noninvasive cardiac output measurement. Microvasc. Res., 4: 438, 1972.

McLaurin, L., et al.: A new technique for the study of left ventricular pressure-volume relations in man. Circulation, 48: 56, 1973.

Mariani, M., et al.: Validity and limitations of the echocardiographic method for measuring left ventricular volumes; comparison with the angiocardiographic method and with the ventricular wash-out curves. J. Nucl. Med. Allied Sci., 23: 35, 1979.

Martin, M.: Assessment of correction formula for echocardiographic estimations of left ventricular volumes. Br. Heart J., 40: 294, 1978.

Murray, J., et al.: Echocardiographic determination of left ventricular dimensions, volumes and performance. Am. J. Cardiol., 30: 252, 1972.

Pombo, J., et al.: Comparison of stroke volume and cardiac output determination by ultrasound and dye dilution in acute myocardial infarction. Am. J. Cardiol., 27: 630, 1971.

Pombo, J., et al.: Left ventricular volumes and ejection fraction by echocardiography. Circulation, 43: 480, 1971.

Popp, R., et al.: Ultrasonic cardiac echography for determining stroke volume and valvular regurgitation. Circulation, 41: 493, 1970.

Popp, R., et al.: Sources of error in calculations of left ventricular volumes by echography. Am. J. Cardiol., 31: 152, 1973.

Prewitt, T., et al.: The "rapid filling wave" of the apexcardiogram: its relation to echocardiographic and cineangiographic measurements of ventricular filling. Br. Heart J., 37: 1256, 1975.

Rasmussen, S., et al.: Stroke volume calculated from the mitral valve echogram in patients with and without ventricular dyssynergy. Circulation, 58: 125, 1978.

Ratshin, R., et al.: Serial evaluation of left ventricular volumes and posterior wall movement in the acute phase of myocardial infarction using diagnostic ultrasound. Am. J. Cardiol., 29: 286, 1972.

Ratshin, R., et al.: The accuracy of ventricular volume analysis by quantitative echocardiography in patients with coronary artery disease with and without wall motion abnormalities. Am. J. Cardiol., 33: 164, 1974.

Ratshin, R., et al.: Determination of left ventricular preload and afterload by quantitative echocardiography in man. Cir. Res., 34: 711, 1974.

Redwood, D., et al.: Evaluation of the ability of echocardiography to measure acute alterations in left ventricular volume. Circulation, 50: 901, 1974.

Schiller, N., et al.: Left ventricular volume from paired biplane two-dimensional echocardiography. Circulation, 60: 547, 1979.

Silverman, N., et al.: Determination of left ventricular volume in children: echocardiographic and angiographic comparisons. Circulation, 62: 548, 1980.

Stefadouros, M., et al.: The effect of isometric exercises on the left ventricular volume in normal man. Circulation, 44: 1185, 1974.

Sweet, R., et al.: Relationship between echocardiography, cardiac output and abnormally contracting segments in patients with ischemic heart disease. Circulation, 52: 634, 1975.

Teichholz, L., et al.: Problems in echocardiographic volume determinations: echocardiographic-angiographic correlations in the presence or absence of asynergy. Am. J. Cardiol., 37: 7, 1976.

TenCate, F., et al.: Dimensions and volumes of left atrium and ventricle determined by single beam echocardiography. Br. Heart J., 36: 737, 1974.

Toshima, H., et al.: Correlations between electrocardiographic, vectorcardiographic and echocardiographic findings in patients with left ventricular volume overload. Am. Heart J., 94: 547, 1977.

Wyatt, H., et al.: Cross-sectional echocardiography. Analysis of mathematic models for quantifying volume of the formalin-fixed left ventricle. Circulation, 61: 1119, 1980.

7

Abnormal Mitral Valve

Abnormal M-mode echocardiographic mitral valve motion provides clues to the identity of specific cardiac lesions when auscultatory or physical manifestations are not prominent. Calcific and fibrotic mitral valve disease is readily detected from the abnormal leaflet motion and the excessive echoes reflected from the valve. Pre- and postoperative echograms are useful to assess the immediate success of mitral commissurotomy and for the long-term evaluation of restenosis. Identification of normal mitral valve motion in the presence of an Austin Flint murmur excludes mitral stenosis. The etiology of auscultatory mitral insufficiency becomes clear when echographic patterns of mitral valve prolapse, hypertrophic cardiomyopathy, left atrial tumor, or ruptured chordae tendineae or calcification of the mitral annulus are recorded. Mitral valve motion is influenced by the filling characteristics of the left ventricle. Fluttering mitral leaflets may be the first indication of the impending disruption of an aortic leaflet infected with bacterial endocarditis.

MITRAL VALVE OBSTRUCTION

Obstruction to blood flow between the left atrium and the left ventricle is most often caused by mitral stenosis secondary to rheumatic fever. Obstruction may also result from left atrial tumor, vegetations, thrombus, cor triatriatum, and mitral orifice hypoplasia or atresia.

Mitral Stenosis

Clinical symptoms often appear on an echocardiographic requisition without any reference to the potential diagnosis of mitral stenosis. If the echocardiographer is aware of the implication of a patient's symptoms, a more thorough examination of the mitral valve, left atrium, and left ventricle can be undertaken.

These clinical findings may include a history of rheumatic fever, systemic embolization, shortness of breath, orthopnea, atrial fibrillation, fatigue, opening snap, diastolic rumble, congestive heart failure, tricuspid incompetence, pulmonary edema, and hemoptysis. Clinical symptoms are not always typical of mitral stenosis. Patterns of motion representing mitral stenosis have been discovered in patients unaware of their heart disease. The opening snap could be inaudible to auscultation, or associated aortic or mitral regurgitation could obscure an opening snap.

An obstructed mitral valve's echogram becomes more box-like and no longer resembles the normal "M" pattern. Both cusps of the mitral valve move toward the transducer at the onset of diastole and remain in this abnormal forward position throughout diastole (Figs. 7–1 to 7–3). Figures 7–4 and 7–5 show the roughened surfaces of a severely calcified and fibrosed mitral valve that reflected many high-intensity echoes even at low levels of amplification. Calcification and fibrosis may involve all or part of a valve (Figs. 7–6 and 7–7). Stiffened leaflets move poorly, and their mobility is further diminished with thickening and fusion of the valve's commissural edges and chordae tendineae. Long-axis, two-dimensional echocardiography (see Fig. 8–1) is most useful to identify the actual site of the mitral stenosis (Fig. 7–8). Short-axis, two-dimensional echocardiography then identifies the narrowest orifice through which left atrial blood must pass[1] (Fig. 7–9).

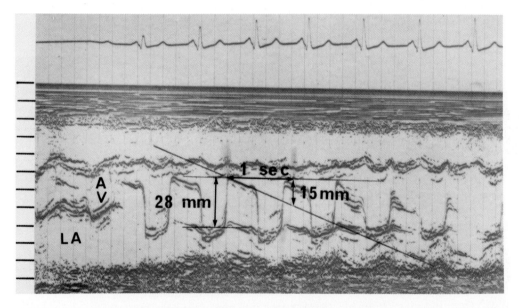

Fig. 7–1. A representative pattern of motion seen with mitral stenosis. The anterior mitral valve amplitude increased as the transducer was angled toward the left atrium (LA). The maximum opening excursion was achieved near the atrioventricular junction, where the posterior mitral leaflet motion almost disappeared. The early diastolic anterior leaflet closing velocity was characteristically decreased at 15 mm/sec; the opening excursion was 28 mm, indicating good leaflet pliability. Leaflets stiffened with fibrosis or calcium are less mobile. The following data were obtained at cardiac catheterization: mitral valve area, 1.2 cm²; cardiac index, 3.7 L/min/m²; transmitral gradient, 40 mm Hg. There was no mitral regurgitation. AV, aortic valve motion.

(Text continues on page 225.)

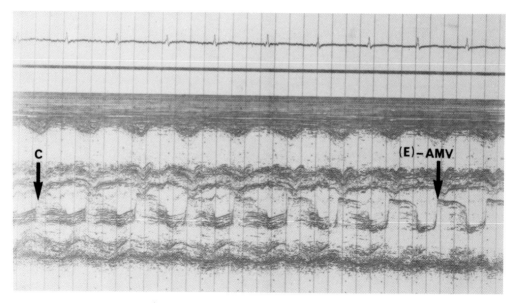

Fig. 7–2. A 62-year-old male patient with mitral stenosis. In this scan of the mitral valve, from its chordal attachment at the free edges of the leaflet to the mid-section of the leaflet, leaflet excursion was most restricted along the free edges. The markedly reduced early diastolic closing velocity was indicative of elevated left atrial pressure. (See Figs. 7–8 and 7–9.) C, level of chordae tendineae; (E)-AMV, maximum open position of anterior mitral leaflet or E-point.

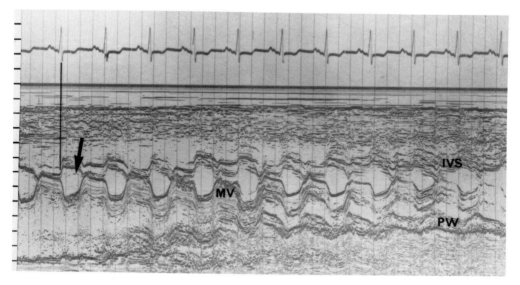

Fig. 7–3. A 28-year-old male patient who had had rheumatic fever at age 14 and who was discharged from the armed services at age 21 because of easy fatigability and an inability to keep up with physical exercise. In this incomplete scan from the left ventricular outflow tract to the left ventricle, the arrow marks an illusionary aortic valve created by coaptation of the septum and the mitral valve during diastole. The mitral valve was stenotic and heavily calcified. (See Fig. 7–10.) MV, mitral valve motion; IVS, interventricular septum; PW, posterior left ventricular wall.

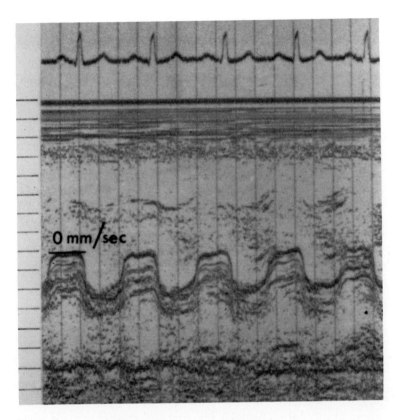

Fig. 7–4. A 55-year-old male patient with ''heart trouble'' of 13 years' duration. The mitral valve remained in the open position throughout diastole, secondary to leaflet rigidity and high left atrial pressure. Multiple echoes were seen in diastole and systole representing leaflet thickening, fibrosis, and calcification. The posterior mitral leaflet movement was almost indistinguishable. The following data were obtained at cardiac catheterization: mitral valve area, 0.72 cm²; mitral valve gradient, 18 mm Hg; cardiac index, 2.33 L/min/m²; pulmonary artery, 33 mm Hg (mean); pulmonary wedge, 40 mm Hg (mean); pulmonary vascular resistance, 1.2 units.

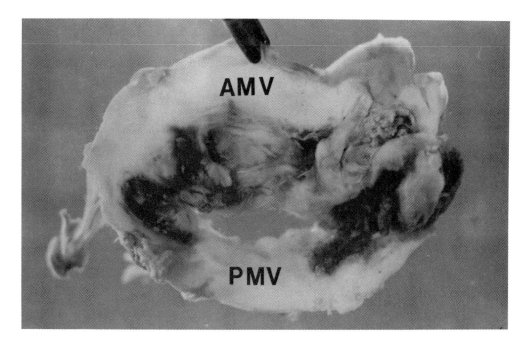

Fig. 7–5. The excised mitral valve from same patient whose mitral echogram appears in Figure 7–4. Pathology: the atrial surface of the valve displayed an annular rim of normal valvular tissue with marked calcification and thickening near the orifice with areas of excoriation. The ventricular surface displayed some atheromatous deposition, particularly along commissures. The chordae tendineae ranged from thin and delicate to thickened and fused. The valve orifice measured approximately 0.7 cm². AMV, anterior mitral leaflet; PMV, posterior mitral leaflet.

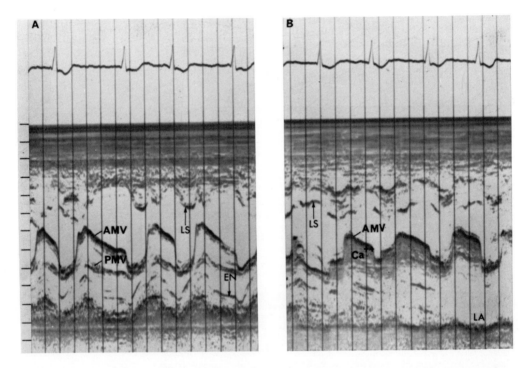

Fig. 7–6. *A,* Mitral stenosis without evidence of calcification. *B,* The same valve, recorded from a more superior plane as the transducer was directed toward the left atrium. Signal amplification was not altered. Dense echoes under the anterior mitral leaflet movement (AMV) represented areas of localized calcification (ca^{++}). PMV, posterior mitral leaflet motion; LS, left septum-blood interface; EN, endocardium-blood interface of posterior left ventricular wall; LA, left atrium. (From Dillon, J., Feigenbaum, H., Knoecke, L., Davis, R., and Chang, S.: Echocardiographic manifestations of valvular vegetations. Am. Heart J., *86*: 698, 1973.)

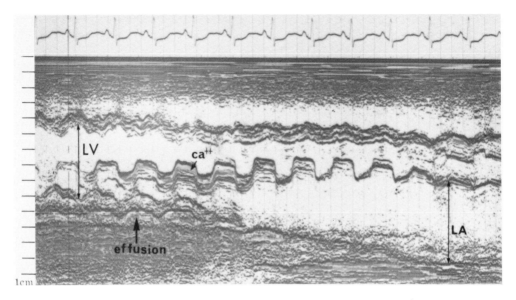

Fig. 7-7. A scan demonstrating the relation of the stenotic mitral valve to the left ventricle, left atrium, and aorta. The mitral valve was heavily calcified and opened poorly. The following data were obtained at cardiac catheterization: severe mitral stenosis, moderate mitral insufficiency. Pulmonary artery pressures were elevated at rest, rising to systemic levels during exercise. LV, left ventricle; ca^{++}, calcium; LA, left atrium.

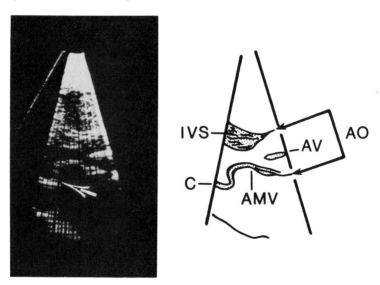

Fig. 7-8. A still frame and its diagram from a parasternal, long-axis, two-dimensional echocardiogram. This patient's M-mode mitral valve echogram appears in Figure 7-2. During diastole, the body of the mitral leaflet billowed anteriorly toward the transducer. The free edges of the leaflet were restricted (arrow) and full leaflet opening could not be accomplished. IVS, interventricular septum; C, chordae tendineae; AMV, anterior mitral valve; AV, aortic valve; AO, aorta.

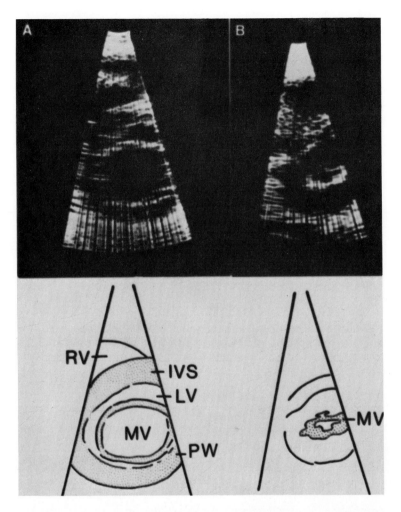

Fig. 7–9. *A,* A still frame and its diagram from a parasternal, short-axis, two-dimensional echocardiogram of a normal mitral valve. The leaflets opened widely into the left ventricular cavity. *B,* A still frame and its diagram from a parasternal, short-axis, two-dimensional echocardiogram from a patient with severe mitral stenosis whose M-mode echogram appears in Figure 7–2; the long-axis, two-dimensional echogram appears in Figure 7–8. The transducer was positioned near the aorta and was angled inferiorly until the *smallest* mitral orifice could be identified. Signal amplification was increased just enough to visualize the circumferential orifice. Rapid estimates of orifice size were obtained by tracing the inner boundaries of the orifice onto electrocardiographic paper. The number of squares contained within the orifice were divided by the number of squares in a square centimeter measured from distance calibrations recorded simultaneously with the photograph. This estimate of mitral orifice size is not influenced by mitral regurgitation. RV, right ventricle; IVS, interventricular septum; LV, left ventricular cavity; MV, open mitral valve; PW, posterior left ventricular wall.

M-mode echographic scans of the mitral valve should always be extended to the aortic valve. Figure 7–3 demonstrates an incomplete scan, terminated at the left ventricular outflow tract. Because this patient had significant tricuspid regurgitation, the septum moved paradoxically, coapting with the open mitral valve during diastole. During systole, the septum moved anteriorly as the mitral valve closed, forming a pattern resembling that of aortic valve motion. By continuing the scan superiorly and medially toward the right shoulder, real aortic valve motion was recorded (Fig. 7–10).

One should experiment with different gain settings during examination of the mitral leaflets. If excessive echoes are present, even at low signal amplification, evidence for calcification, fibrosis, or leaflet thickening should be considered. The intensity of echoes returned from diseased leaflets often interferes with resolution of the separate cusps (Fig. 7–5). Less amplification is seldom helpful. One should scan the valve from the chordae tendineae to the leaflet's annular attachment to identify individual leaflet motion (Fig. 7–7).

Early diastolic closing velocity of the anterior mitral leaflet should increase, and the posterior leaflet motion should be normalized, after an open mitral commissurotomy (Fig. 7–11). Relief of the mitral stenosis lowers left atrial pressure, and blood flows more freely from the left atrium to the left ventricle. Figure 7–12 shows one patient whose anterior mitral leaflet exhibited restricted anterior leaflet movement

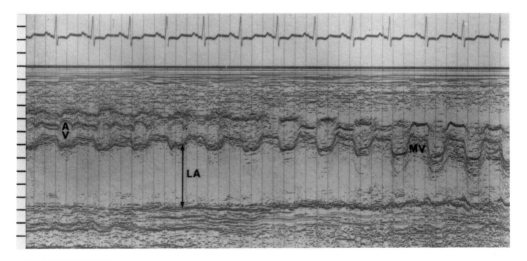

Fig. 7–10. A tracing from the patient in Figure 7–3. In this scan from the true aortic valve inferiorly toward the left ventricular outflow tract, the left atrial dimension was markedly dilated. No significant mitral insufficiency was noted on the cineangiogram. The following data were obtained at catheterization: pulmonary artery, 110/66 mm Hg; right ventricle, 110/20 mm Hg; mitral valve gradient, 30 mm Hg; moderate aortic insufficiency. AV, aortic valve motion; LA, left atrium; MV, stenotic and calcified mitral valve.

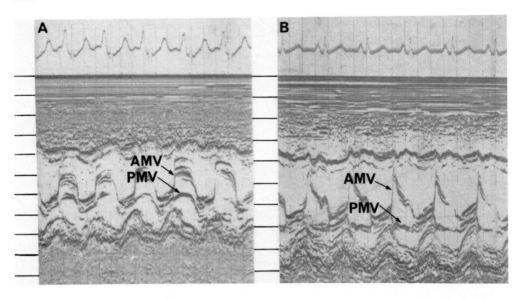

Fig. 7–11. *A,* Mitral stenosis before surgical intervention. The closing velocity of the mitral valve was greatly reduced during diastole. *B,* Postoperative mitral valve echogram prior to the patient's discharge from the hospital. The diastolic closing velocity was improved; posterior leaflet movement was normalized. AMV, anterior mitral leaflet motion; PMV, posterior mitral leaflet motion.

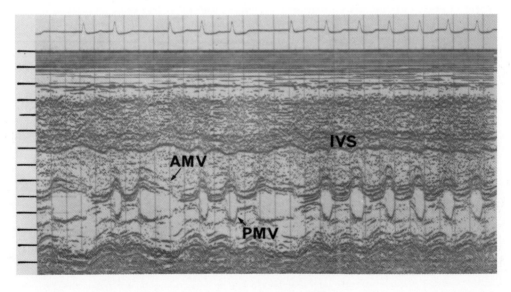

Fig. 7–12. A postoperative tracing of the mitral valve showing the normal motion of the posterior leaflet and the typical pattern of mitral stenosis exhibited by the anterior mitral leaflet. Preoperative tracings were not available. A closed mitral commissurotomy was performed in 1962. With the exception of atrial fibrillation, this patient was asymptomatic in 1972 when this tracing was recorded. IVS, interventricular septum; AMV, anterior mitral valve motion; PMV, posterior mitral valve motion.

and normal posterior leaflet movement ten years after a closed mitral commissurotomy. Although restricted blood flow was suggested, the patient was asymptomatic.

Annular Calcification

Mitral valve obstruction can occur without actually involving the mitral leaflets. Severe calcification of the mitral annulus narrows the mitral orifice, particularly along the posterior aspect of the valve. Calcium appears as a mass of echoes between the posterior mitral leaflet and the posterior wall of the atrioventricular junction. Calcification of the annulus is common in the geriatric patient (Fig. 7–13).

False Mitral Valve Obstruction

M-mode echocardiographic patterns of motion often suggest disease or anatomic structures that are incorrect or do not exist. Before completing any examination, one should be certain that all anatomic motion has been correctly identified. Figure 7–14 was recorded as soon as the transducer was placed on the patient's chest along the parasternum. At first, the patient was thought to have mitral stenosis with a normally moving tricuspid valve. However, further examination did not disclose posterior mitral leaflet motion, and left ventricular

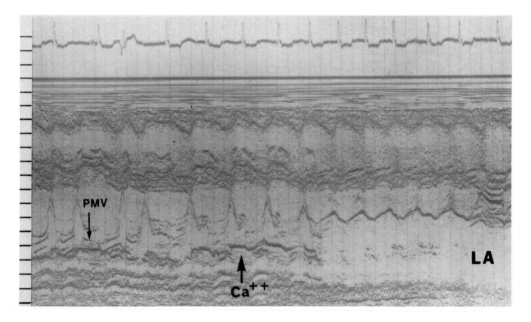

Fig. 7–13. A 66-year-old female patient with mitral regurgitation secondary to calcification of the mitral valve annulus. The anterior and posterior mitral leaflets exhibited normal motion and were not unusually echo-reflective; these findings were compatible with normal leaflet thickness. PMV, posterior mitral leaflet motion; Ca^{++}, calcium deposited in mitral annulus; LA, left atrium.

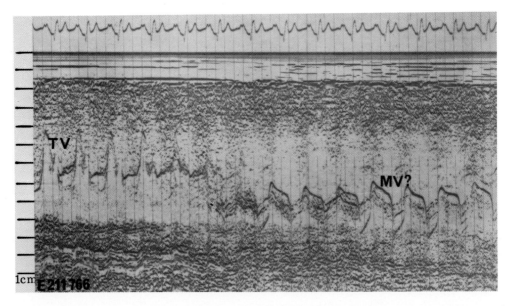

Fig. 7–14. A 19-year-old male patient with transposition and dextroversion. The initial recording suggested mitral stenosis and normal tricuspid valve motion. The posterior mitral leaflet motion could not be identified in this tracing, recorded along the left parasternum. TV, questionable tricuspid valve; MV?, questionable mitral valve. (See Fig. 7–15.)

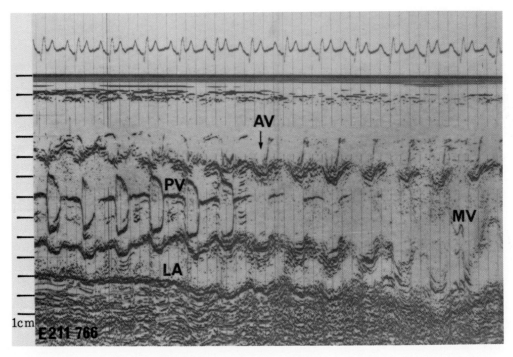

Fig. 7–15. A final tracing from the patient in Figure 7–14. The pattern of motion originally thought to represent mitral stenosis was actually a record of the left pulmonary leaflet motion. This scan was recorded from the right parasternum with angulation of the transducer from the left shoulder toward the right flank. AV, aortic valve motion; PV, pulmonary valve motion; LA, left atrium; MV, mitral valve motion.

wall motion could not be located. There was a short interlude while the hospital chart was consulted, and the presence of dextroversion was noted. The transducer was then positioned along the right parasternum and directed superiorly and laterally toward the left shoulder. Normal mitral valve motion was recorded from this position (Fig. 7–15). What was previously believed to be mitral valve motion was actually left pulmonary valve motion. Aortic valve motion was recorded directly superior to this movement. The patient had transposition of the great vessels as well as dextroversion.

Left Atrial Myxoma and Thrombus

Patients with unsuspected left atrial tumors have been diagnosed as having primary pulmonary hypertension, primary cardiomyopathy, mitral stenosis, mitral regurgitation, infective endocarditis, and congestive heart failure. Many of the symptoms are similar to those seen with mitral stenosis and may be listed on the echocardiographic consultation request form.

M-mode echocardiograms were obtained from 22 patients with left atrial myxoma. Over half the cases were clinically unsuspected. Twenty were confirmed by angiography, and 2 patients refused cardiac catheterization. All 22 tumors were

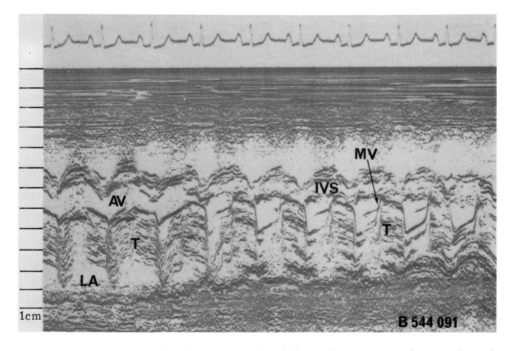

Fig. 7–16. A 50-year-old female patient with a left atrial myxoma. In this scan from the aorta and left atrium inferiorly to the mitral valve, the tumor was seen in the left atrium during systole, moving into the mitral orifice during diastole. AV, aortic valve motion; LA, left atrium; IVS, interventricular septum; MV, anterior mitral leaflet motion; T, tumor.

surgically excised. Left atrial myxoma recurred in 2 patients within 3 months and 3 years, respectively, after initial diagnosis and surgical removal. The most interesting feature of the echocardiograms was their variability from each other, yet each one was characteristic enough to establish a definitive diagnosis. Six examples of left atrial myxoma, with related laboratory or surgery data, are shown in Figures 7–16 to 7–24.

In each case of left heart myxoma, the diastolic phase of the mitral valve's motion was filled with a mass of echoes that persisted even at low signal amplification. Most of the tumors were large enough to block the mitral valve orifice. This blocking resulted in a mitral valve pattern of motion similar to patterns produced by mitral stenosis.

If a tumor was not attached to the mitral leaflet, it had to travel from the left atrial cavity to the mitral orifice during diastole. Hence, most tracings show some delay between the time when the mitral valve opened until the mass entered the mitral orifice (Figs. 7–16, 7–17, 7–19, and 7–21).

When a tumor is attached to the mitral leaflet, diagnosis becomes more difficult. Figure 7–24 shows a myxoma that was attached to the left atrial side of the mitral leaflet. Echoes from the tumor never left the mitral valve area, but remained persistently in the atrioventricular area throughout systole.

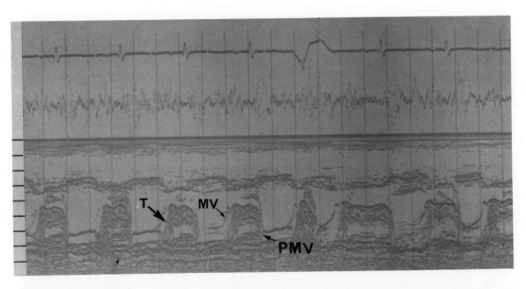

Fig. 7–17. A 44-year-old female patient with a left atrial myxoma, clinically unsuspected. The patient had intermittent heart failure of 15 years' duration. On this hospital admission, the patient exhibited severe pulmonary hypertension and a loud diastolic rumble. An echocardiogram was ordered to exclude mitral stenosis. The myxoma was surgically excised following cardiac catheterization. The specimen was soft, yellowish-white, and encapsulated, weighing 75 g and measuring 9.0 × 6.0 × 2.5 cm. There was evidence of hemorrhage, but no necrosis. T, tumor; PMV, posterior mitral leaflet motion; MV, anterior mitral leaflet motion.

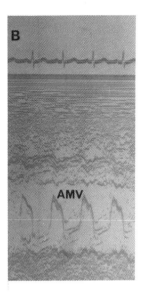

Fig. 7–18. A 48-year-old male patient with an acute embolus to the left femoral artery. *A,* A preoperative echogram of an "extremely friable, gelatinous tumor" measuring 5.0 × 3.0 × 1.6 cm, weighing 18 g. The structure was homogeneous on microscopic examination. The tumor was attached to the left atrial wall close to the posterior mitral leaflet. The pedicle was approximately 1 cm wide. *B,* A postoperative echogram demonstrated nonobstructed mitral leaflet motion. AMV, anterior mitral leaflet motion; T, tumor; PV, posterior mitral leaflet motion.

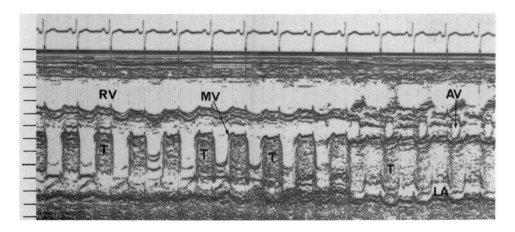

Fig. 7–19. A 24-year-old female patient with a left atrial myxoma. Amplification had been reduced to levels adequate to visualize the septum and the posterior left ventricular wall without difficulty. Note the slight delay between the maximum diastolic opening of the mitral valve and the entry of the myxoma into the mitral orifice. The posterior mitral leaflet motion was obscured by the density of the tumor. RV, right ventricle; T, tumor; MV, mitral valve diastolic motion; AV, aortic valve motion; LA, left atrium.

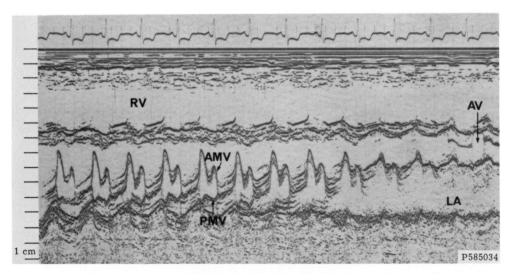

Fig. 7–20. A postoperative scan of the mitral valve following the removal of the left atrial myxoma seen in Figure 7–19. The anterior and posterior mitral valve motion were entirely normal. RV, right ventricle; AMV, anterior mitral leaflet motion; PMV, posterior mitral leaflet motion; LA, left atrium; AV, aortic valve motion.

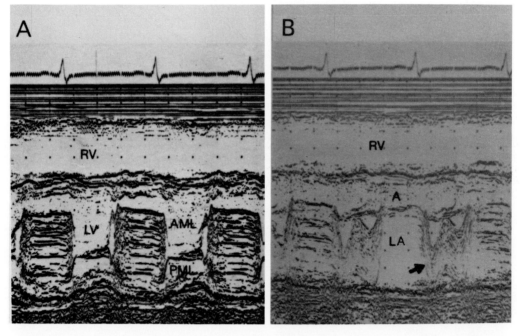

Fig. 7–21. A 66-year-old female patient. *A,* A left atrial myxoma entered the mitral valve orifice shortly after the onset of diastole. *B,* During diastole, the tumor was flung back into the left atrium, rebounded in mid-systole, and moved toward the posterior left atrial wall prior to the next diastolic period. The following data were obtained at catheterization: pulmonary artery, 60 mm Hg (mean); pulmonary wedge, 36 mm Hg (mean); left ventricle, 156/15 mm Hg; mitral valve gradient, 20 mm Hg. RV, right ventricle; LV, left ventricle; AML, anterior mitral leaflet motion; PML, posterior mitral leaflet motion; arrow, early systolic entry of tumor into left atrium. (From Alvarez, H.: Valor de la ecocardiografía en el diagnóstico del mixoma de la aurícula izquierda. Arch. Inst. Nac. Cardiol. Mex., *48*:667, 1978.)

232

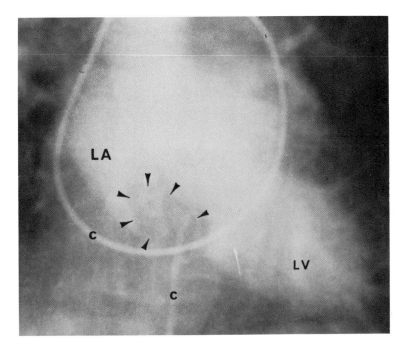

Fig. 7–22. A levophase right anterior oblique angiogram from the patient in Figures 7–21 and 7–23. The systolic position of the tumor in the left atrium is indicated by arrowheads. C, catheter; LA, left atrium; LV, left ventricle. (From Alvarez, H.: Valor de la ecocardiografía en el diagnóstico del mixoma de la aurícula izquierda. Arch. Inst. Nac. Cardiol. Mex., *48*:667, 1978.)

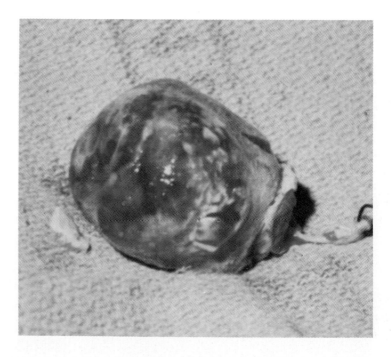

Fig. 7–23. The left atrial myxoma from the patient seen in Figures 7–21 and 7–22. The specimen measured 5.0 × 4.0 × 3.0 cm and was attached by a short pedicle to the muscular portion of the atrial septum and the inferior posterior left atrial wall. The appearance of the cut surface was glistening, gelatinous, red, and yellow. Microscopic examination revealed calcium within many vascular structures. (From Alvarez, H.: Valor de la ecocardiografía en el diagnóstico del mixoma de la aurícula izquierda. Arch. Inst. Nac. Cardiol. Mex., *48*:667, 1978.)

The movements of several masses within the left atrium are shown in Figures 7–16, 7–19, 7–21, 7–24, 7–25, and 7–26. Only the mass shown in Figures 7–26 was presumed (and proved) to be a thrombus secondary to mitral stenosis and atrial fibrillation. In one patient (Fig. 7–18), echoes from the tumor were not detected within the left atrium from either the parasternal or the suprasternal examination site. Individual echocardiographers performed the examination at two different hospitals on different echographs. This lack of echo-reflectiveness from the tumor suggested that either the tumor was not intercepted by the sound beam within the left atrium, or the tumor's density was so similar to the density of blood that an acoustic mismatch failed to occur as sound waves passed from the left atrial blood into the tumor. Pathologic examination revealed a friable tumor of gelatinous, homogeneous consistency. Figure 7–27 shows a deceptive tracing. Severe mitral stenosis and high signal amplification mimicked a left atrial mass even though a mass did not exist. The movement of the echoes within the mitral orifice and behind the posterior aortic wall was similar to the motion of a true atrial myxoma (Fig. 7–25).

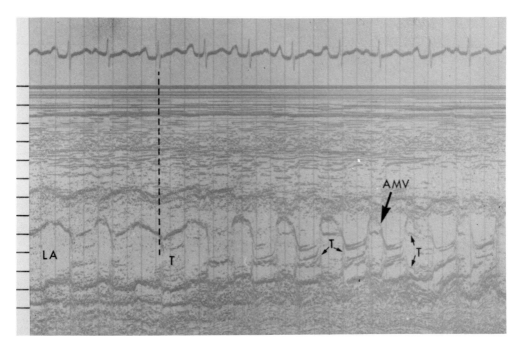

Fig. 7–24. A 52-year-old female patient with a recurrent left atrial myxoma three years after surgical removal of a similar lesion. At the onset of diastole, the tumor moved simultaneously with the opening mitral leaflet. There was a 12-mm Hg end-diastolic pressure gradient across the mitral valve. Surgeons found the tumor to be attached to the posterior mitral leaflet. LA, left atrium; T, tumor; AMV, anterior mitral leaflet motion. (See Fig. 7–47B, cineangiogram of myxoma.)

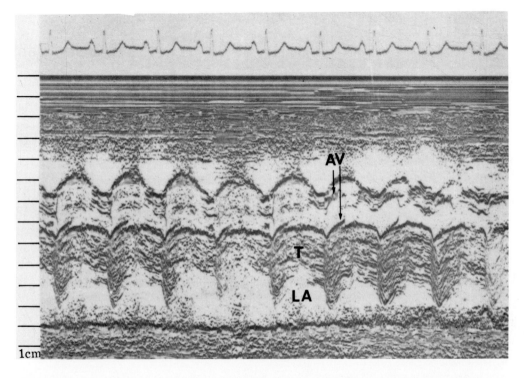

Fig. 7–25. The left atrial position of the tumor seen in Figure 7–16. The tumor was closely applied to the anterior aspect of the left atrium. During surgical exploration, this myxoma was found to be large, with restricted mobility. The pedicle was short, attached to the intra-atrial wall. AV, aortic valve motion during systole; T, tumor; LA, left atrium.

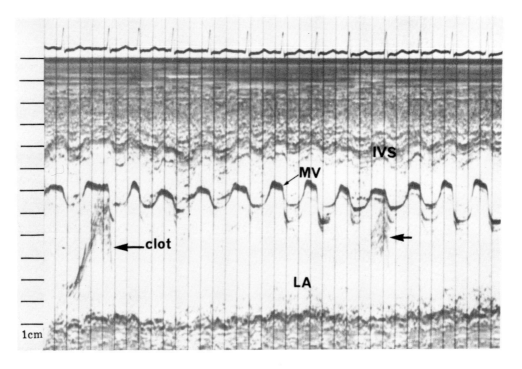

Fig. 7–26. A free-floating thrombus in the left atrium. The size of the thrombus exceeded the mitral orifice and prevented its entry into the left ventricle. The transducer had been angled toward the left ventricular outflow tract and had been held motionless. The thrombus periodically passed in and out of the sound beam. The surgically excised specimen measured 2.0 × 4.0 cm; the mitral valve orifice was 1.3 cm². MV, characteristic motion of stenotic mitral valve; IVS, interventricular septum; LA, left atrium.

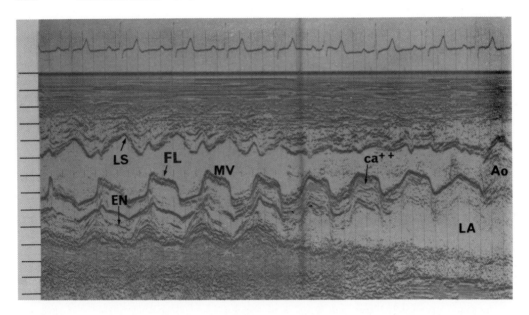

Fig. 7–27. A 39-year-old female patient with severe calcific mitral stenosis and regurgitation and moderate aortic regurgitation. The mild echographic fluttering (FL) of the mitral chordae tendineae was consistent with aortic regurgitation. The excessive echo-reflectiveness of the mitral valve was consistent with severe calcification or fibrosis, but these echoes could be mistaken for tumor or thrombus. The following catheterization data were obtained: pulmonary artery, 40 mm Hg (mean); pulmonary wedge, 27 mm Hg (mean); mitral valve gradient, 17 mm Hg; cardiac index, 4.0 L/min/m². At operation, the mitral valve was found to be substantially calcified. No thrombi were present in the left atrium. LS, left septum; EN, endocardial surface of posterior left ventricular wall; MV, anterior mitral valve motion; ca++, calcium; LA, left atrium; Ao, aorta. (From Feigenbaum, H.: Echocardiography, 2nd Ed. Philadelphia, Lea & Febiger, 1976.)

SYSTOLIC ANTERIOR MITRAL MOTION (SAM)

Figure 7–28 demonstrates a convex, systolic displacement of some portion of the anterior and posterior mitral leaflets or chordae tendineae. Systolic anterior displacement of the mitral valve (SAM) is neither a symptom nor a disease. It is an abnormal motion of parts of the mitral apparatus in the presence of a narrowed left ventricular outflow tract and vigorous systolic ejection. This movement has been observed in normal persons with small left ventricles. Although SAM is one characteristic of idiopathic hypertrophic subaortic stenosis, it is not pathognomonic for this disease. Some patients with concentric myocardial hypertrophy secondary to aortic stenosis or severe systemic hypertension have shown abnormal mitral valve displacement. Two patients, one with aortic regurgitation (Fig. 7–29) and one with atrial septal defect (Fig. 7–30), showed pronounced systolic mitral valve displacement on their echocardiograms. At cardiac catheteriza-

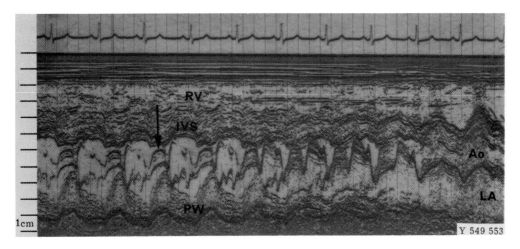

Fig. 7–28. A 27-year-old male patient with idiopathic hypertrophic subaortic stenosis (IHSS). The presenting symptom was a grade V/VI, long, harsh murmur along the left parasternum, accompanied by a left ventricular heave and thrill. The electrocardiogram showed nonspecific ST-T wave changes; cardiac fluoroscopy suggested aortic stenosis.

Hypertrophic cardiomyopathy was suggested by the systolic apposition of the mitral valve (arrow) with the thick septum. The following data were obtained during catheterization: pulmonary artery, 11 mm Hg (mean); pulmonary wedge, 8 mm Hg (mean); left ventricle, apical, 200/16 mm Hg; left ventricle, outflow tract, 110/16 mm Hg; simultaneous aortic pressure, 110/72 mm Hg. Pressure gradients: rest, 90 mm Hg; post PVC, 170 mm Hg; Valsalva maneuver, 130 mm Hg. Cardiac index, 2.8 L/min/m². RV, right ventricle; Ao, aorta; LA, left atrium; IVS, interventricular septum; PW, posterior left ventricular wall.

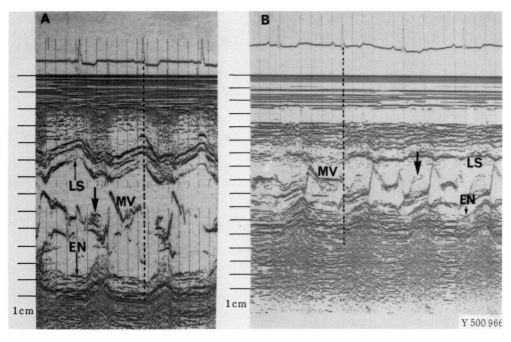

Fig. 7–29. A 37-year-old male patient with moderately severe aortic regurgitation. *A,* A preoperative tracing showed diastolic flutter of the mitral valve and systolic anterior motion of the mitral valve (arrow). *B,* In the postoperative tracing following aortic valve replacement, the abnormal systolic mitral valve displacement persisted. Passive to paradoxical septal motion was a common observance following open heart operations by sternal split. LS, left septum; EN, endocardial surface of posterior left ventricular wall; MV, mitral valve motion.

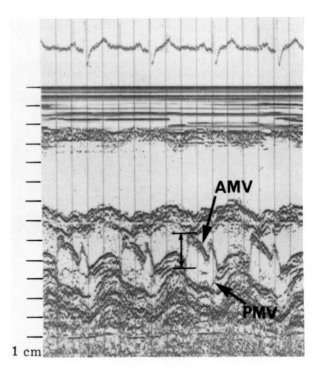

Fig. 7–30. A 48-year-old female patient with an unsuspected atrial septal defect. Although there was some systolic anterior displacement of the mitral valve, there was no apposition between the anterior septum and the valve. AMV, anterior mitral valve motion; PMV, posterior mitral valve motion.

tion, provocation with amyl nitrite, hyperventilation, Valsalva maneuver, and isoproterenol infusion did not produce any pressure gradients within the left ventricles or their outflow tracts.

The systolic anterior motion of the mitral valve should be evaluated at the level of the free edges of the mitral valve. If the transducer is angled too superiorly toward the anterior mitral annulus and atrioventricular junction, an impression of SAM arises from spurious echoes from the posterior aortic wall (Fig. 7–31).

Some means of provocation may be useful in an attempt to accentuate latent systolic mitral obstruction when hypertrophic cardiomyopathy is suspected. Provocation may take place while both mitral leaflets are being recorded. If a technologist is initiating these procedures, a physician should be available, since serious side effects have been known to occur (Table 7–1).

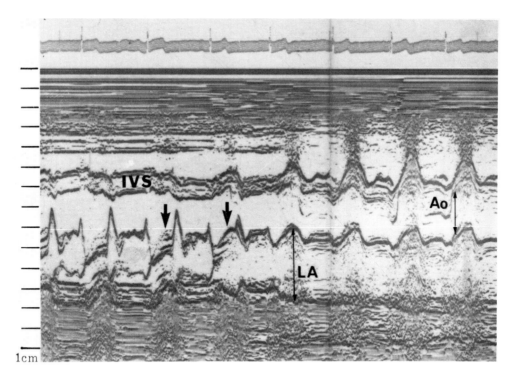

Fig. 7–31. A scan from the normal mitral valve to the aorta. Owing to poor lateral resolution, the transducer received echoes from both the anterior mitral leaflet and the aortic root; these echoes gave a false impression of systolic anterior mitral leaflet displacement (arrows). Ao, aorta; LA, left atrium; IVS, interventricular septum.

Table 7–1.
Provocative Maneuvers to Accentuate Latent Systolic Obstruction

Provocation method	Side effects
Amyl nitrite inhalation	Increased heart rate, dizziness, peripheral flushing, seizures, fainting, and headache
Hyperventilation	Dizziness, fainting, increased heart rate, anxiety, and tingling in fingers
Carotid massage to provoke premature ventricular contractions	Slowing of heart rate, fainting, and cardiac arrest

FLUTTERING MITRAL VALVE

Diastole

High-frequency diastolic oscillations of the mitral valve are most commonly produced by aortic regurgitation (Figs. 7–32 to 7–37). Ventricular septal defect, congenital mitral stenosis (Fig. 7–38), and ruptured chordae tendineae (Fig. 7–40) similarly alter early diastolic mitral valve motion. High-frequency leaflet oscillation is most obvious when signal amplification is low. Too much amplification blurs the fine diastolic undulations of the leaflet.

Thickened and calcified mitral leaflets have not fluttered in the presence of even significant aortic regurgitation. However, if the chordae tendineae have remained pliable and have not become fused or thickened, they may flutter, indicating the presence of aortic regurgitation (Fig. 7–37). The echographic appearance of high-frequency mitral leaflet vibration, secondary to aortic regurgitation, is different from the slow, coarse leaflet oscillations caused by atrial flutter (Fig. 7–39).

Acute aortic regurgitation rarely produces fluttering mitral leaflets because the valve closes before atrial or ventricular depolarization. When the echocardiogram is recorded, one

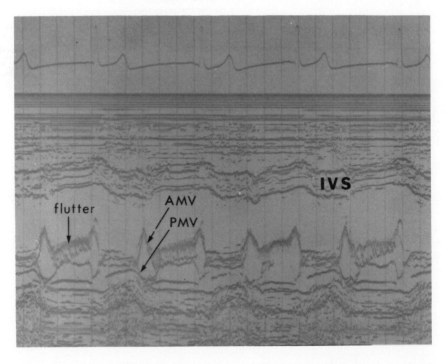

Fig. 7–32. An 18-year-old male patient with moderate aortic regurgitation secondary to a bicuspid aortic valve. Mitral fluttering was most remarkable between rapid left ventricular filling and atrial contraction. AMV, anterior mitral leaflet motion; PMV, posterior mitral leaflet motion; IVS, interventricular septum.

(Text continues on page 250.)

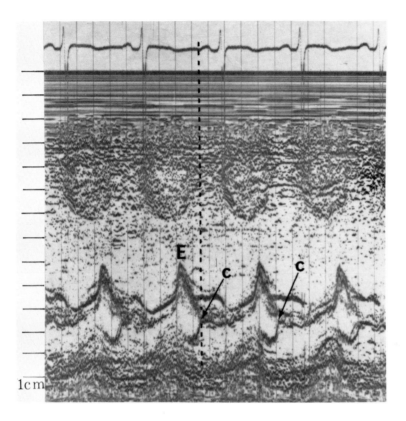

Fig. 7–33. A 35-year-old male patient with acute aortic regurgitation secondary to myxomatous degeneration of a bicuspid aortic valve. The mitral valve closed before the onset of ventricular depolarization. The valve did not reopen in response to the left atrial contraction. E, maximum diastolic excursion of anterior mitral leaflet; c, premature closure of mitral valve.

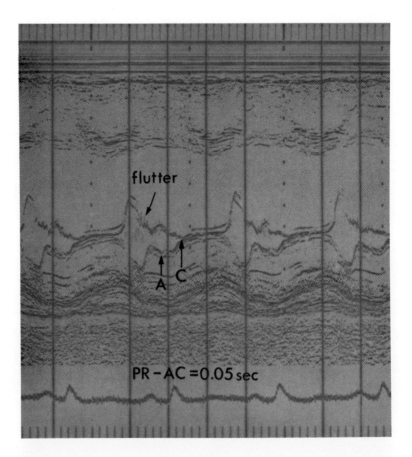

Fig. 7–34. A 65-year-old male patient with severe aortic insufficiency secondary to bacterial endocarditis. The fluttering of the mitral valve was consistent with aortic regurgitation. The following data were obtained at catheterization: Aorta, 120/55 mm Hg; left ventricle, 120/30 mm Hg. The markedly elevated left ventricular end-diastolic pressure was reflected in the abnormally long A-C interval. A, peak atrial contraction; C, closure of anterior and posterior mitral leaflets; PR–AC, difference between A-C interval from mitral valve and P-R interval on electrocardiogram. The normal difference should exceed 0.06 sec.

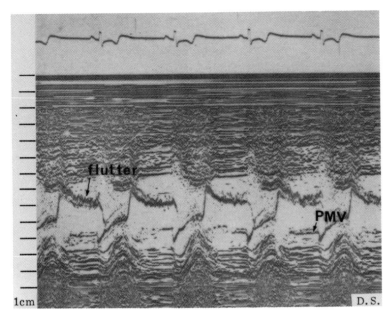

Fig. 7-35. Diastolic mitral valve motion mimicking mitral stenosis. The fluttering anterior mitral leaflet was indicative of aortic insufficiency. The normal posterior mitral leaflet motion and the general lack of excessive echoes reflected from the mitral valve excluded mitral thickening and obstruction. An Austin Flint murmur was heard during auscultation. PMV, posterior mitral valve motion.

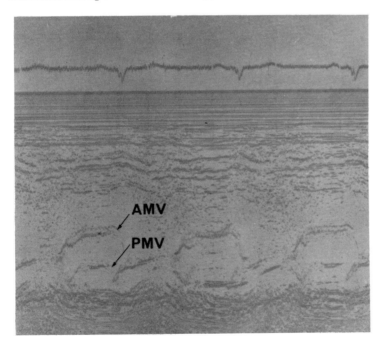

Fig. 7-36. A 65-year-old male patient with moderately severe aortic regurgitation secondary to a markedly dilated aortic root. The mitral leaflets were not unusually echo-reflective, and the posterior mitral leaflet motion was normal. No mitral stenosis was demonstrated at catheterization. AMV, anterior mitral leaflet motion; PMV, posterior mitral leaflet motion.

245

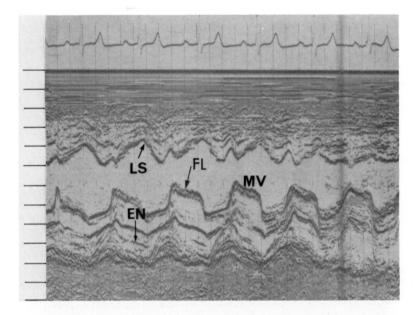

Fig. 7–37. A 39-year-old female patient with severe, calcific mitral stenosis and regurgitation and moderate aortic regurgitation. The mild fluttering of the chordae tendineae was consistent with aortic regurgitation. (See Fig. 7–20.) At operation, the entire anterior mitral leaflet was rigid with calcium. The chordae tendineae were free of calcification and were not thickened. LS, left septal-blood interface; EN, endocardial-blood interface of posterior left ventricular wall; FL, fluttering chordae tendineae; MV, mitral leaflet motion. (From Feigenbaum, H.: Echocardiography, 2nd Ed. Philadelphia, Lea & Febiger, 1976.)

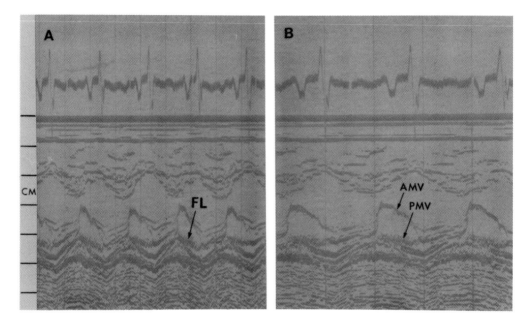

Fig. 7–38. A 21-day-old infant weighing 3.29 kg with a ventricular septal defect and congenital mitral stenosis. The fluttering of the posterior mitral leaflet raised the suspicion of a possible congenital mitral obstruction. Poor left atrial emptying was demonstrated during a levophase cineangiogram. FL, fluttering posterior mitral leaflet (PMV); AMV, anterior mitral leaflet motion. *A,* Paper recording speed, 50 mm/sec. *B,* Paper recording speed, 97 mm/sec.

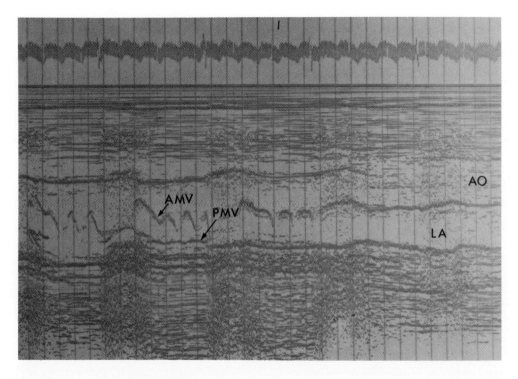

Fig. 7–39. A postoperative tracing from the patient in Figure 7–19. The coarse undulations of the mitral valve are due to atrial flutter. The posterior mitral leaflet was relatively passive, but this could have been an artifact. The tracing was obtained five days postoperatively, and the patient could not be positioned for optimal examination. AMV, anterior mitral valve motion; PMV, posterior mitral valve motion; AO, aorta; LA, left atrium.

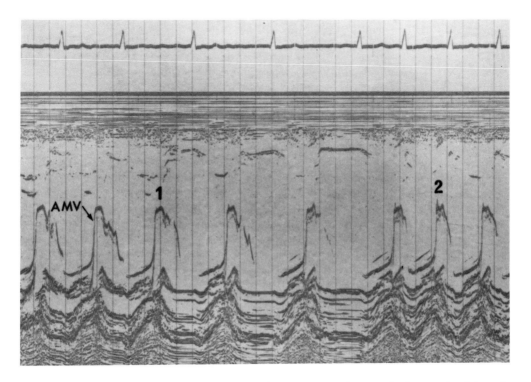

Fig. 7–40.   An 18-year-old male patient with severe mitral regurgitation and mild aortic regurgitation who had rheumatic fever at age 15. Pansystolic murmur, thrill, and loud S_3 were heard at the apex. (1), E-point was blunted; (2), E-point was followed by an abrupt, high-velocity posterior displacement of the anterior mitral leaflet suggesting an untethering of the anterior mitral leaflet. The following data were obtained at catheterization: left ventricle, 115/18 mm Hg; pulmonary artery, 35 mm Hg (mean); pulmonary wedge, 27 mm Hg (mean). (See Fig. 7–41.) AMV, anterior mitral leaflet motion.

must be certain that premature mitral valve closure is not an artifact introduced by a peculiar relationship between the sound beam and the mitral leaflets (see Fig. 2–12). Bradycardia may also allow the valve to drift closed before the onset of ventricular depolarization.

Systole

Systolic fluttering of the mitral valve occurs when the midportion of the mitral apparatus is separated from its restraining chordae tendineae or papillary muscle. With the onset of systole, the untethered portion of the leaflet is forcefully displaced toward the left atrium. Regurgitant blood passes this loose tissue and causes it to vibrate (Figs. 7–41 to 7–43).

PROLAPSED MITRAL VALVE

The echocardiographic consultation request form may list the symptoms of chest pain, midsystolic click–late systolic

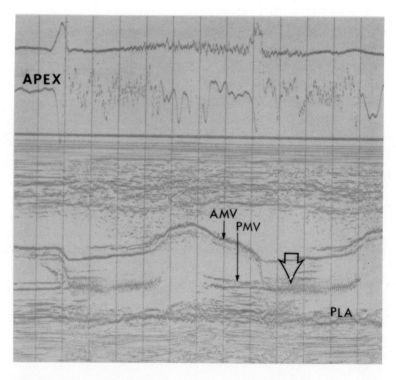

Fig. 7–41. A tracing from the patient in Figure 7–40. High-frequency systolic vibrations of the mitral apparatus were consistent with an untethered mitral leaflet (arrow). The posterior mitral leaflet appeared slightly thickened and passive during diastole. A phonocardiogram demonstrated a pansystolic murmur at the apex. AMV, anterior mitral valve motion; PMV, posterior mitral valve motion; PLA, posterior left atrial wall.

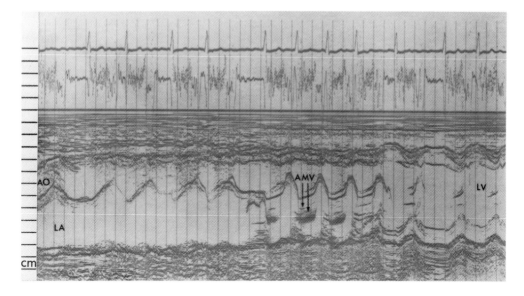

Fig. 7–42. A tracing from the patient in Figures 7–40 and 7–41. In this compressed scan from the aorta to the left ventricle, portions of the mitral valve collapsed into the left atrium and vibrated throughout systole. The recording speed was approximately 16 mm/sec. AMV, anterior mitral leaflet motion; AO, aorta; LV, left ventricle; LA, left atrium.

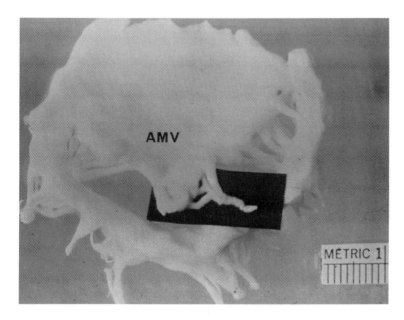

Fig. 7–43. The excised mitral valve from the patient in Figure 7–42. Black paper highlights the central portion of the anterior mitral leaflet, which was thickened, elongated and flail. The posterior leaflet was narrowed and thickened. All posterior mitral leaflet chordae tendineae were intact prior to surgical excision.

murmur (Barlow's syndrome), shortness of breath, dizziness, and syncope.

Mitral valve prolapse has many names: floppy valve, billowing valve, and ballooned valve. The physician may hear single or multiple systolic clicks with holosystolic, midsystolic, or late-systolic murmurs. The valve may be silent, having neither click nor murmur, and yet may demonstrate classic prolapsing on the echocardiogram.

Patterns of Motion

Mitral valve prolapse commonly occurs in mid- to late systole (Figs. 7–44 to 7–48). An unusual variant of prolapse is shown in Figure 7–49. There was an abrupt, early-systolic posterior displacement of the valve, followed by a midsystolic prolapse, proved at cardiac catheterization.

Some prolapsed valves have been erroneously identified as left atrial tumors (Figs. 7–45 and 7–46). Redundant leaflet tissue intercepts the sound beam during diastole, mimicking motion patterns of a left atrial myxoma. Multiple scans of the valve between the atrioventricular junction and the lower posterior left atrial wall are necessary to distinguish the echographic pattern of mitral valve prolapse from an atrial tumor.

In the presence of a large pericardial effusion, the mitral valve could appear to prolapse, but this motion is secondary to total cardiac displacement as the heart moves freely within a

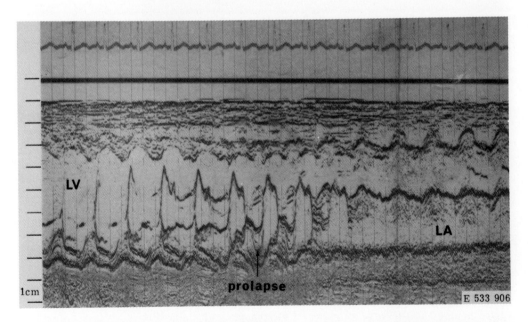

Fig. 7–44. An asymptomatic 9-year-old female patient with a prolapsed mitral valve visualized at the atrioventricular junction. LV, left ventricle; LA, left atrium.

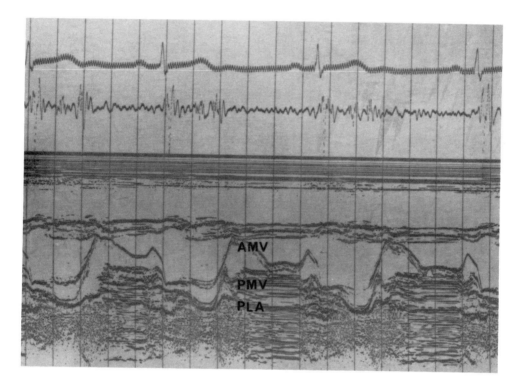

Fig. 7–45. A 29-year-old female patient with severe prolapse of the mitral valve that had been diagnosed as a left atrial tumor at another hospital. Minute transducer angulations were necessary to record the complete motion of the posterior mitral leaflet throughout the complete cardiac cycle. An apex phonocardiogram demonstrated a midsystolic click. AMV, anterior mitral leaflet motion; PMV, posterior mitral leaflet motion; PLA, posterior left atrial wall.

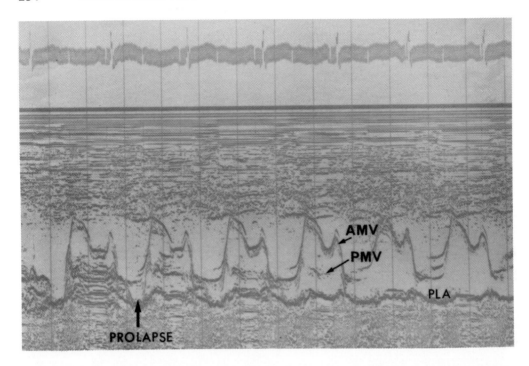

Fig. 7–46. A tracing from the patient in Figure 7–45. The transducer was angled slightly superiorly to demonstrate the prolapse of the posterior mitral leaflet into the left atrium. The absence of echo-reflective tissue in the left atrium and the rapid, early diastolic closure of the anterior mitral leaflet was evidence against the presence of a left atrial tumor. AMV, anterior mitral leaflet motion; PMV, posterior mitral leaflet motion; PLA, posterior left atrial wall.

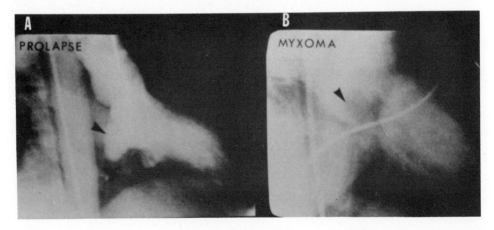

Fig. 7–47. *A,* A frame from a cineangiogram, right anterior oblique projection, from the patient in Figures 7–45 and 7–46 that demonstrates a marked prolapse of the mitral leaflet (arrowhead). *B,* A frame from a cineangiogram, right anterior oblique projection, from the patient in Figure 7–19 with a left atrial myxoma. A large, radiolucent mass (arrowhead) was found to be adherent to the posterior mitral leaflet at the time of operation.

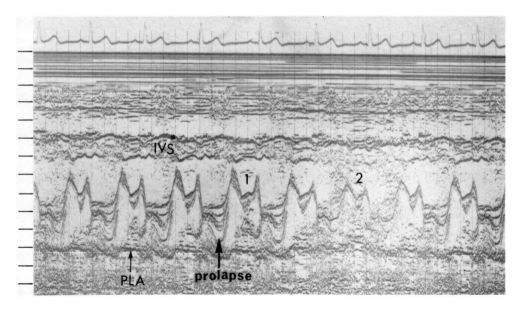

Fig. 7–48. A prolapsed mitral valve recorded from one higher intercostal space than the remainder of the study. The prolapsed mitral valve was not evident from lower intercostal spaces. During expiration, the opening excursion of the mitral valve was greater than during inspiration. Systolic excursion of the mitral valve prolapse was less during inspiration, although the onset of the prolapse did not appear to be altered. (1), expiration; (2), inspiration. IVS, interventricular septum; PLA, posterior left atrial wall.

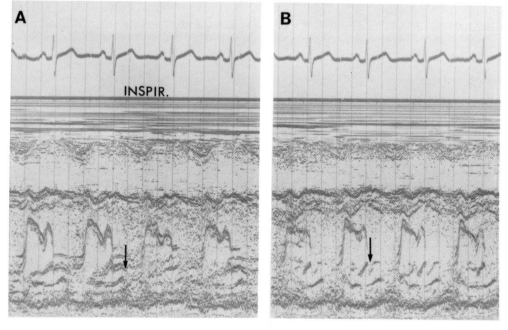

Fig. 7–49. A 39-year-old male patient with mitral valve prolapse. *A,* The transducer was positioned over the mitral valve near the sternum. The onset of the prolapse (arrow) was well defined when the patient inhaled. *B,* This shows an abrupt, early systolic posterior displacement of the mitral valve (arrow). The transducer had been shifted slightly laterally, away from the left parasternum. Midsystolic prolapse was not seen as well from this examination site.

255

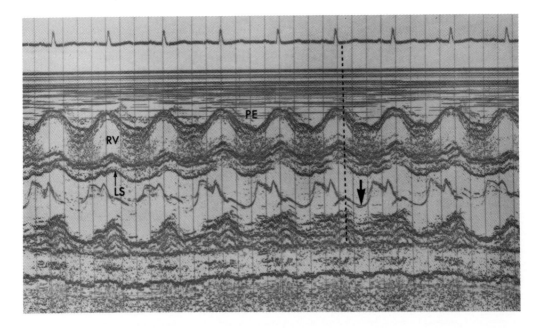

Fig. 7–50. A 66-year-old female patient with idiopathic, chronic pericardial effusion. The quantity of exudate was so great that the entire heart moved freely within the fluid (swinging heart). The anterior right ventricular wall and the septum and the mitral valve moved in unison. The mitral valve "prolapse" pattern (arrow) was abolished when the effusion was removed. PE, anterior pericardial effusion. The echo-free space behind the left atrium probably represented the descending aorta. RV, right ventricle; LS, left septum.

large volume of fluid (Fig. 7–50). When the quantity of effusion is decreased, the mitral valve resumes its normal systolic motion.

Recording Technique

There are three approaches to recording mitral valve prolapse with M-mode echocardiography. The most common method uses a full scan of the mitral valve. The patient is initially supine, but the most adequate tracings have been obtained from patients positioned in a partial left lateral decubitus plane. One should center the transducer over the mitral valve and angle it from the free edges of the mitral leaflets to the annular attachment. The prolapse is best visualized at the atrioventricular junction (see Fig. 7–44). The main disadvantage with this approach is that the mid- to late-systolic motion of the posterior mitral leaflet is often obscured by posterior left ventricular wall motion.

The second approach is to record mitral valve motion from one higher intercostal space. This may necessitate angling the transducer inferiorly and medially until motion of both leaflets is clearly outlined against the posterior left atrial wall. This

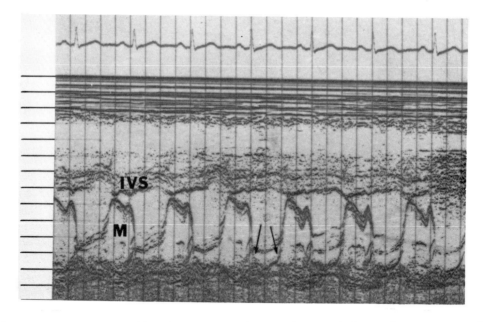

Fig. 7–51. A 51-year-old male patient with a grade III/VI holosystolic murmur at the apex, transmitted diffusely over the precordium and laterally to the left axilla and posterior chest. The echocardiogram revealed a slight thickening of the anterior mitral leaflet with the holosystolic collapse of the posterior mitral leaflet (arrows). The left atrial dimension was only slightly increased. The electrocardiogram and the chest roentgenogram were normal. The patient experienced minimal dyspnea without chest pain during multistaged treadmill exercise (4.2 MPH, 20°, 12 min). Continuous electrocardiograms were stable, except for rare, unifocal ventricular extrasystoles. No further diagnostic procedures or medical therapy were indicated. The patient has been followed with regular physical examinations and echocardiography. IVS, interventricular septum; M, mitral leaflet motion during diastole.

transducer position should be noted on the tracing, since holosystolic hammocking or sagging of the mitral valve may be recorded from this position (Fig. 7–51). I have not been able to record an artificially produced midsystolic prolapse from this transducer position.

A third approach is to record anterior and posterior systolic leaflet motion. Then one should carefully *slide* the transducer medially or laterally across the intercostal space and thus across the leaflets (see Fig. 7–49).

Provocation of Latent Prolapse

Sometimes one sees a variation in the opening amplitude of the prolapsing valve with respiration (see Figs. 7–48 and 7–49). The systolic excursion of the prolapse decreases, but the onset of the prolapse does not appear to be altered.

Since a physician is rarely available when echocardiograms are recorded, I do not use amyl nitrite to provoke latent prolapses. I prefer to have the patient perform mild leg exercise or sit-ups. Hyperventilation and Mueller's maneuver have also been successful.

1. Hyperventilation. The patient breathes deeply and rapidly for 30 seconds. This breathing is sufficient to raise the heart rate enough to stimulate some latent prolapses, usually of a minor, late-systolic type. Since the heart rate increases and the left ventricular stroke volume decreases proportionately, the "prolapse" may be secondary to changes in the left ventricular volume rather than indicative of a real valvular disorder.

2. Mueller's Maneuver. The patient is instructed first to inhale, then to exhale until he feels comfortable. Then he is instructed to bear down against tightened abdominal muscles without expelling any further air. A practice session acquaints the patient with the procedure and its effect upon his feeling of well-being. A control tracing of systolic mitral valve motion is recorded before the maneuver begins. Continuous recording of mitral valve motion is maintained during the 5- to 15-second maneuver and after the patient is instructed to relax and to breathe normally. This maneuver has an advantage over the Valsalva maneuver in that the lungs are not inflated and do

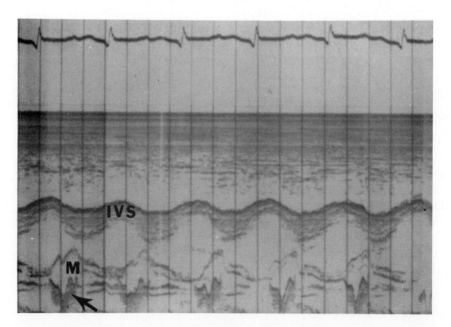

Fig. 7-52. An elderly male patient with infective endocarditis. The posterior mitral leaflet exhibited shaggy echoes (arrow) inscribed below the leaflet's movement. These echoes were reflected from vegetations that did not interfere with the leaflet's diastolic mobility. The abnormal anterior mitral leaflet motion was due to ruptured chordae tendineae. (See Fig. 7-53.) IVS, interventricular septum; M, mitral leaflet motion. (From Dillon, J., Feigenbaum, H., Knoecke, L., Davis, R., and Chang, S.: Echocardiographic manifestations of valvular vegetations. Am. Heart J., 86: 698, 1973.)

not interfere with the quality of the echocardiogram. While some latent mitral prolapses have been demonstrated during and after the Mueller maneuver, they may be due to a decreased ventricular volume during this procedure and not to a real valvular disorder. I tend to be conservative in the echographic diagnosis of mitral valve prolapse; this caution results in a better fit to the clinical findings.

INFECTIVE ENDOCARDITIS

Mitral valve vegetations secondary to infective endocarditis are seen as "shaggy" echoes located *under* the inscribed leaflet motion (Figs. 7–52 to 7–55). An absence of echographic evidence of vegetations on the cardiac valves does not exclude a diagnosis of infective endocarditis. Normal valvular motion and tissue thickness simply imply that large vegetations are not present. Serial echocardiograms of the infected patient

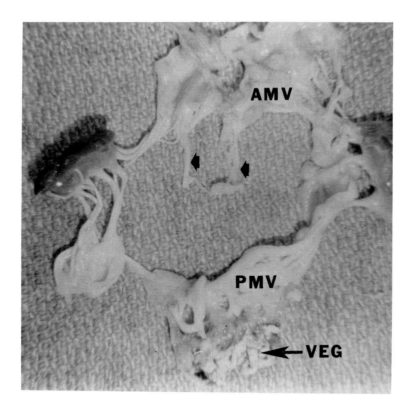

Fig. 7–53. An excised mitral valve from the patient in Figure 7–52. Several chordae tendineae were ruptured (small arrows). There was a large hole in the anterior mitral leaflet (AMV). A vegetative mass was attached to the posterior mitral leaflet (PMV). VEG, vegetation. (From Dillon, J., Feigenbaum, H., Knoecke, L., Davis, R., and Chang, S.: Echocardiographic manifestations of valvular vegetations. Am. Heart J., *86*: 698, 1973.)

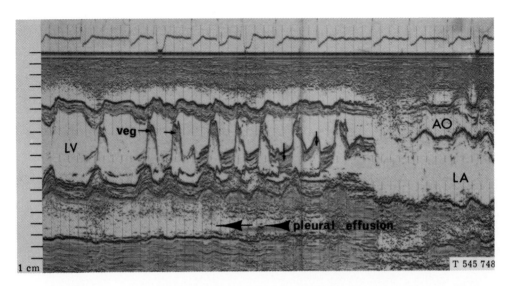

Fig. 7–54. A 63-year-old male patient with mitral regurgitation and infective endocarditis. The leaflets were unusually echo-reflective during diastole and systole, but leaflet motion was not restricted. At operation, the mitral valve's surface was rough, with markedly thickened and irregular leaflet edges covered by pinkish brown, friable vegetation. Some areas of the valve were fused, although this restriction was not noted on the echocardiogram. A large quantity of left pleural fluid was aspirated. There was no pericardial effusion. LV, left ventricle; veg, vegetation; AO, aorta, LA, left atrium.

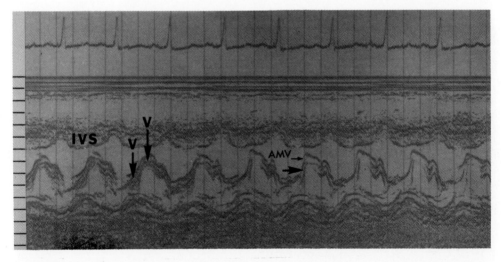

Fig. 7–55. A 63-year-old female patient with aortic and mitral regurgitation and infective endocarditis. The mitral leaflets were unusually echo-reflective, a finding consistent with old rheumatic valve disease or vegetations (V). At low signal amplification, there appeared to be a delay between the anterior mitral leaflet excursion and the entry of other echoes into the orifice (horizontal arrow). Scans into the left atrium did not reveal any echoes suggesting atrial tumor. At operation, the thin, white anterior mitral leaflet tissue was extremely friable. Irregular, tan-white vegetations were adherent to the leaflet tissue. IVS, interventricular septum; AMV, anterior mitral leaflet motion.

may disclose the late appearance or enlargement of valvular vegetations or a disruption of normal leaflet motion secondary to leaflet degeneration. Two-dimensional echocardiography is more sensitive to vegetations.[2-4]

REFERENCES

1. Martin, R., et al.: Reliability and reproducibility of two-dimensional echocardiograph measurement of the stenotic mitral valve orifice area. Am. J. Cardiol., *43*: 560, 1979.
2. Gilbert, B., et al.: Two-dimensional echocardiographic assessment of vegetative endocarditis. Circulation, *55*: 346, 1977.
3. Mintz, G., et al.: Comparison of two-dimensional and M-mode echocardiography in the evaluation of patients with infective endocarditis. Am. J. Cardiol., *43*: 738, 1979.
4. Wann, L., et al.: Comparison of M-mode and cross-sectional echocardiography in infective endocarditis. Circulation, *60*: 728, 1979.

BIBLIOGRAPHY

ANNULAR CALCIFICATION

Curati, W., et al.: Ultrasonic features of mitral annulus calcification. A report of 21 cases. Radiology, *122*: 215, 1977.

Dashkoff, D., et al.: Echocardiographic features of mitral annulus calcification. Circulation (Suppl.), *52*: 34, 1975.

D'Cruz, I., et al.: Clinical manifestations of mitral annulus calcification with emphasis on its echocardiographic features. Am. Heart J., *94*: 367, 1977.

de Bono, D., et al.: Mitral-annulus calcification and cerebral or retinal ischaemia. Lancet, *2*: 383, 1979.

Fulkerson, P., et al.: Calcification of the mitral annulus: etiology, clinical associations, complications and therapy. Am. J. Med., *66*: 967, 1979.

Gabor, G., et al.: Echocardiographic and clinical spectrum of mitral annular calcification. Am. J. Cardiol., *38*: 836, 1976.

Hakki, A., et al.: Obstruction to left ventricular inflow secondary to combined mitral annular calcification and idiopathic hypertrophic subaortic stenosis. Cathet. Cardiovasc. Diagn., *6*: 191, 1980.

Hirschfeld, D., et al.: Echocardiogram in calcified mitral annulus. Am. J. Cardiol., *36*: 354, 1975.

Howard, P., et al.: The echocardiographic diagnosis of calcified mitral annulus. Am. J. Med. Sci., *273*: 267, 1977.

Kronzon, I., et al.: Mitral ring calcification in idiopathic hypertrophic subaortic stenosis. Am. J. Cardiol., *42*: 60, 1978.

Kronzon, I., et al.: Two-dimensional echocardiography in mitral annulus calcification. A.J.R., *134*: 220, 1979.

McLean, J., et al.: The echocardiographic association of mitral valve prolapse and mitral annulus calcification. Clin. Cardiol., *2*: 220, 1979.

Schott, C., et al.: Mitral annular calcification. Clinical and echocardiographic correlations. Arch. Intern. Med., *137*: 1143, 1977.

Tanabe, J., et al.: Echocardiographic findings of mitral annulus calcification. Special emphasis on clinical usefulness. *In* Noninvasive Cardiovascular Diagnosis. Edited by E. B. Diethrich. Baltimore, University Park Press, 1978.

Wanderman, K., et al.: Coexistence of hypertrophic obstructive cardiomyopathy and mitral annulus calcification: proposed etiologic relationship. Isr. J. Med. Sci., *15*: 422, 1979.

Zoneraich, S., et al.: Conduction disturbances in patients with calcified mitral annulus diagnosed by echocardiography. J. Electrocardiol., *12*: 137, 1979.

ENDOCARDITIS

Alam, M., et al.: Echocardiographic features of mitral obstruction due to bacterial endocarditis. Chest, *76*: 331, 1979.

Andy, J., et al.: Echocardiographic observations in opiate addicts with active infective endocarditis. Frequency of involvement of the various valves and comparison of echocardiographic features of right and left sided cardiac valve endocarditis. Am. J. Cardiol., *40*: 17, 1977.

Bamrah, V., et al.: Haemophilus parainfluenzae mitral valve vegetation without hemodynamic abnormality. Demonstration by angiography and serial echocardiography. Am. J. Med., *66*: 543, 1979.

Becker, R., et al.: Surgery for mitral valve endocarditis. Chest, *75*: 314, 1979.

Bell, R., et al.: Posterior mitral valve vegetation. J. Tenn. Med. Assoc., *70*: 657, 1977.

Bender, R., et al.: Echocardiographic diagnosis of bacterial endocarditis of the mitral valve in a neonate. Am. J. Dis. Child., *131*: 746, 1977.

Boucher, C., et al.: The value and limitations of echocardiography in recording mitral valve vegetations. Am. Heart J., *94*: 37, 1977.

Chandraratna, P., et al.: Limitations of the echocardiogram in diagnosing valvular vegetations in patients with mitral valve prolapse. Circulation, *56*: 436, 1977.

Child, J., et al.: Noninvasive detection of fungal endocarditis (editorial). Chest, *75*: 539, 1979.

Child, J., et al.: Coronary ostial embolus and mitral vegetation simulating a left atrial myxoma: a case of probable cryptococcal valvulitis. Clin. Cardiol., *2*: 43, 1979.

Clements, S., et al.: The M-mode echocardiogram and endocarditis. J. Med. Assoc., *68*: 321, 1979.

Copeland, J., et al.: Acute mitral valvular obstruction from infective endocarditis: echocardiographic diagnosis and report of the second successfully treated case. J. Thorac. Cardiovasc. Surg., *78*: 128, 1979.

DeSilva, M., et al.: Haemophilus paraphrophilus endocarditis in a prolapsed mitral valve. Am. J. Clin. Pathol., *66*: 922, 1976.

Dillon, J., et al.: Echocardiographic manifestations of valvular vegetations. Am. Heart J., *86*: 698, 1973.

Dillon, J.: Echocardiography in valvular vegetations. Am. J. Med., *62*: 856, 1977.

Egeblad, H., et al.: Mitral valve replacement in infective endocarditis as prophylaxis against embolism. Eur. J. Cardiol., *10*: 369, 1979.

Estevez, C., et al.: Serial echocardiographic abnormalities in nonbacterial thrombotic endocarditis of the mitral valve. Chest, *69*: 801, 1976.

Gregoratos, G., et al.: Infective endocarditis. Diagnosis and management. Med. Clin. North Am., *63*: 173, 1979.

Horowitz, M., et al.: Vegetative bacterial endocarditis on the prolapsing mitral valve. Echocardiographic evaluation. Arch. Intern Med., *137*: 788, 1977.

Kinney, E., et al.: The echocardiogram in scleroderma endocarditis of the mitral valve. Arch. Intern. Med., *139*: 1179, 1979.

Markiewicz, W., et al.: Echocardiography in infective endocarditis. Lack of specificity in patients with valvular pathology. Eur. J. Cardiol., *10*: 247, 1979.

Matula, G., et al.: Mitral obstruction from staphylococcal endocarditis, corrected surgically. J.A.M.A., *233*: 58, 1975.

Miller, M., et al.: Infective endocarditis: new diagnostic techniques. Am. Heart J., *96*: 123, 1978.

Naik, D., et al.: The role of echocardiography in suspected infective endocarditis. Clin. Radiol., *29*: 381, 1978.

Nicholson, M., et al.: Mitral valve vegetations in bacterial endocarditis resembling left atrial myxoma. Aust. N.Z. J. Med., *10*: 327, 1980.

Nomeir, A., et al.: Bacterial endocarditis. Echocardiographic and clinical evaluation during therapy. J. Clin. Ultrasound, *4*: 23, 1976.

Pasternak, R., et al.: Echocardiographic diagnosis of large fungal verruca attached to mitral valve. Br. Heart J., *38*: 1209, 1976.

Roy, P., et al.: Spectrum of echocardiographic findings in bacterial endocarditis. Circulation, *53*: 474, 1976.

Schoolmeester, W., et al.: Multivalvular vegetations in a patient with enterococcal endocarditis diagnosed by echocardiography. South. Med. J., *71*: 644, 1978.

Thomson, K., et al.: The reliability of echocardiography in the diagnosis of infective endocarditis. Radiology, *125*: 473, 1977.

Wann, L., et al.: Echocardiography in bacterial endocarditis. N. Engl. J. Med., *295*: 135, 1976.

Wann, L.: Echocardiography in the management of bacterial endocarditis. Compr. Ther., *5*: 43, 1979.

Weyman, A., et al.: Loeffler's endocarditis presenting as mitral and tricuspid stenosis. Am. J. Cardiol., *40*: 438, 1977.

FLUTTERING MITRAL VALVE

Botvinick, E., et al.: Echocardiographic demonstration of early mitral valve closure in severe aortic insufficiency. Circulation, *51*: 836, 1975.

Ciraulo, D.: Mitral valve fluttering: an echocardiographic feature of left atrial myxoma. Chest, *76*: 95, 1979.

Craige, E., et al.: Studies on mitral valve motion in the presence of the Austin Flint murmur. Trans. Am. Clin. Climatol Assoc., *83*: 209, 1972.

DeMaria, A., et al.: Echography and phonocardiography of acute aortic regurgitation in bacterial endocarditis. Ann. Intern. Med., *82*: 329, 1975.

Fortuin, N., et al.: On the mechanism of the Austin Flint murmur. Circulation, *45*: 558, 1972.

Fujii, J., et al.: Dual echocardiographic determination of atrial contraction sequence in atrial flutter and other related atrial arrhythmias. Circulation, *58*: 314, 1978.

Glasser, S.: Late mitral valve opening in aortic regurgitation. Chest, *70*: 70, 1976.

Gray, K., et al.: Echocardiographic assessment of severity of aortic regurgitation. Br. Heart J., *37*: 691, 1975.

Joyner, C., et al.: Behavior of the anterior mitral leaflet of the mitral valve in patients with the Austin Flint murmur. Clin. Res., *14*: 251, 1966.

Jsowig, B., et al.: Flutter of the mitral valve associated with a diastolic murmur in the absence of disease. Am. Heart J., *97*: 635, 1979.

Meyer, J., et al.: Systolic flutter, an echocardiographic clue to the diagnosis of ruptured chordae tendineae. Am. Heart J., *93*: 3, 1977.

Pridie, R., et al.: Echocardiography of the mitral valve in aortic valve disease. Br. Heart J., *33*: 296, 1971.

Skorton, D., et al.: Accuracy of the echocardiographic diagnosis of aortic regurgitation. Am. J. Med., *69*: 377, 1980.

Tye, K., et al.: Anemia producing mitral valve flutter on the echocardiogram. Angiology, *30*: 291, 1979.

Winsberg, F., et al.: Fluttering of the mitral valve in aortic insufficiency. Circulation, *41*: 225, 1970.

Zoneraich, O., et al.: Atrial flutter: electrocardiographic, vectorcardiographic and echocardiographic correlation. Am. Heart J., *96*: 286, 1978.

LEFT ATRIAL MYXOMA AND THROMBUS

Abdulla, A., et al.: Left atrial myxoma: echocardiographic diagnosis and determination of size. J.A.M.A., *238*: 510, 1977.

Asinger, R., et al.: Left atrial myxoma presenting as shock—diagnosis by echocardiography. Minn. Med., *62*: 723, 1979.

Attar, S., et al.: Cardiac myxoma. Ann. Thorac. Surg., *29*: 397, 1980.

Bass, N., et al.: Left atrial myxoma diagnosed by echocardiography, with observations on tumor movement. Br. Heart J., *35*: 1332, 1973.

Beran, R., et al.: The neurological aspects of atrial myxoma. Clin. Exp. Neurol., *16*: 105, 1979.

Berning, J., et al.: The diagnostic challenge of left atrial myxoma. Importance of echocardiographic screening. Acta Med. Scand., *206*: 115, 1979.

Bodenheimer, M., et al.: Echocardiographic features of experimental left atrial tumor. Am. Heart J., *88*: 615, 1974.

Borgren, H., et al.: Imaging procedures in the detection of cardiac tumors, with emphasis on echocardiography: A review. Cardiovasc. Intervent. Radiol., *3*: 107, 1980.

Bourdillon, P., et al.: Left atrial myxoma with aortic regurgitation. Br. Heart J., *40*: 575, 1978.

Buchanan, R., et al.: Left atrial myxoma mimicking vasculitis: echocardiographic diagnosis. Can. Med. Assoc. J., *120*: 1540, 1979.

Bulkley, B., et al.: Atrial myxomas: a fifty year review. Am. Heart J., 97: 639, 1979.

Bulkley, B., et al.: Atrial myxomas: triumph of machine over man (editorial). Chest, 75: 537, 1979.

Chadda, K., et al.: Nonprolapsing atrial myxoma; clinical, echocardiographic and angiographic correlations. Angiology, 29: 179, 1978.

Croxson, F., et al.: Long-term follow-up of atrial myxoma. Br. Heart J., 34: 1018, 1972.

Dodd, M., et al.: Echocardiography in left atrial myxoma: relation to the findings in mitral stenosis. Aust. N.Z. J. Med., 2: 124, 1972.

Edmands, R., et al.: Atrial myxoma: a curable disorder. J. Indiana State Med. Assoc., 67: 903, 1974.

Effert, S., et al.: The diagnosis of intra-atrial tumors and thrombi by the ultrasonic echo method. German Med. Monthly, 4: 1, 1959.

Farah, M.: Familial atrial myxoma. Ann. Intern. Med., 83: 358, 1975.

Finegan, R., et al.: Diagnosis of left atrial myxoma by echocardiography. N. Engl. J. Med., 282: 1022, 1970.

Fortuin, N.: Echocardiogram of the month: atrial myxoma. Med. Times, 108: 45, 1980.

Furuse, A., et al.: Echocardiography and angiography for detection of left atrial thrombosis. Jpn. Heart J., 17: 163, 1976.

Gabelman, C., et al.: Surgical treatment of recurrent primary malignant tumor of the left atrium. J. Thorac. Cardiovasc. Surg., 77: 914, 1979.

Giuliani, E., et al.: Unusual echocardiographic findings in a patient with left atrial myxoma. Mayo Clin. Proc., 53: 469, 1978.

Graboys, T., et al.: Echocardiographic diagnosis of left atrial thrombus: a case report. J. Clin. Ultrasound, 5: 284, 1977.

Graham, H., et al.: Infected atrial myxoma. Am. J. Cardiol., 38: 658, 1976.

Gustafson, A., et al.: Left atrial myxoma diagnosed by ultrasound cardiography. Angiology, 24: 554, 1973.

Hamer, J., et al.: Left atrial myxoma moving from right atrium to left ventricle. Noninvasive and invasive techniques and surgical findings. Acta Med. Scand., 205: 527, 1979.

Hepp, A., et al.: Left atrial metastasis of chorion carcinoma, presenting as mitral stenosis. Br. Heart J., 39: 1154, 1977.

Hibi, N., et al.: Realtime observation of left atrial myxoma with high speed B mode echocardiography. J. Clin. Ultrasound, 7: 34, 1979.

Huggins, T., et al.: Left atrial myxoma: computed tomography as a diagnostic modality. J. Comput. Assist. Tomogr., 4: 253, 1980.

Huston, K., et al.: Left atrial myxoma simulating peripheral vasculitis. Mayo Clin. Proc., 53: 752, 1978.

Imperio, J., et al.: The distribution patterns of biatrial myxomas. Ann. Thorac. Surg., 29: 469, 1980.

Johnson, M., et al.: Echocardiographic diagnosis of a left atrial myxoma found attached to the free left atrial wall. J. Clin. Ultrasound, 1: 75, 1973.

Kerber, R., et al.: Left atrial myxoma. Am. J. Cardiol., 34: 838, 1974.

Kostis, J., et al.: Echocardiographic diagnosis of left atrial myxoma. Chest, 58: 550, 1970.

Kounis, N.: Left atrial myxoma presenting with intermittent claudication and Raynaud's phenomenon: echocardiographic patterns of the tumor size. Angiology, 30: 356, 1979.

Lee, Y., et al.: Nonprolapsing left atrial tumor. The M-mode echocardiographic diagnosis. Chest, 78: 332, 1980.

Lewis, B., et al.: Diagnostic value of cross-sectional echocardiography in atrial myxoma. Isr. J. Med. Sci., 15: 426, 1979.

Lortscher, R., et al.: Left atrial myxoma presenting as rheumatic fever. Chest, 66: 302, 1974.

Martinez, E., et al.: Echocardiographic diagnosis of left atrial myxoma. Am. J. Cardiol., 33: 281, 1974.

Mikell, F., et al.: Two-dimensional echocardiographic demonstration of left atrial thrombi in patients with prosthetic mitral valves. Circulation, 60: 1183, 1979.

Millman, A., et al.: Left atrial myxoma: two-dimensional echocardiographic, angiographic, and pathological correlations. J. Med. Soc. N.J., 76: 749, 1979.

Morgan, D., et al.: Left heart myxomas. Am. J. Cardiol., *40*: 611, 1977.

Moscovitz, H., et al.: Simulated left atrial tumor. A hemodynamic, echocardiographic and cineangiographic study. Am. J. Cardiol., *34*: 63, 1974.

Nasser, W., et al.: Part II: Phonocardiographic, echocardiographic, hemodynamic and angiographic features in nine cases. Am. Heart J., *83*: 810, 1972.

Nicholson, M., et al.: Mitral valve vegetations in bacterial endocarditis resembling left atrial myxoma. Aust. N.Z. J. Med., *10*: 327, 1980.

Parashar, S.: Echocardiographic diagnosis of left atrial myxoma. Indian Heart J., *31*: 50, 1979.

Petsas, A., et al.: Echocardiographic diagnosis of left atrial myxoma; usefulness of suprasternal approach. Br. Heart J., *38*: 627, 1976.

Poehlmann, H., et al.: Left atrial thrombus detected by ultrasound. J. Clin. Ultrasound, *3*: 65, 1975.

Popp, R., et al.: Ultrasound for the diagnosis of atrial tumor. Ann. Intern. Med., *71*: 785, 1969.

Pridie, R.: Left atrial myxomas in childhood. Presentation with emboli and diagnosis by ultrasonics. Thorax, *27*: 759, 1972.

Rajpal, R., et al.: Infected left atrial myxoma with bacteremia simulating infective endocarditis. Arch. Intern. Med., *139*: 1176, 1979.

Rees, J., et al.: Lentiginosis and left atrial myxoma. Br. Heart J., *35*: 874, 1973.

Rogers, E., et al.: Left atrial myxoma infected with Histoplasma capsulatum. Am. J. Med., *64*: 683, 1978.

St. John Sutton, M., et al.: Atrial myxomas: a review of clinical experience in 40 patients. Mayo Clin. Proc., *55*: 371, 1980.

Sandok, B., et al.: CNS embolism due to atrial myxoma: clinical features and diagnosis. Arch. Neurol., *37*: 485, 1980.

Schattenberg, T.: Echocardiographic diagnosis of left atrial myxoma. Mayo Clin. Proc., *43*: 620, 1968.

Siltanen, P., et al.: Atrial myxoma in a family. Am. J. Cardiol., *38*: 252, 1976.

Spangler, R., et al.: Echocardiographic demonstration of a left atrial thrombus. Chest, *67*: 716, 1975.

Spencer, W., et al.: Detection of left atrial myxoma by echocardiography. Arch. Intern. Med., *128*: 787, 1971.

Srivastava, T., et al.: Echocardiogram in left atrial myxoma. Am. J. Med., *54*: 136, 1973.

Steinmetz, E., et al.: Left atrial myxoma as a neurological problem: a case report and review. Stroke, *4*: 451, 1973.

Stewart, J., et al.: Left atrial myxoma: false negative echocardiographic findings in a tumor demonstrated by coronary arteriography. Am. Heart J., *98*: 228, 1979.

Sunagawa, K., et al.: Left atrial ball thrombus diagnosed by two-dimensional echocardiography. Am. Heart J., *100*: 89, 1980.

Sung, R., et al.: Hemodynamic features of prolapsing and nonprolapsing left atrial myxoma. Circulation, *51*: 342, 1975.

Tallury, V., et al.: Ultrasound cardiography in the diagnosis of left atrial thrombosis. Chest, *59*: 501, 1971.

Tanabe, J., et al.: Left atrial myxoma: association with acute coronary embolization in an 11-year-old boy. Pediatrics, *63*: 778, 1979.

Vengsarkar, A., et al.: Phantom echoes resembling a myxoma in mitral valve prolapse. (A case report.) J. Postgrad. Med., *25*: 237, 1979.

Wolfe, S., et al.: Diagnosis of atrial tumors by ultrasound. Circulation, *39*: 615, 1969.

Yuste, P.: Myxoma of the left atrium: pre- and post-operative echocardiographic study of a case. Rev. Esp. Cardiol., *38*: 169, 1975.

OTHER CARDIAC-RELATED TUMORS AND THROMBUS

Acrcilla, R., et al.: Right ventricular mass estimation by angioechocardiography. Cathet. Cardiovasc. Diagn., *2*: 125, 1976.

Atsuchi, Y., et al.: Echocardiographic diagnosis of prolapsing right atrial myxoma. Jpn. Heart J., *17*: 798, 1976.

Bender, F., et al.: Diagnosis of primary tumors of the heart. Minerva Med., *64*: 1692, 1973.

Broadbent, J., et al.: Thrombus of inferior vena cava presenting as right atrial tumor. Roentgenographic, phono-echocardiographic, angiographic and surgical findings. J. Thorac. Cardiovasc. Surg., 72: 422, 1976.

Casolo, F., et al.: Heart tumors. A review of 29 operated cases. Ann. Radiol. (Paris), 21: 331, 1978.

Chandraratna, P., et al.: Echocardiographic, angiocardiographic and surgical correlations in right ventricular myxoma simulating valvar pulmonic stenosis. Circulation, 55: 619, 1977.

Chandraratna, P., et al.: Echocardiographic evaluation of extracardiac masses. Br. Heart J., 40: 741, 1978.

Child, J., et al.: Echocardiographic differentiation of mediastinal tumors from cardiac disease. Chest, 67: 108, 1975.

Cohen, J., et al.: Echocardiographic features of a calcified pericardial tumor. J. Med. Soc. N.J., 77: 587, 1980.

DeJoseph, R., et al.: Echocardiographic diagnosis of intraventricular clot. Chest, 71: 417, 1977.

DeMaria, A., et al.: Left ventricular thrombi identified by cross-sectional echocardiography. Ann. Intern. Med., 90: 14, 1979.

Farooki, Z., et al.: Ultrasonic pattern of ventricular rhabdomyoma in two infants. Am. J. Cardiol., 34: 842, 1974.

Farooki, Z., et al.: Echocardiographic diagnosis of right atrial extension of Wilms' tumor. Am. J. Cardiol., 36: 363, 1975.

Farooki, Z., et al.: Echocardiographic pattern of right atrial tumor motion. Br. Heart J., 38: 580, 1976.

Farooki, Z., et al.: Echocardiographic differentiation of a cystic and a solid tumor of the heart. Am. J. Cardiol., 39: 107, 1977.

Foote, W., et al.: False-positive echocardiographic diagnosis of pericardial effusion. Result of tumor encasement of the heart simulating constrictive pericarditis. Chest, 71: 546, 1977.

Gelfard, E., et al.: Melanotic malignant schwannoma of the right atrium. J. Thorac. Cardiovasc. Surg., 74: 808, 1977.

Goldschoager, S., et al.: Right atrial myxoma with right to left shunt and polycythemia presenting as congenital heart disease. Am. J. Cardiol., 30: 82, 1972.

Gottdiener, J., et al.: Posterior cardiac displacement by anterior mediastinal tumor. Chest, 77: 784, 1980.

Gustafson, A., et al.: Bilateral atrial myxomas diagnosed by echocardiography. Acta Med. Scand., 201: 391, 1977.

Harbold, N., et al.: Echocardiographic diagnosis of right atrial myxoma. Mayo Clin. Proc., 48: 284, 1973.

Horgan, J., et al.: Primary and secondary right atrial tumors detected by echocardiography. J. Clin. Ultrasound, 5: 92, 1977.

Isner, J., et al.: Cardiac sarcoma causing "ASH" and simulating coronary heart disease. Am. J. Med., 66: 1025, 1979.

Kaminsky, M., et al.: Atrial myxoma mimicking a collagen disorder. Chest, 75: 93, 1979.

Kendrick, M., et al.: Ventricular pacemaker wire simulating a right atrial mass. Chest, 72: 649, 1977.

Koch, P., et al.: Displacement of the heart by a giant mediastinal cyst. Am. J. Cardiol., 40: 445, 1977.

Levisman, J., et al.: Echocardiographic diagnosis of a mobile, pedunculated tumor in the left ventricular cavity. Am. J. Cardiol., 36: 957, 1975.

Mahar, L., et al.: Primary cardiac myxosarcoma in a child. Mayo Clin. Proc., 54: 261, 1979.

Melendez, L., et al.: Right ventricular tumor demonstrated by echocardiography. Can. Med. Assoc. J., 118: 62, 1978.

Meller, J., et al.: Left ventricular myxoma; echocardiographic diagnosis and review of the literature. Am. J. Med., 63: 816, 1977.

Meyers, S., et al.: Right atrial myxoma with right to left shunting and mitral valve prolapse. Am. J. Med., 62: 308, 1977.

Nanda, N., et al.: Echocardiographic features of right ventricular outflow tumor prolapsing into pulmonary artery. Am. J. Cardiol., 40: 272, 1977.

Oliva, P., et al.: Left ventricular outflow obstruction produced by pedunculated fibroma in a newborn: clinical, angiographic, echocardiographic and surgical observations. Chest, 74: 590, 1978.

O'Neil, M., et al.: Cardiac myxomas: a clinical diagnostic challenge. Am. J. Surg., 138: 68, 1979.

Panella, J., et al.: Angiosarcoma of the heart. Diagnosis by echocardiography. Chest, 76: 221, 1979.

Pernod, J., et al.: Right atrial myxoma: an echocardiographic study. Br. Heart J., 40: 201, 1978.

Ports, T., et al.: Echocardiography of right ventricular tumors. Circulation, 56: 439, 1977.

Ports, T., et al.: Echocardiography of left ventricular masses. Circulation, 58: 528, 1978.

Powers, J., et al.: Familial cardiac myxoma: emphasis on unusual clinical manifestations. J. Thorac. Cardiovasc. Surg., 77: 782, 1979.

Rees, A., et al.: Echocardiographic evidence of left ventricular tumor in a neonate. Chest, 73: 433, 1978.

Roelandt, J., et al.: Ultrasonic demonstration of right ventricular myxoma. J. Clin. Ultrasound, 5: 191, 1977.

Sasaki, S., et al.: Primary intracavitary cardiac tumors; a review of 11 surgical cases. J. Cardiovasc. Surg., 18: 15, 1977.

Shah, A., et al.: Echocardiographic features of cardiac compression by mediastinal pancreatic pseudocyst. Chest, 77: 440, 1980.

Slovis, T., et al.: Wilms' tumor to the heart: clinical and radiographic evaluation. A.J.R., 131: 263, 1978.

Snyder, S.: Massive pericardial coelomic cyst. Diagnostic features and unusual presentation. Chest, 71: 100, 1977.

Spence, M., et al.: Angiokeratoma corporis diffusum (Anderson-Fabry disease) in a single large family in Nova Scotia. J. Med. Genet., 15: 428, 1978.

Tripton, B., et al.: Embolism to the central nervous system from cardiac myxoma. Report of two cases. J. Neurosurg., 47: 937, 1977.

van den Bos, A., et al.: Progressive development of a left ventricular thrombus. Chest, 74: 307, 1978.

Yabek, S., et al.: Cardiac fibroma in a neonate presenting with severe congestive heart failure. J. Pediatr., 91: 310, 1977.

Yuste, P., et al.: Echocardiogram in right atrial myxoma. Chest, 69: 94, 1976.

Zajtchuk, R., et al.: Bilateral atrial myxomas. Pre-operative diagnosis and successful removal. J. Thorac. Cardiovasc. Surg., 69: 291, 1975.

MITRAL VALVE OBSTRUCTION

Ambrose, J., et al.: Changing diastolic closure rates (E-F slopes) in a patient with mitral stenosis: a case report. Angiology, 30: 62, 1979.

Andres, R., et al.: Echocardiographic manifestation of "false" mitral stenosis that was. Ann. Intern. Med., 83: 503, 1975.

Armstrong, T., et al.: Noninvasive observations on initial low frequency vibrations of the first heart sound—correlation with the "presystolic" murmur in mitral stenosis. Br. Heart J., 40: 750, 1978.

Bellin, H., et al.: Ultrasonic-cardiographic long-term observations in patients with operated stenosis of the mitral valve. Bibl. Cardiol., 33: 191, 1975.

Berman, N., et al.: Mitral stenosis with posterior diastolic movement of posterior leaflet. Can. Med. Assoc. J., 112: 976, 1975.

Cachera, J., et al.: Surgery for mitral stenosis: comparative evaluation of the different procedures. In The Mitral Valve. Edited by D. Kalmanson. Acton, Mass., Publishing Sciences Group, 1976.

Chandraratna, P., et al.: Echocardiographic assessment of the mitral valve area in noncalcific mitral stenosis. In Noninvasive Cardiovascular Diagnosis. Edited by E. Diethrich. Baltimore, University Park Press, 1978.

Chang, S., et al.: Mitral stenosis and ruptured mitral chordae: an unusual echocardiographically detectable combination. Med. Ultrasound, 2: 27, 1978.

Collins-Nakai, R., et al.: Congenital mitral stenosis: a review of 20 years' experience. Circulation, 56: 1039, 1977.

Cope, G., et al.: A reassessment of the echocardiogram in mitral stenosis. Circulation, 52: 664, 1975.

Driscoll, D., et al.: Echocardiographic features of congenital mitral stenosis. Am. J. Cardiol., 42: 259, 1978.

Duchak, J., et al.: The posterior mitral valve echo and the echocardiographic diagnosis of mitral stenosis. Am. J. Cardiol., 29: 628, 1972.

Fisher, M., et al.: Assessment of severity of mitral stenosis by echocardiographic leaflet separation. Arch. Intern. Med., *139*: 402, 1979.

Flaherty, J., et al.: Atypical posterior leaflet motion in echocardiogram in mitral stenosis. Am. J. Cardiol., *35*: 675, 1975.

Forman, H., et al.: Lutembacher's syndrome: recognition by echocardiography. J. Clin. Ultrasound, 7: 53, 1979.

Fortuin, N., et al.: Echocardiographic studies of genesis of mitral diastolic murmurs. Br. Heart J., *35*: 75, 1973.

Freeman, J., et al.: Mitral leaflet velocity in the determination of mitral stenosis. Med. Res. Eng., *11*: 4, 1972.

Fukukawa, K., et al.: Use of digitized left ventricular echocardiograms in assessment of mitral stenosis. Br. Heart J., *42*: 176, 1979.

Garcia, J., et al.: Echocardiography in the diagnosis of Lutembacher syndrome. Cathet. Cardiovasc. Diagn., *4*: 283, 1978.

Glasser, S., et al.: Posterior leaflet motion in mitral stenosis. Chest, *71*: 87, 1977.

Godman, M., et al.: Echocardiography in evaluation of congenital mitral valve disease in infants and children. Br. Heart J., *37*: 783, 1975.

Henry, W., et al.: Measurement of mitral orifice area in patients with mitral valve disease by real-time, two-dimensional echocardiography. Circulation, *51*: 827, 1975.

Henry, W., et al.: Echocardiographic evaluation of patients with mitral stenosis. Am. J. Med., *62*: 813, 1977.

Inoh, T., et al.: Evaluation of mitral valvular lesion of mitral stenosis by M-mode echocardiography: with special reference to the indication for commissurotomy. Kobe J. Med. Sci., *26*: 127, 1980.

Koyanagi, S., et al.: The change in the left atrial dimension during diastole. Echocardiographic assessment of mitral stenosis. Jpn. Heart J., *21*: 17, 1980.

Krueger, S., et al.: Echocardiographic diagnosis of silent mitral stenosis. Nebr. Med. J., *60*: 159, 1975.

LeGalley, T., et al.: Exercising pulmonary blood flow in mitral stenosis with anomalous pulmonary venous connection. Chest, *71*: 400, 1977.

Levisman, J., et al.: Posterior mitral leaflet motion in mitral stenosis. Circulation, *51*: 511, 1975.

Lundström, N.: Ultrasoundcardiographic studies of the mitral valve region in young infants with mitral atresia, mitral stenosis, hypoplasia of the left ventricle and cor triatriatum. Circulation, *45*: 324, 1972.

Lundström, N.: Echocardiography in the diagnosis of congenital mitral stenosis and an evaluation of the results of mitral valvotomy. Circulation, *46*: 44, 1972.

McLaurin, L., et al.: An appraisal of mitral valve echocardiograms mimicking mitral stenosis in conditions with right ventricular pressure overload. Circulation, *48*: 797, 1973.

Martin, R., et al.: Reliability and reproducibility of two-dimensional echocardiograph measurement of the stenotic mitral valve orifice area. Am. J. Cardiol., *43*: 560, 1979.

Millward, D., et al.: Echocardiographic studies to explain opening snaps in presence of nonstenotic mitral valves. Am. J. Cardiol., *31*: 64, 1973.

Moss, A., et al.: Echocardiography in congenital heart disease. West. J. Med., *124*: 102, 1976.

Motro, M., et al.: Should patients with pure mitral stenosis undergo cardiac catheterization? Am. J. Cardiol., *46*: 515, 1980.

Naccarelli, G., et al.: Echocardiographic assessment of mitral stenosis by the left atrial emptying index. Chest, *76*: 668, 1979.

Naito, M., et al.: Rheumatic mitral stenosis: cross-sectional echocardiographic analysis. Am. Heart J., *100*: 34, 1980.

Nichol, P., et al.: Two-dimensional echocardiographic assessment of mitral stenosis. Circulation, *55*: 120, 1977.

Nicolosi, G., et al.: Sensitivity and specificity of echocardiography in the assessment of valve calcification in mitral stenosis. Am. Heart J., *98*: 171, 1979.

Nicolosi, G., et al.: Echocardiographic evaluation of mitral stenosis in predicting mitral valve replacement vs. commissurotomy. Relation to hemodynamic measurements. Chest, *77*: 147, 1980.

Nathan, M., et al.: Idiopathic hypertrophic subaortic stenosis and mitral stenosis. Ann. Thorac. Surg., *12*: 191, 1971.

Palomo, A., et al.: Echo-phonocardiographic determination of left atrial and left ventricular filling pressures with and without mitral stenosis. Circulation, *61*: 1043, 1980.

Pernod, J., et al.: Contribution of ultrasonic echocardiography to the diagnosis of mitral valve disease. *In* The Mitral Valve. Edited by D. Kalmanson. Acton, Mass., Publishing Sciences Group, 1976.

Petty, T., et al.: The problem of mitral stenosis and chronic obstructive pulmonary disease. Chest, *75*: 716, 1979.

Raj, M., et al.: Echocardiographic assessment of mitral valve calcification. Br. Heart J., *38*: 81, 1976.

Salerni, R., et al.: Pressure and sound correlates of the mitral valve echocardiogram in mitral stenosis. Circulation, *58*: 119, 1978.

Shabetai, R., et al.: Asymmetrical hypertrophic cardiomyopathy simulating mitral stenosis. Circulation, *45*: 37, 1972.

Shah, L., et al.: Congenital mitral stenosis. (A case report.) J. Postgrad. Med., *25*: 239, 1979.

Shah, L., et al.: False negative mitral valve echo in the case of Lutembacher's syndrome. J. Postgrad. Med., *25*: 243, 1979.

Shiu, M.: Mitral valve closure index: echocardiographic index of severity of mitral stenosis. Br. Heart J., *39*: 839, 1977.

Shiu, M., et al.: Echocardiographic analysis of posterior mitral leaflet movement in mitral stenosis. Br. Heart J., *40*: 372, 1978.

Snider, A., et al.: Congenital left ventricular inflow obstruction evaluated by two-dimensional echocardiography. Circulation, *61*: 848, 1980.

Strunk, B., et al.: The assessment of mitral stenosis and prosthetic mitral valve obstruction, using the posterior aortic wall echocardiogram. Circulation, *55*: 885, 1977.

Toutouzas, P., et al.: End-diastolic amplitude of mitral valve echogram in mitral stenosis. Br. Heart J., *39*: 73, 1977.

Toutouzas, P., et al.: Noninvasive study of early diastole in mitral stenosis. Circulation, *57*: 708, 1978.

Toutouzas, P., et al.: Early diastole in mitral valve disease. Bibl. Cardiol., *37*: 142, 1979.

Toutouzas, P., et al.: Double diastolic murmur in mitral stenosis with atrial fibrillation and complete heart block. Br. Heart J., *43*: 92, 1980.

Umeda, T., et al.: M-mode and cross-sectional echocardiographic evaluation of rheumatic mitral valve disease. Jpn. Circ. J., *43*: 297, 1979.

Vengsarkar, A., et al.: Cor triatriatum: echocardiographic error in diagnosis. (A case report.) J. Postgrad. Med., *25*: 233, 1979.

Wann, L., et al.: Determination of mitral valve area by cross-sectional echocardiography. Ann. Intern. Med., *88*: 337, 1978.

Wise, J., Jr., et al.: Echocardiographic evaluation of mitral stenosis using diastolic posterior left ventricular wall motion. Circulation, *61*: 1037, 1980.

MITRAL REGURGITATION

Ahmad, S., et al.: The echocardiographic diagnosis of rupture of a papillary muscle. Chest, *73*: 232, 1978.

Antman, E., et al.: Demonstration of the mechanisms by which mitral regurgitation mimics aortic stenosis. Am. J. Cardiol., *42*: 1044, 1978.

Bartall, H., et al.: "Push-up palpitations": unusual presentation of ruptured chordae tendineae: a case report. Angiology, *30*: 347, 1979.

Burgess, J., et al.: Echocardiographic findings in different types of mitral regurgitation. Circulation, *48*: 97, 1973.

Chandraratna, P., et al.: Incident of ruptured chordae tendineae in the mitral valvular prolapse syndrome: an echocardiographic study. Chest, *75*: 334, 1979.

Child, J., et al.: M-mode and cross-sectional echocardiographic features of flail posterior mitral leaflets. Am. J. Cardiol., *44*: 1383, 1979.

Cosby, R., et al.: The echocardiogram in the nonrheumatic mitral insufficiency. Chest, *66*: 642, 1974.

Giles, T., et al.: Value of exploratory "scanning" in the echocardiographic diagnosis of ruptured chordae tendineae. Circulation, *49*: 678, 1974.

Gross, C., et al.: Echocardiography in chronic rheumatic mitral valve disease. Chest, 68: 569, 1975.

Guy, F., et al.: Mitral valve prolapse as a cause of hemodynamically important mitral regurgitation. Can. J. Surg., 23: 166, 1980.

Humphries, W., et al.: Echocardiographic equivalents of a flail mitral leaflet. Am. J. Cardiol., 40: 802, 1977.

Kim, H., et al.: An attempt to correlate the mitral valve echogram with the hemodynamics of patients with pure mitral insufficiency. Jpn. Circ. J., 37: 403, 1973.

Levisman, J.: Echocardiographic diagnosis of mitral regurgitation in congestive cardiomyopathy. Am. Heart J., 93: 33, 1977.

Meyer, J., et al.: Systolic flutter, an echocardiographic clue to the diagnosis of ruptured chordae tendineae. Am. Heart J., 93: 3, 1977.

Millward, D., et al.: Echocardiographic studies of the mitral valve in patients with congestive cardiomyopathy and mitral regurgitation. Am. Heart J., 85: 413, 1973.

Mintz, G., et al.: Two-dimensional echocardiographic recognition of ruptured chordae tendineae. Circulation, 57: 244, 1978.

Mintz, G., et al.: Two-dimensional echocardiographic evaluation of patients with mitral insufficiency. Am. J. Cardiol., 44: 670, 1979.

Mintz, G., et al.: Statistical comparison of M-mode and two-dimensional echocardiographic diagnosis of flail mitral leaflets. Am. J. Cardiol., 45: 253, 1980.

Morcerf, F., et al.: Echocardiographic determination of the etiology of severe mitral regurgitation. Clev. Clin. Q., 43: 163, 1976.

Ogawa, S., et al.: Flail mitral valve in rheumatic heart disease. Chest, 71: 88, 1978.

Ogawa, S., et al.: The role of cross-sectional echocardiography in the diagnosis of flail mitral leaflets. Clin. Cardiol., 1: 85, 1978.

Pathak, L.: Diagnostic ultrasound in mitral regurgitation. Indian Heart J., 29: 192, 1977.

Popp, R.: New trends in noninvasive ultrasonic diagnosis of mitral valve disease. In The Mitral Valve. Edited by D. Kalmanson. Acton, Mass., Publishing Sciences Group, 1976.

Pridie, R., et al.: Mechanism of mitral regurgitation in hypertrophic obstructive cardiomyopathy. Br. Heart J., 32: 203, 1970.

Rashid, A., et al.: Papillary muscle rupture following nonpenetrating chest trauma: report of a case with hemodynamic and serial echocardiographic findings and successful surgical treatment. Heart Lung, 7: 647, 1978.

Sasayama, S., et al.: Dynamic geometry of the left atrium and left ventricle in acute mitral regurgitation. Circulation, 60: 177, 1979.

Sweatman, T., et al.: Echocardiographic diagnosis of ruptured chordae tendineae. Am. J. Cardiol., 26: 661, 1970.

Sweatman, T., et al.: Echocardiographic diagnosis of mitral regurgitation due to ruptured chordae tendineae. Circulation, 46: 580, 1972.

Sze, K., et al.: Systolic flutter of the mitral valve. Am. Heart J., 96: 157, 1978.

Winters, W., et al.: Abnormal mitral valve motion as demonstrated by the ultrasound technique in apparent pure mitral insufficiency. Am. Heart J., 77: 196, 1969.

PROLAPSED MITRAL VALVE

Allen, H., et al.: Significance and prognosis of an isolated late systolic murmur: a 9–22 year followup. Br. Heart J., 36: 525, 1974.

Appelblatt, N., et al.: Ten to forty-year followup of 69 patients with systolic click and without apical late systolic murmur. Am. J. Cardiol., 35: 119, 1975.

Barlow, J., et al.: The problem of non-ejection systolic clicks and associated mitral systolic murmur; emphasis on the billowing mitral leaflet syndrome. Am. Heart J., 90: 636, 1975.

Barnett, H., et al.: Further evidence relating mitral valve prolapse to cerebral ischemic events. N. Engl. J. Med., 302: 139, 1980.

Bartall, H., et al.: Influence of Müller's maneuver on mitral valve prolapse: correlation with external carotid pulse tracing and echocardiogram. Chest, 74: 654, 1978.

Belardi, F.: Mitral valve prolapse in a family practice setting. J. Fam. Pract., 6: 511, 1978.

Bisset, G., et al.: Clinical spectrum and long-term follow-up of isolated mitral valve prolapse in 119 children. Circulation, 62: 423, 1980.

Bloch, A., et al.: Echocardiographic spectrum of posterior systolic motion of the mitral valve in the general population. J. Clin. Ultrasound, 5: 243, 1977.

Boudoulas, H., et al.: Metabolic studies in mitral valve prolapse syndrome. A neuroendocrine-cardiovascular process. Circulation, 61: 1200, 1980.

Boughner, D.: Correlation of echocardiographic and angiographic abnormalities in mitral valve prolapse. In Ultrasound in Medicine. Edited by D. White. New York, Plenum Press, 1975.

Campbell, R., et al.: Ventricular arrhythmias in syndrome of balloon deformity of mitral valve; definition of possible high risk group. Br. Heart J., 38: 1053, 1976.

Chandraratna, P.: On the frequency of early systolic clicks in mitral valve prolapse. Cardiology, 62: 315, 1977.

Chandraratna, P., et al.: Incident of ruptured chordae tendineae in the mitral valvular prolapse syndrome: an echocardiographic study. Chest, 75: 334, 1979.

Clements, S., et al.: The echocardiographic correlate of a systolic click appearing after open mitral commissurotomy. J. Clin. Ultrasound, 6: 395, 1978.

Cobbs, B., et al.: Ventricular buckling: a factor in the abnormal ventriculogram and peculiar hemodynamics associated with mitral valve prolapse. Am. Heart J., 93: 741, 1977.

Cohen, M.: Double mitral leaflet prolapse: echocardiographic-phonocardiographic correlation. Am. Heart J., 91: 168, 1976.

Cohen, M., et al.: Angiographic-echocardiographic correlation in mitral valve prolapse. Am. Heart J., 97: 43, 1979.

Criley, J., et al.: Prolapsed mitral leaflet syndrome. Cardiovasc. Clin., 10: 213, 1979.

Darsee, J., et al.: Prevalence of mitral valve prolapse in presumably healthy young men. Circulation, 59: 619, 1979.

Darsee, J., et al.: Mitral valve prolapse and ophthalmoplegia: a progressive, cardioneurologic syndrome. Ann. Intern. Med., 92: 735, 1980.

deLeon, A.: Mitral valve prolapse; etiology, diagnosis, management. Postgrad. Med., 67: 66, 1980.

DeMaria, A., et al.: The variable spectrum of echocardiographic manifestations of the mitral valve prolapse syndrome. Circulation, 50: 33, 1974.

DeMaria, A., et al.: "Silent" mitral prolapse. Circulation, 50: 1284, 1974.

DeMaria, A., et al.: Echocardiographic identification of the mitral valve prolapse syndrome. Am. J. Med., 62: 819, 1977.

Desser, K., et al.: Apexcardiographic-echocardiographic correlation in mitral valve prolapse. Chest, 70: 68, 1976.

Devereux, R., et al.: Mitral valve prolapse. Circulation, 54: 3, 1976.

Dillon, J., et al.: Use of echocardiography in patients with prolapsed mitral valve. Circulation, 43: 503, 1971.

Ebel, T.: Mitral valve prolapse. Adv. Pediatr., 25: 263, 1978.

Engel, P., et al.: Mitral valve prolapse—a review. Aviat. Space Environ. Med., 51: 273, 1980.

Felner, J., et al.: Systolic honks in young children. Am. J. Cardiol., 20: 206, 1977.

Fontana, M., et al.: Postural changes in left ventricular and mitral valve dynamics in the systolic click-late systolic murmur syndrome. Circulation, 51: 165, 1975.

Fortuin, N.: Echocardiogram of the month: mitral valve prolapse. Med. Times, 108: 124, 1980.

Fortuin, N., et al.: Mitral valve prolapse. Md. State Med. J., 26: 101, 1977.

Gardin, J., et al.: Pseudo-ischemic "false positive" S-T segment changes induced by hyperventilation in patients with mitral valve prolapse. Am. J. Cardiol., 45: 952, 1980.

Gelfand, M., et al.: Mitral valve systolic click syndrome. Am. Fam. Physician, 21: 135, 1980.

Guy, F., et al.: Mitral valve prolapse as a cause of hemodynamically important mitral regurgitation. Can. J. Surg., *23*: 166, 1980.

Harbi, N., et al.: Clinical, noninvasive, and invasive findings in fifty patients with mitral valve prolapse. *In* Noninvasive Cardiovascular Diagnosis. Edited by E. Diethrich. Baltimore, University Park Press, 1978.

Howard, P., et al.: Systolic retraction of the aortic valve in mitral valve prolapse. Echocardiographic correlation with external pulse tracings. Chest, *71*: 659, 1977.

Inoh, T., et al.: Diagnosis and classification of the mitral valve prolapse by the ultrasoundcardiotomography and the evaluation of the M-mode technic. Jpn. Circ. J., *43*: 305, 1979.

Jacobs, W., et al.: Echocardiogram of month: palpitations and late systolic murmur in a young man. Arch. Intern. Med., *137*: 911, 1977.

Jeresaty, R., et al.: "Silent" mitral valve prolapse. Am. J. Cardiol., *35*: 146, 1975.

Jeresaty, R.: Sudden death in the mitral valve prolapse-click syndrome. Am. J. Cardiol., *37*: 317, 1976.

Kantor, J., et al.: Mitral valve prolapse syndrome in agoraphobic patients. Am. J. Psychiatry, *137*: 467, 1980.

Kerber, R., et al.: Echocardiographic patterns in patients with the syndrome of systolic click and late systolic murmur. N. Engl. J. Med., *284*: 691, 1971.

Kerin, N., et al.: Echocardiographic source of early anterior systolic motion in late systolic mitral valve prolapse. Chest, 77: 567, 1980.

Kleid, J., et al.: Systolic time intervals in the syndrome of mid-systolic click and late systolic murmur. Chest, *71*: 65, 1977.

Kounis, N.: Mitral valve prolapse: whiplike motion of the posterior mitral leaflet detected by two-dimensional echocardiography. Angiology, *31*: 198, 1980.

Laiken, S., et al.: Instantaneous transmitral blood flow and anterior mitral leaflet motion in man. Circulation, *59*: 476, 1979.

LeWinter, M., et al.: Phenylephrine-induced atypical chest pain in patients with prolapsing mitral valve leaflets. Am. J. Cardiol., *34*: 12, 1974.

Liedtke, J., et al.: Geometry of left ventricular contraction in the late systolic click syndrome. Circulation, *47*: 27, 1973.

Liedtke, A., et al.: Mitral valve echoes in patients with mitral valve prolapse syndrome. Am. Heart J., *97*: 286, 1979.

Luisada, A., et al.: Systolic click and late systolic murmur in a young woman. Chest, *66*: 292, 1974.

McLarin, C., et al.: Echocardiographically determined mitral valve prolapse in male patients. South. Med. J., *72*: 1416, 1979.

Markiewicz, W., et al.: Mitral valve prolapse in one hundred presumably healthy young females. Circulation, *53*: 464, 1976.

Marshall, C., et al.: Sudden death and the ballooning posterior leaflet syndrome. Arch. Pathol., *98*: 134, 1974.

Mathey, D., et al.: The determinants of onset of mitral valve prolapse in the systolic click, late systolic murmur syndrome. Circulation, *53*: 872, 1976.

Mathey, D., et al.: Abnormal left ventricular contraction pattern in the systolic click, late systolic murmur syndrome. Circulation, *56*: 311, 1977.

Mills, P., et al.: Long-term prognosis of mitral valve prolapse. N. Engl. J. Med., *297*: 13, 1977.

Naggar, C., The mitral valve prolapse syndrome. Spectrum and therapy. Med. Clin. North Am., *63*: 337, 1979.

O'Rourke, R., et al.: Prolapsing mitral valve leaflet syndrome. West. J. Med., *122*: 217, 1975.

O'Rourke, R., et al.: The systolic click-murmur syndrome. Clinical recognition and management. Curr. Probl. Cardiol., *1*: 1, 1976.

Perloff, J.: Systolic click and late systolic murmur (editorial). West, J. Med., *122*: 248, 1975.

Pomerance, A.: Ballooning deformity (mucoid degeneration) of atrioventricular valve. Br. Heart J., *31*: 343, 1969.

Popp, R., et al.: Echocardiographic abnormalities in the mitral valve prolapse syndrome. Circulation, *49*: 428, 1974.

Procacci, P., et al.: Prevalence of clinical mitral valve prolapse in 1169 young women. N. Engl. J. Med., *294*: 1086, 1976.

Reiffel, J., et al.: Augmentation of auscultatory and echocardiographic mitral valve prolapse by atrial premature depolarizations. Am. Heart J., *93*: 533, 1977.

Rippe, J., et al.: Mitral valve prolapse in adults with congenital heart disease. Am. Heart J., *97*: 561, 1979.

Ruwitch, J., et al.: Insensitivity of echocardiography in detecting mitral valve prolapse in older patients with chest pain. Am. J. Cardiol., *40*: 686, 1977.

Saffro, R., et al.: Transient ischemic attack associated with mitral systolic clicks. Arch. Intern. Med., *139*: 693, 1979.

Sahn, D., et al.: Echocardiographic spectrum of mitral valve motion in children with and without mitral valve prolapse; the nature of false positive diagnosis. Am. J. Cardiol., *39*: 422, 1977.

Sbarbaro, J., et al.: Prospective study of mitral valvular prolapse in young men. Chest, *75*: 555, 1979.

Schmaltz, A., et al.: Clinical and angio- and echocardiographic findings in 45 children with mitral valve prolapse syndrome. Eur. J. Cardiol., *7*: 49, 1978.

Schreiber, T., et al.: Effect of atrial septal defect repair on left ventricular geometry and degree of mitral valve prolapse. Circulation, *61*: 888, 1980.

Shappell, S., et al.: Sudden death and the familiar occurrence of mid-systolic click, late systolic murmur syndrome. Circulation, *48*: 1128, 1973.

Shell, W., et al.: The familial occurrence of the syndrome of mid-late systolic click and late systolic murmur. Circulation, *39*: 327, 1967.

Sherman, E., et al.: Myxomatous transformation of the mitral valve producing mitral insufficiency: floppy valve syndrome. Am. J. Dis. Child., *119*: 171, 1970.

Smith, E., et al.: Angiographic diagnosis of mitral valve prolapse; correlation with echocardiography. Am. J. Cardiol., *40*: 165, 1977.

Terasawa, Y., et al.: Mechanism of production of midsystolic click in a prolapsed mitral valve. Jpn. Heart J., *18*: 652, 1977.

Towne, W., et al.: A midsystolic ejection click. Chest, 77: 223, 1980.

Trent, J., et al.: Morphology of a prolapsed posterior mitral valve leaflet. Am. Heart J., *79*: 539, 1970.

Tresch, D., et al.: Mitral valve prolapse in the elderly. J. Am. Geriatr. Soc., *27*: 421, 1979.

Udoshi, M., et al.: Incident of mitral valve prolapse in subjects with thoracic skeletal abnormalities—a prospective study. Am. Heart J., *97*: 303, 1979.

Venkatesh, A., et al.: Mitral valve prolapse in anxiety neurosis (panic disorder). Am. Heart J., *100*: 302, 1980.

Weiss, A., et al.: Echocardiographic detection of mitral valve prolapse; exclusion of false positive diagnosis and determination of inheritance. Circulation, *52*: 1091, 1975.

Winkle, R., et al.: Simultaneous echocardiographic, phonocardiographic recordings at rest and during amyl nitrite administration in patients with mitral valve prolapse. Circulation, *51*: 522, 1975.

Winkle, R., et al.: Arrhythmias in patients with mitral valve prolapse. Circulation, *52*: 73, 1975.

Winkle, R., et al.: Life threatening arrhythmias in the mitral valve prolapse syndrome. Am. J. Med., *60*: 961, 1976.

Associated with Other Disease

Aranda, J., et al.: Mitral valve prolapse and coronary artery disease. Clinical, hemodynamic and angiographic correlations. Circulation, *52*: 245, 1975.

Barnett, H., et al.: Further evidence relating mitral valve prolapse to cerebral ischemic events. N. Engl. J. Med., *302*: 139, 1980.

Betriu, A., et al.: Prolapse of the posterior mitral leaflet of the mitral valve associated with secundum atrial septal defect. Am. J. Cardiol., *35*: 363, 1975.

Brown, O., et al.: Aortic root dilatation and mitral valve prolapse in Marfan's syndrome. Circulation, *52*: 651, 1975.

Cabeen, W., et al.: Mitral valve prolapse and conduction defects in Ehlers-Danlos syndrome. Arch. Intern. Med., *137*: 1227, 1977.

Chandraratna, P., et al.: Echocardiographic observations on the association between mitral valve prolapse and asymmetric septal hypertrophy. Circulation, *55*: 622, 1976.

Desser, K., et al.: Clicks secondary to pneumothorax confounding the diagnosis of mitral valve prolapse. Chest, *71*: 523, 1977.

Freed, C., et al.: Echocardiographic findings in Marfan's syndrome. West. J. Med., *126*: 87, 1977.

Gooch, A., et al.: Arrhythmias and left ventricular asynergy in the prolapsing mitral leaflet syndrome. Am. J. Cardiol., *29*: 611, 1972.

Gottdiener, J., et al.: Mid-systolic click and mitral valve prolapse following mitral commissurotomy. Am. J. Med., *64*: 295, 1978.

Kay, J., et al.: Surgical correction of severe mitral prolapse without mitral insufficiency but with pronounced cardiac arrhythmia. J. Thorac. Cardiovasc. Surg., *78*: 259, 1979.

Levisman, J., et al.: Abnormal motion of the mitral valve with pericardial effusion: pseudo-prolapse of the mitral valve. Am. Heart J., *91*: 18, 1976.

Lopes, V., et al.: Left posterior hemiblock: a new cause of mitral valve prolapse. Adv. Cardiol., *19*: 120, 1977.

Meyers, S., et al.: Right atrial myxoma with right to left shunting and mitral valve prolapse. Am. J. Med., *62*: 308, 1977.

Miller, A., et al.: Prolapsed mitral valve associated with the Holt-Oram syndrome. Chest, *67*: 230, 1975.

Payvandi, M., et al.: Cardiac, skeletal and ophthalmologic abnormalities in relatives of patients with the Marfan syndrome. Circulation, *55*: 797, 1977.

Pocock, W., et al.: An association between the billowing posterior mitral leaflet syndrome and congenital heart disease, particularly atrial septal defect. Am. Heart J., *81*: 720, 1971.

Raizada, V., et al.: Mitral valve prolapse in patients with coronary artery disease. Echocardiographic-angiographic correlation. Br. Heart J., *39*: 53, 1977.

Salomon, J., et al.: Thoracic skeletal abnormalities in idiopathic mitral leaflet syndrome. Circulation, *48*: 287, 1973.

Scampardonis, G., et al.: Left ventricular abnormalities in prolapsed mitral leaflet syndrome. Circulation, *48*: 287, 1973.

Thomason, H., Jr., et al.: Congenital complete atrioventricular block and prolapsing mitral valve. Chest, *70*: 539, 1976.

Victorica, B., et al.: Ostium secundum atrial septal defect associated with balloon mitral valve in children. Am. J. Cardiol., *33*: 668, 1974.

Weinrauch, L., et al.: Mitral valve prolapse in rheumatic mitral stenosis. Chest, *72*: 752, 1977.

SYSTOLIC ANTERIOR MOTION (SAM)

Awdeh, M., et al.: Systolic anterior motion of the mitral valve caused by sarcoid involving the septum. South. Med. J., *71*: 969, 1978.

Bulkley, B., et al.: Systolic anterior motion of the mitral valve without asymmetric septal hypertrophy. Chest, *69*: 694, 1976.

Come, P., et al.: Hypercontractile cardiac states simulating hypertrophic cardiomyopathy. Circulation, *55*: 901, 1977.

Cooperberg, P., et al.: Parachute accessory anterior mitral valve leaflet causing left ventricular outflow tract obstruction. Circulation, *53*: 908, 1976.

Falicov, R., et al.: Hypertrophic cardiomyopathy with mid-ventricular obstruction associated with mitral stenosis. Cathet. Cardiovasc. Diagn., *3*: 247, 1977.

Greenwald, J., et al.: Echographic mitral systolic motion in left ventricular aneurysm. Br. Heart J., *37*: 684, 1975.

Kerin, N., et al.: Echocardiographic source of early anterior systolic motion in late systolic mitral valve prolapse. Chest, *77*: 567, 1980.

King, J., et al.: Markedly abnormal mitral valve motion without simultaneous interventricular pressure gradient due to uneven mitral-septal contact in idiopathic hypertrophic subaortic stenosis. Am. J. Cardiol., *34*: 360, 1974.

Maron, B., et al.: Left ventricular outflow tract obstruction due to systolic anterior motion of the anterior mitral leaflet in patients with concentric left ventricular hypertrophy. Circulation, *57*: 527, 1978.

Maron, B., et al.: Hypertrophic cardiomyopathy. Recent observations regarding the specificity of three hallmarks of the disease: asymmetric septal hypertrophy, septal disorganization and systolic anterior motion of the anterior mitral leaflet. Am. J. Cardiol., 45: 141, 1980.

Mintz, G., et al.: Systolic anterior motion of the mitral valve in the absence of asymmetric hypertrophy. Circulation, 57: 256, 1978.

Nathan, M., et al.: Idiopathic hypertrophic subaortic stenosis and mitral stenosis. Ann. Thorac. Surg., 12: 191, 1971.

Nimura, Y., et al.: An unusual pattern of the mitral echocardiogram observed in cases of congestive cardiomyopathy and other myocardial diseases. Jpn. Heart J., 16: 500, 1975.

Pridie, R., et al.: Ultrasonic mitral echograms in the assessment of treatment in hypertrophic obstructive cardiomyopathy. Recent Adv. Stud. Cardiac Struct. Metab., 2: 817, 1973.

Rodger, J.: Motion of mitral apparatus in hypertrophic cardiomyopathy with obstruction. Br. Heart J., 38: 732, 1976.

Termini, B., et al.: Systolic anterior motion of the mitral valve following annuloplasty. Vasc. Surg., 11: 55, 1977.

Udoshi, M., et al.: Systolic anterior motion of the mitral valve with and without asymmetric septal hypertrophy. Role of left ventricular posterior wall motion. Cardiology, 66: 147, 1980.

SURGICAL EVALUATION

Clements, S., et al.: The echocardiographic correlate of a systolic click appearing after open mitral commissurotomy. J. Clin. Ultrasound, 6: 395, 1978.

Danilowicz, D., et al.: Echocardiographic patterns after mitral annuloplasty. Cardiology, 65: 129, 1980.

Ikäheimo, M., et al.: Echocardiography after mitral valvotomy and in the diagnosis of mitral restenosis. Ann. Clin. Res., 9: 201, 1977.

Johnson, M., et al.: Usefulness of echocardiography in patients undergoing mitral valve surgery. J. Thorac. Cardiovasc. Surg., 64: 922, 1972.

Leutenegger, F., et al.: Progression of mild mitral stenosis and incidence of restenosis after open commissurotomy: a study using echocardiography. Am. Heart J., 98: 562, 1979.

Lundström, N.: Echocardiography in the diagnosis of congenital mitral stenosis and evaluation of the results of mitral valvulotomy. Circulation, 46: 44, 1972.

Mary, D., et al.: Study with reflected ultrasound of patients with mitral valve repair. Br. Heart J., 35: 480, 1973.

Nanda, N., et al.: Mitral commissurotomy versus replacement: pre-operative evaluation by echocardiography. Circulation, 51: 263, 1975.

Nicolosi, G., et al.: Echocardiographic evaluation of mitral stenosis in predicting mitral valve replacement vs. commissurotomy. Relation to hemodynamic measurements. Chest, 77: 147, 1980.

Pathak, L., et al.: Pre- and post-operative evaluation of mitral stenosis by echocardiography. Indian Heart J., 28: 158, 1976.

Selzer, A., et al.: Immediate and long range results of valvuloplasty for mitral regurgitation due to ruptured chordae tendineae. Circulation (Suppl.), 45: 52, 1972.

Shiu, M., et al.: Echocardiographic and exercise evaluation of results of mitral valvotomy operations. Br. Heart J., 41: 139, 1979.

Shu, T., et al.: Significance of echocardiographic evaluation on surgery to mitral stenosis. Jpn. Heart J., 18: 751, 1977.

Silver, W., et al.: The echocardiogram in a case of mitral stenosis before and after surgery. Am. Heart J., 78: 811, 1969.

Tatmichi, K.: The ultrasono-cardiographic criterion for the operative procedures of mitral valvular disease. Jpn. Circ. J., 37: 473, 1973.

Thomas, R., et al.: Echocardiographic pattern of posterior mitral valve leaflet movement after mitral valve repair. Br. Heart J., 41: 399, 1979.

Tsuchioka, H., et al.: Standardization of parameters in follow-up study after mitral commissurotomy. J. Cardiovasc. Surg., 20: 137, 1979.

Yazawa, Y., et al.: Echocardiographic proof of improved posterior wall motion of the left ventricle after surgery to correct mitral stenosis. In Noninvasive Cardiovascular Diagnosis. Edited by E. Diethrich. Baltimore, University Park Press, 1978.

Yuste, P., et al.: Ultrasonic analysis of mitral stenosis: pre- and post-operative studies. Rev. Esp. Cardiol., 26: 85, 1973.

8

Abnormal Aortic Root and Aortic Valve

Echocardiography is useful for the initial detection and confirmation of diseases affecting the aortic root and its valve. Symptoms and clinical findings secondary to disease of these structures are sometimes nondiagnostic. Patients complain of dizziness, fainting, shortness of breath, chest pain, and an irregular heartbeat. Physicians hear systolic ejection murmurs and clicks. The diastolic murmur of aortic regurgitation may be confused with the diastolic rumble of mitral stenosis. Some murmurs are present from birth. Others appear following acute febrile illnesses or chest trauma.

An enlarged heart may or may not be related to disease of the aorta or the aortic valve. To exclude occult narrowing, thickening, dilatation, or disruption of the aortic apparatus, examination of the left ventricular outflow tract, aortic valve, and proximal ascending aorta should be a routine part of an echocardiographic examination. When indicated, two-dimensional suprasternal examination of the transverse and proximal descending aorta should be performed to exclude the presence of aortic hypoplasia or coarctation.

AORTIC ROOT DILATATION

Symmetrical enlargement of the aortic root can occur secondary to Marfan's syndrome, cystic medial necrosis, dissection of the aortic root, intra-annular abscesses, and aortic regurgitation. Moderate and moderately severe aortic stenosis is often accompanied by an enlargement of the aorta just distal to the valve (poststenotic dilatation).

Long-axis, two-dimensional echocardiography is most suitable to document the longitudinal length of aortic root dilatation extending into the proximal ascending aorta (Figs. 8–1 and 8–2). Normally, the walls of the ascending aorta are parallel, and the diameter of the aortic lumen is equal to, or larger than, the diameter of the aortic annulus.

The dimension of the aortic annulus must be appropriate for the patient's body size. Dilatation of the aortic root and aorta is detected with M-mode echocardiography as an extraordinary divergence of the aortic walls when the transducer is angled

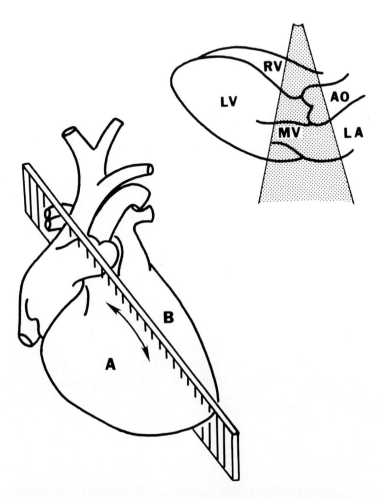

Fig. 8–1. A diagram of a parasternal, long-axis view of the left ventricular outflow tract and the aortic root. The transducer was positioned over the aortic root with the sound beam aligned in a plane between the right shoulder and the left flank. Imagine that section B on the lower diagram has been removed. The upper right diagram presents the cut surface of section A as seen on a preview monitor. RV, right ventricle; LV, left ventricle; MV, mitral valve; AO, aorta; LA, left atrium.

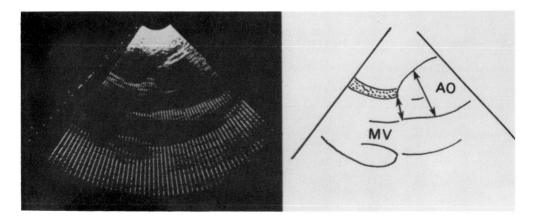

Fig. 8–2. A 40-year-old male patient with chest pain and cardiomegaly. The diastolic dimension of the dilated proximal ascending aorta (large arrow) is shown on a single frame (with diagram) from a parasternal, long-axis, two-dimensional echocardiogram. The diameter of the aortic annulus was normal (small arrow). AO, aorta; MV, mitral valve. (From Chang, S., and Chang, J.: Recent echocardiographic evaluation of the great vessels and their valves. In Progress in Medical Ultrasound. Vol. 1. Edited by A. Kurjak. Amsterdam, Excerpta Medica, 1980.)

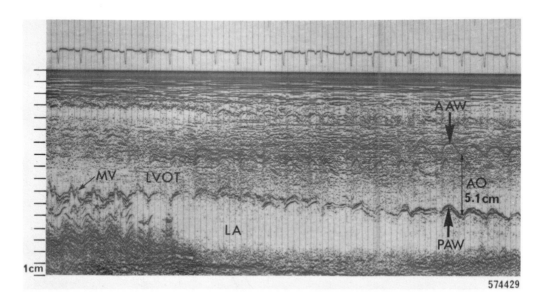

Fig. 8–3. A 51-year-old male patient with severe aortic regurgitation and a markedly dilated aorta extending to the proximal aortic arch. The widening of the aorta steadily increased during the scan from the left ventricular outflow tract (LVOT) to the proximal ascending aorta (AO). MV, mitral valve; LA, left atrium; AAW, anterior aortic wall; PAW, posterior aortic wall.

superiorly from the left ventricular outflow tract to the ascending aorta (Fig. 8–3). The diameter of the proximal ascending aorta is at least 12% greater than the diameter of the aortic annulus. An abrupt change in the aorta's diameter is consistent with an aneurysm or an aortic root dissection (Fig. 8–4).

In the presence of aortic stenosis, M-mode scans should be continued superiorly beyond the sinuses of Valsalva into the ascending aorta to detect poststenotic aortic dilatation. Mild dilatation is difficult to distinguish from the slight widening of the aorta one commonly sees as the interrogating sound beam traverses obliquely through the proximal ascending aorta. This artificial widening of the aorta may be minimized by locating the transducer as perpendicularly as possible over the ascending aorta. If interference from the lung precludes a satisfactory recording, one should turn the patient toward a

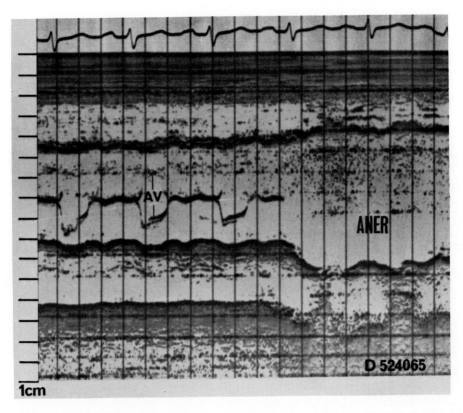

Fig. 8–4. A 39-year-old female patient with Marfan's syndrome. There was a massive dilatation of the aorta with a large dissection, extending from the origin of the aortic valve to the aortic arch, and minimal aortic regurgitation The scan was superior to and medial from the area of aortic leaflet motion. The posterior aortic wall was aneurysmal and showed discordant movement impinging upon the left atrium during systole (ANER). AV, aortic valve motion. (From Feigenbaum, H.: Echocardiography. 2nd Ed. Philadelphia, Lea & Febiger, 1976.)

partial left lateral decubitus position and have the patient exhale and hold his breath intermittently while the echocardiographer searches for the aorta. If the aorta has been displaced rightward for any reason, the dimensions of the aortic root may be obtained from the right parasternum. In these cases, rotation of the patient toward a partial right lateral position displaces the aorta further to the right and also displaces the right lung. This maneuver has been particularly helpful in children with congenital aortic stenosis.

OBSTRUCTED FLOW INTO THE AORTA

Subvalvular Aortic Stenosis and Its Mimics

The aortic valve's diastolic and systolic movement can be influenced by disease not directly related to the aortic valve itself. The aortic valve opens when a volume of blood is forcibly ejected through it during systole. Any sudden interruption of the blood's forward movement allows partial closure of the aortic leaflets (Fig. 8–5). Whereas intrasystolic aortic valve closure is sensitive to dynamic subvalvular

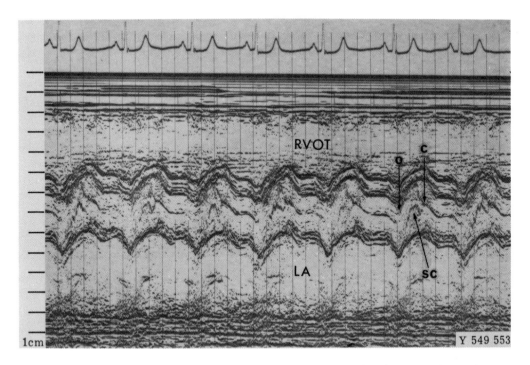

Fig. 8–5. A 27-year-old male patient with severe idiopathic hypertrophic subaortic stenosis. The midsystolic closure of the posterior aortic leaflet indicated a significant dynamic obstruction to forward blood flow. At cardiac catheterization, the subaortic pressure gradients were: rest, 90 mm Hg; post-PVC, 170 mm Hg; post-Valsalva maneuver, 130 mm Hg. RVOT, right ventricular outflow tract; LA, left atrium; o, initial opening of aortic valve; sc, intrasystolic valve closure; c, end-systolic closure of aortic valve.

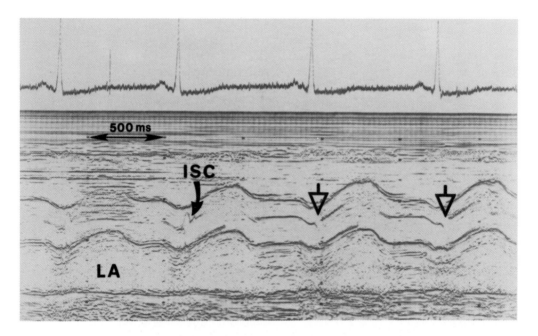

Fig. 8–6. A nine-year-old female patient with membranous subaortic obstruction. ISC, early intrasystolic closure of the anterior aortic valve. Open arrows, a poorly recorded early systolic closing movement of the anterior aortic leaflet. This caused the false appearance of eccentric anterior leaflet mobility. At catheterization, there was a subaortic pressure gradient of 70 mm Hg. (See Figure 8–7.) LA, left atrium; ms, milliseconds.

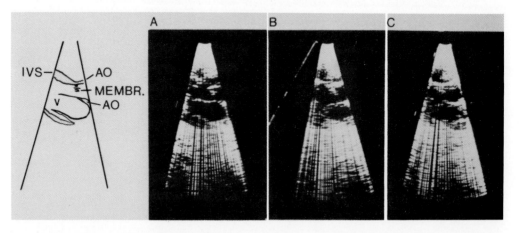

Fig. 8–7. Single frames, with diagram, of subaortic membrane from the patient in Figure 8–6. Serial frames were selected from a parasternal, long-axis, two-dimensional echocardiogram. A, Diastole; a subaortic membrane (MEMBR) was localized in the left ventricular outflow tract. B and C, Early and late systole; the obstructive subaortic membrane was pushed toward the aorta during ejection. At operation, a membranous ring of subaortic tissue was excised. The membrane was positioned just below the aortic root. AO, aorta; IVS, interventricular septum; v, open mitral valve.

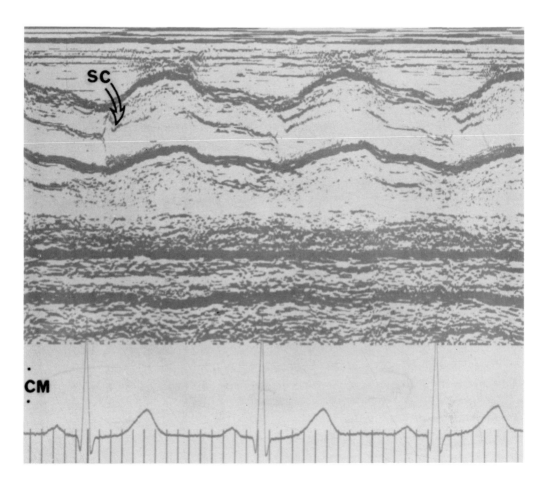

Fig. 8–8. A four-year-old female patient with an aneurysm of the membranous ventricular septum with a ventricular septal defect. SC, Early systolic closure of the anterior aortic leaflet secondary to an interrupted forward flow through the aortic valve as blood was shunted to the right ventricle. (See Fig. 8–9.) (From Chang, S., and Chang, J.: Recent echocardiographic evaluation of the great vessels and their valves. *In* Progress in Medical Ultrasound. Vol. 1. Edited by A. Kurjak. Amsterdam, Excerpta Medica, 1980.)

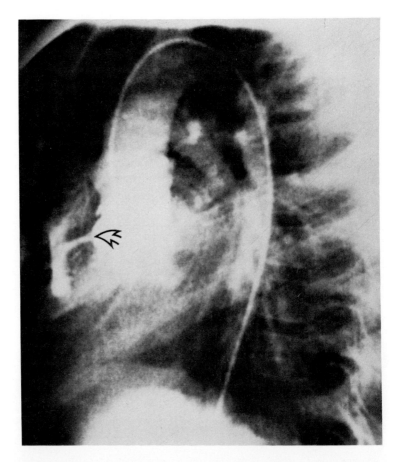

Fig. 8–9. A cineangiogram, lateral projection, from the patient in Figure 8–8. The contrast media entered the right ventricle through the membranous ventricular septal defect (arrow). (From Chang, S., and Chang, J.: Recent echocardiographic evaluation of the great vessels and their valves. *In* Progress in Medical Ultrasound. Vol 1. Edited by A. Kurjak. Amsterdam, Excerpta Medica, 1980.)

obstruction, as with idiopathic hypertrophic subaortic stenosis, early valve closure is not pathognomonic for this condition. A membranous subvalvular obstruction and a membranous septal aneurysm with a ventricular septal defect produce similar patterns of motion (Figs. 8–6 to 8–9).

Valvular Aortic Stenosis

Obstruction to blood flow through the aortic valve can result from tissue fibrosis and calcification or from congenital malformation of the leaflets. Rough, irregular leaflet surfaces are more echo-reflective than the smooth surfaces of a normal aortic valve. Systolic leaflet separation is more difficult to record and to interpret. Diseased aortic leaflet motion is easier to record if the transducer is moved leftward, nearer the left ventricular apex and angled toward the throat or the right shoulder. Amplification should be low, since overamplification obscures leaflet separation and movement (Fig. 8–10).

Leaflet fibrosis and calcification without obstruction are not uncommon in patients with a history of rheumatic heart disease or in elderly patients (Figs. 8–11 and 8–12). In these persons, the significance of abnormal aortic leaflet "thickening" must be correlated with other echocardiographic, clinical, and phonocardiographic findings.

The clinical severity and aortic pressure gradient across a congenitally obstructed aortic valve cannot be determined from isolated aortic valve echocardiograms. Commissural fusion of the aortic leaflets forms a dome during systole (Fig. 8–13). If the sound beam passes through the base of the domed valve, M-mode echocardiographic aortic leaflet separation appears normal (Fig. 8–14). Long-axis, two-dimensional echocardiography is more suitable to demonstrate valvular doming and poststenotic dilatation of the proximal aorta (Fig. 8–15).

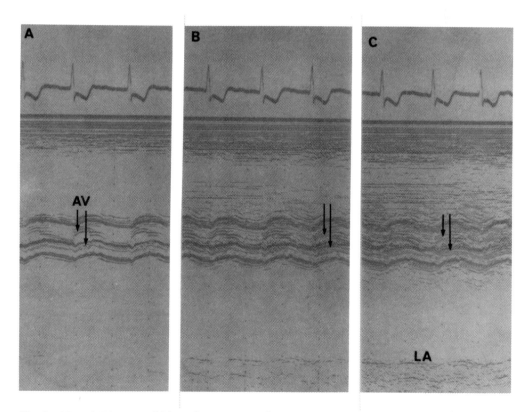

Fig. 8–10. A 76-year-old female patient with aortic stenosis. *A*, Systolic leaflet separation was visualized best with low amplification. *B* and *C*, The amplification progressively increased, resulting in poor definition of leaflet separation and thickness. AV, aortic valve; LA, left atrium.

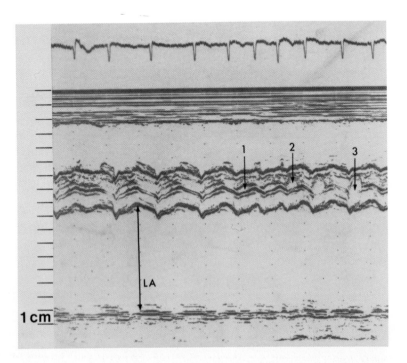

Fig. 8–11. A 48-year-old male patient with severe calcific mitral stenosis without regurgitation and with moderate aortic regurgitation. A beat-to-beat variation of systolic aortic leaflet separation was noted. The increased echo-reflectiveness from complexes 1 and 2 was consistent with leaflet thickening or rolling. At the time of operation, the aortic leaflets were thin, with rolling and calcification of the leaflet margins. LA, enlarged left atrium. (From Chang, S., Clements, S., and Chang, J.: Aortic stenosis: echocardiographic cusp separation and surgical description of aortic valve in 22 patients. Am. J. Cardiol., 39: 499, 1977.)

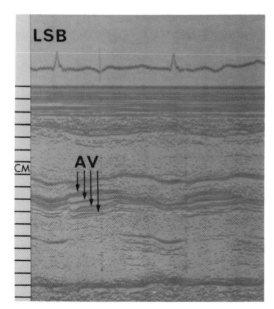
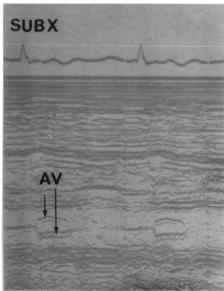

Fig. 8–12. A 76-year-old male patient with chronic obstructive lung disease, coronary artery disease, and congestive heart failure. The patient was sitting during the echocardiographic examination to alleviate breathing difficulties. A, The increased echo-reflectiveness of the aortic leaflets was consistent with leaflet fibrosis and/or calcification. B, Systolic leaflet fluttering and more leaflet separation were recorded from the subcostal examination site. Localized or diffuse leaflet thickening is not unusual in geriatric patients. The significance of leaflet thickening must be determined from the remainder of the echogram and other clinical findings. AV, aortic valve; LSB, left sternal border; SUBX, subcostal examination site.

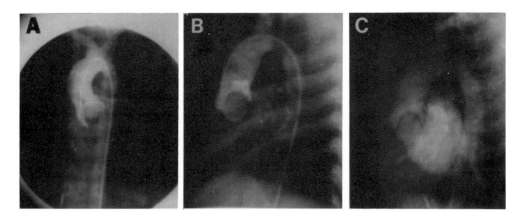

Fig. 8–13. A 16-month-old male patient with severe aortic stenosis. A and B, An aortogram showing doming of the aortic valve in frontal and lateral projections, respectively. C, A levophase cineangiogram showing aortic leaflet thickening and systolic doming. The catheter did not traverse the aortic valve, and percutaneous puncture was not attempted to obtain left ventricular pressure. Pressures obtained at cardiac catheterization: right ventricle, 29/0 mm Hg; pulmonary artery, 21/11 mm Hg; right pulmonary artery, 16/9 mm Hg; left pulmonary artery, 19/10 mm Hg; aorta, 80/58 mm Hg. The patient is scheduled for an aortic valve commissurotomy. (See Fig. 8–15.)

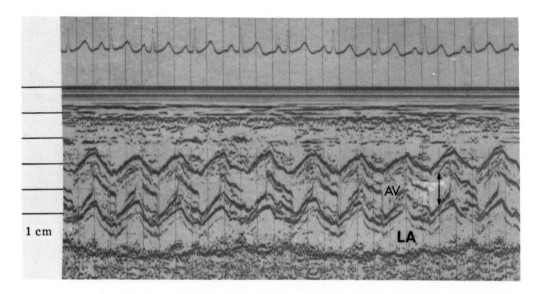

Fig. 8–14. A four-year-old male patient with congenital aortic stenosis. Although the aortic leaflets appear to open widely (arrow), this valve was severely obstructed, with an 85-mm Hg transaortic gradient. AV, aortic valve; LA, left atrium.

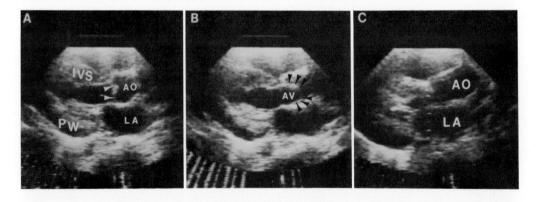

Fig. 8–15. A long-axis, two-dimensional echocardiogram from the patient shown in Figure 8–13. *A,* The diastolic frame showed a markedly thickened left ventricle and closed anterior and posterior aortic leaflets. *B,* The systolic frame showed the domed appearance of the open aortic leaflets. The aortic valve could not be traversed by catheter. *C,* Post-stenotic aortic dilatation. The transducer was moved superiorly on the chest to a position perpendicular to the proximal ascending aorta. This was not a good position from which to monitor septal-aortic continuity; a lower intercostal space would have been more suitable.

Supravalvular Aortic Stenosis

Echocardiographic identification of supravalvular aortic stenosis requires angulation of the sound beam from the aortic valve superiorly into the ascending aorta. Narrowing of the proximal ascending aorta is pathognomonic for supravalvular aortic stenosis (Figs. 8–16 to 8–18). The echocardiographer must be sure that synchronously moving anterior and posterior aortic walls have been recorded as far above the aortic root as possible. The obstructive segment's length and location are accurately assessed by long-axis, two-dimensional echocardiography (Fig. 8–19).

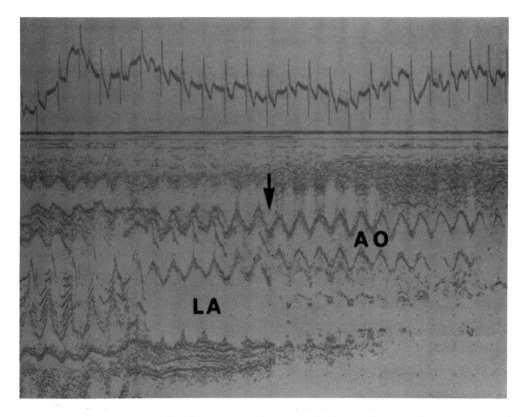

Fig. 8–16.   A two-year-old male patient with supravalvular aortic stenosis. A compressed scan from the left ventricle to the proximal ascending aorta showed an initial area of narrowing (arrow). The anterior and posterior aortic walls moved synchronously throughout the cardiac cycle. (See Fig. 8–18.) AO, aorta; LA, left atrium. (From Chang, S., and Chang, J.: Recent echocardiographic evaluation of the great vessels and their valves. *In* Progress in Medical Ultrasound. Vol. 1. Edited by A. Kurjak. Amsterdam, Excerpta Medica, 1980.)

(Text continues on page 295.)

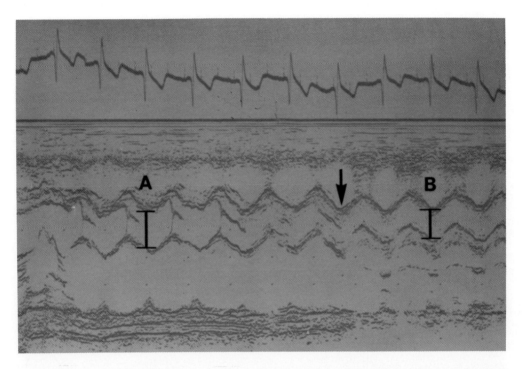

Fig. 8–17. A tracing from the patient in Figure 8–16 recorded at a faster paper speed from videotape to facilitate the measurement of the aortic annulus *(A)* and the area of supravalvular stenosis *(B)*. The arrow corresponds to the initial area of narrowing identical to that in Figure 8–16. The percentage of narrowing may be estimated by the following method: subtract the diameter of the obstructed segment from the diameter of the annulus; divide the remainder by the diameter of the annulus and multiply the result by 100. (From Chang, S., and Chang, J.: Recent echocardiographic evaluation of the great vessels and their valves. *In* Progress in Medical Ultrasound. Vol. 1. Edited by A. Kurjak. Amsterdam, Excerpta Medica, 1980.)

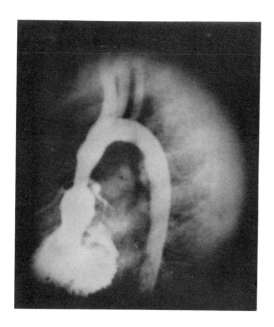

Fig. 8–18. A cineangiogram, lateral projection, of the patient in Figures 8–16 and 8–17 that demonstrates the hourglass narrowing of the aorta distal to the valve. There was a 45-mm Hg pressure gradient at the site of obstruction. There was a small aneurysm in the proximal aspect of the circumflex artery. (From Chang, S., and Chang, J.: Recent echocardiographic evaluation of the great vessels and their valves. *In* Progress in Medical Ultrasound. Vol. 1. Edited by A. Kurjak. Amsterdam, Excerpta Medica, 1980.)

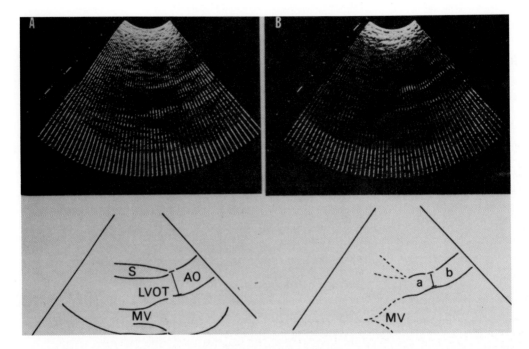

Fig. 8–19. Two long-axis, two-dimensional still frames and matching diagrams of the left ventricular outflow tract *(A)* and the proximal ascending aorta *(B)* from the patient in Figures 8–16 to 8–18. Note the diameter of the aortic annulus in *A* in contrast to the decreased dimension of the aorta distal to the valve in *B*. LVOT, left ventricular outflow tract; MV, mitral valve; AO, aorta; a, aortic root; b, proximal ascending aorta; S, interventricular septum. (From Chang, S., and Chang, J.: Recent echocardiographic evaluation of the great vessels and their valves. *In* Progress in Medical Ultrasound. Vol. 1. Edited by A. Kurjak. Amsterdam, Excerpta Medica, 1980.)

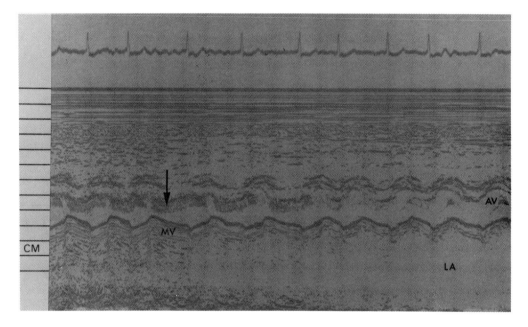

Fig. 8–20. A 40-year-old female patient with severe calcific mitral stenosis and severe aortic regurgitation. An echo-reflective mass (arrow) recorded in the left ventricular outflow tract was thought to be prolapsing aortic leaflet tissue. At operation, all three aortic leaflets were thickened and calcified along the edges; the posterior, noncoronary leaflet prolapsed into the ventricular outflow tract. MV, mitral valve motion; AV, aortic valve motion; LA, left atrium.

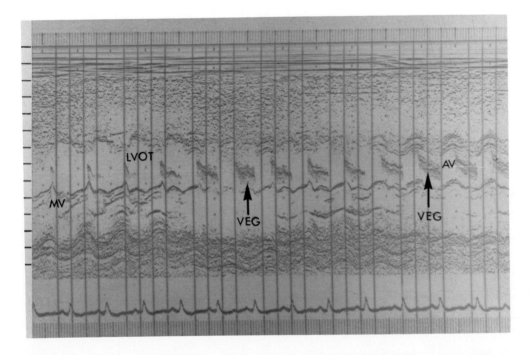

Fig. 8–21. A 65-year-old male patient with severe aortic regurgitation with an aortic annular abscess secondary to staphylococcal endocarditis. A scan from the mitral valve to the aorta showed the aortic leaflet prolapsing into the left ventricular outflow tract. The "shaggy" echo-reflective quality of the aortic leaflets strongly suggested the presence of vegetations, which were confirmed at the time of operation. The right coronary cusp prolapsed into the left ventricular outflow tract. The remaining leaflets were markedly deteriorated and incompetent. MV, mitral valve motion; LVOT, left ventricular outflow tract; VEG, vegetation; AV, aortic valve motion.

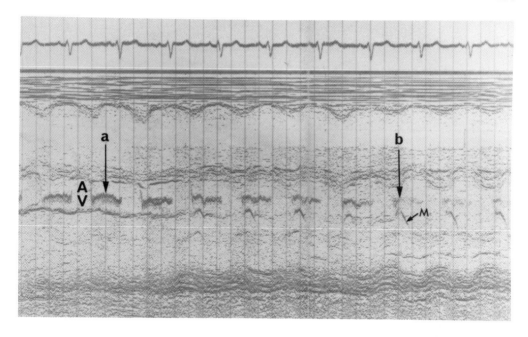

Fig. 8–22. A 55-year-old male patient with severe aortic regurgitation, pulmonary hypertension, severe cirrhosis of liver, and diabetes. Scans from the aortic valve to the left ventricular outflow tract revealed marked diastolic fluttering and prolapse of the aortic leaflet consistent with a flail aortic leaflet. Supravalvular aortography revealed a normal aorta and aortic root without evidence of an aneurysm. The right coronary aortic leaflet prolapsed into the left ventricular outflow tract during diastole. Pullback pressures across the aortic valve were recorded at cardiac catheterization: left ventricle, 123/34 mm Hg; aorta, 123/43 mm Hg. AV, aortic valve motion; a, diastolic leaflet fluttering; b, prolapsed aortic leaflet tissue. (From Chang, S., and Chang, J.: Recent echocardiographic evaluation of the great vessels and their valves. *In* Progress in Medical Ultrasound. Vol. 1. Edited by A. Kurjak. Amsterdam, Excerpta Medica, 1980.)

PROLAPSE OF AORTIC LEAFLET

Myxomatous degeneration, endocarditis, and chest trauma have resulted in prolapse of one or more aortic leaflets into the left ventricular outflow tract. Differentiation between myxomatous degeneration and vegetations is difficult because both conditions reflect "shaggy," "fuzzy" echoes (Figs. 8–20 and 8–21). Diastolic fluttering of an aortic leaflet occurs when the leaflet is flail (Fig. 8–22), but similar patterns of movement have been seen by intact prolapsing leaflets or by vegetations attached to a leaflet.

BIBLIOGRAPHY

AORTIC DILATATION

Brown, O., et al.: Echocardiographic criteria for aortic root dissection. Am. J. Cardiol., 36: 17, 1975.

Candel-Riera, J., et al.: Aortic root dissection. Another cause of early systolic closure of the aortic valve. Br. Heart J., 43: 579, 1980.

Cooperberg, P., et al.: Rupture of a sinus of Valsalva aneurysm. Report of a case diagnosed pre-operatively by echocardiography. Radiology, 113: 171, 1974.

Curati, W., et al.: Echographic demonstration of mobility of the dissecting flap of an aortic aneurysm. Radiology, 123: 173, 1977.

DeMaria, A., et al.: Identification and localization of aneurysms of the ascending aorta by cross-sectional echocardiography. Circulation, 59: 755, 1979.

Di Luzio, V., et al.: Echocardiographic diagnosis of the dissection of the thoracic aorta. G. Ital. Cardiol., 6: 677, 1976.

Kasper, W., et al.: Diagnosis of dissecting aortic aneurysm with suprasternal echocardiography. Am. J. Cardiol., 42: 291, 1978.

Kronzon, I., et al.: Illustrative echocardiogram: aortic root dissection. Chest, 65: 88, 1974.

Krueger, S., et al.: Echocardiographic mimics of aortic root dissection. Chest, 67: 441, 1975.

Krueger, S., et al.: Aortic root dissection: an echocardiographic demonstration of torn intimal flap. J. Clin. Ultrasound, 4: 35, 1976.

Matsumoto, M., et al.: Echocardiographic diagnosis of ruptured aneurysm of sinus of Valsalva: report of two cases. Circulation, 53: 383, 1976.

Matsumoto, M., et al.: Use of kymo-two-dimensional echoaortocardiography for the diagnosis of aortic root dissection and mycotic aneurysm of the aortic root. Ultrasound Med. Biol., 3: 153, 1977.

Matsumoto, M., et al.: A two-dimensional echoaortocardiographic approach to dissecting aneurysms of the aorta to prevent false-positive diagnoses. Radiology, 127: 491, 1978.

Millward, D., et al.: Dissecting aortic aneurysm diagnosed by echocardiography in a patient with rupture of the aneurysm into the right atrium. Am. J. Cardiol., 30: 427, 1972.

Moothart, R., et al.: Echocardiography in aortic root dissection and dilatation. Am. J. Cardiol., 36: 11, 1975.

Nanda, N., et al.: Diagnosis of aortic root dissection by echocardiography. Circulation, 48: 506, 1973.

Roller, D., et al.: Psoriasis, sacroilitis and aortitis: an echocardiographic mimic of aortic root dissection. Chest, 75: 641, 1979.

Rothbaum, D., et al.: Echocardiographic manifestation of right sinus of Valsalva aneurysm. Circulation, 49: 768, 1974.

Schulman, R., et al.: Echocardiographic features of an unruptured aneurysm of the right sinus of Valsalva. Chest, 77: 700, 1980.

Sher, R., et al.: Aneurysm of the sinus of Valsalva: its natural history. Postgrad. Med., 65: 191, 1979.

Waller, B., et al.: Marfan cardiovascular disease without the Marfan syndrome. Fusiform ascending aortic aneurysm with aortic and mitral valve regurgitation. Chest, 77: 533, 1980.

Weyman, A., et al.: Premature pulmonic valve opening following sinus of Valsalva aneurysm rupture into the right atrium. Circulation, 51: 556, 1975.

Wong, B., et al.: Echocardiographic features of an aneurysm of the left sinus of Valsalva. Chest, 73: 105, 1978.

Yoshida, S., et al.: Ruptured sinus of Valsalva aneurysm into the left ventricle. Jpn. Heart J., 19: 954, 1978.

Yuste, P., et al.: Dissecting aortic aneurysm diagnosed by echocardiography. Br. Heart J., 36: 111, 1974.

AORTIC REGURGITATION

Chandraratna, P., et al.: Echocardiography of the "floppy" aortic valve; case report. Circulation, 52: 959, 1975.

Cohen, I., et al.: Pathophysiologic observations on premature opening of the aortic valve utilizing a technique for multiplane echocardiographic analysis. Am. Heart J., 97: 766, 1979.

Corrigall, D., et al.: Phonocardiographic and echocardiographic features of ruptured aortic valvular cusp. Chest, 69: 669, 1976.

Das, G., et al.: Echocardiographic manifestations of ruptured aortic valvular leaflets in the absence of valvular vegetations. Chest, 72: 464, 1977.

El Shahawy, M., et al.: Diagnosis of aortic valvular prolapse by echocardiography. Chest, 69: 411, 1976.

Estevez, C., et al.: Echocardiographic manifestations of aortic cusp rupture in a myxomatous aortic valve. Chest, 69: 685, 1976.

Honig, H., et al.: Severe aortic regurgitation secondary to idiopathic aortitis. Am. J. Med., 63: 623, 1977.

Kleiner, J., et al.: Echocardiographic manifestation of flail right and noncoronary aortic valve leaflets. Chest, 74: 301, 1978.

Krivokapich, J., et al.: Flail aortic valve leaflets: M-mode and two-dimensional echocardiographic manifestations. Am. Heart J., 99: 425, 1980.

Mardelli, T., et al.: Cross-sectional echocardiographic detection of aortic valve prolapse. Am. Heart J., 100: 295, 1980.

Newman, J., et al.: Cardiac abnormalities associated with rheumatoid arthritis: aortic insufficiency requiring valve replacement. J. Rheumatol., 7: 375, 1980.

Perea, R., et al.: Echocardiographic diagnosis of aortic valve prolapse; report of 2 cases. Rev. Esp. Cardiol., 29: 355, 1976.

Pietro, D., et al.: Premature opening of the aortic valve: an index of highly advanced aortic regurgitation. J. Clin. Ultrasound, 6: 170, 1978.

Rolston, W., et al.: Echocardiographic appearance of ruptured aortic cusp. Am. J. Med., 62: 133, 1977.

Strivastava, T., et al.: Echocardiographic features of flail aortic valve. Chest, 73: 90, 1978.

Tajik, A., et al.: Diastolic opening of aortic valve: an echocardiographic observation. Mayo Clin. Proc., 52: 112, 1977.

Venkataraman, K., et al.: Diastolic flutter of aortic valves in aortic regurgitation. A report of seven cases. Angiology, 30: 297, 1979.

Weaver, W., et al.: Mid-diastolic aortic valve opening in severe acute aortic regurgitation. Circulation, 55: 145, 1977.

Whipple, R.: Echocardiographic manifestations of flail aortic valve leaflets. J. Clin. Ultrasound, 5: 417, 1977.

AORTIC STENOSIS

Subvalvular

Berger, M., et al.: Unsuspected hypertrophic subaortic stenosis in the elderly diagnosed by echocardiography. J. Am. Geriatr. Soc., 27: 178, 1979.

Berry, T., et al.: Echocardiographic assessment of discrete subaortic stenosis in childhood. Am. J. Cardiol., 43: 957, 1979.

Caudill, C., et al.: Membranous subaortic stenosis complicated by aneurysm of the membranous septum and mitral valve prolapse. Circulation, 53: 580, 1976.

Chahine, R., et al.: Mid-systolic closure of aortic valve in hypertrophic cardiomyopathy. Echocardiographic and angiographic correlation. Am. J. Cardiol., 43: 17, 1979.

Chandraratna, P., et al.: Pre- and post-operative echocardiographic features of discrete subaortic stenosis. Cardiology, 61: 181, 1976.

Chung, K., et al.: Echocardiography in co-existing hypertrophic subaortic stenosis and fixed left ventricular outflow obstruction. Circulation, 49: 673, 1974.

Cohen, M.: Idiopathic hypertrophic subaortic stenosis: echocardiographic characteristics. J. Med. Soc. N.J., 77: 447, 1980.

Davis, R., et al.: Echocardiographic manifestations of discrete subaortic stenosis. Am. J. Cardiol., 33: 277, 1974.

Hagaman, J., et al.: Early aortic valve closure in combined idiopathic hypertrophic subaortic stenosis and discrete subaortic stenosis. Am. J. Cardiol., 45: 1083, 1980.

Harrison, E., et al.: Coexisting right and left hypertrophic subvalvular stenosis and fixed left ventricular outflow obstruction due to aortic valve stenosis. Am. J. Cardiol., 40: 133, 1977.

Hess, P., et al.: Echocardiographic features of combined membranous subaortic stenosis and acquired calcific aortic valvulopathy. Am. Heart J., 94: 349, 1977.

Johnson, A., et al.: Combined hypertrophic subaortic stenosis and calcific aortic valvular stenosis. Am. J. Cardiol., 35: 706, 1975.

Johnson, M., et al.: Echocardiography of the aortic valve in non-rheumatic left ventricular outflow tract lesions. Radiology, 112: 677, 1974.

Kelly, D., et al.: Discrete subaortic stenosis. Circulation, 46: 309, 1972.

Krajcer, Z., et al.: Early systolic closure of the aortic valve in patients with hypertrophic subaortic stenosis and discrete subaortic stenosis. Correlation with preoperative and postoperative hemodynamics. Am. J. Cardiol., 41: 823, 1978.

Kronzon, I., et al.: Fixed membranous subaortic stenosis. Chest, 67: 473, 1975.

Krueger, S., et al.: Echocardiographic features of combined hypertrophic and membranous subvalvular aortic stenosis: a case report. J. Clin. Ultrasound, 4: 31, 1976.

Krueger, S., et al.: Echocardiography in discrete subaortic stenosis. Circulation, 59: 506, 1979.

Nanda, N., et al.: Echocardiography in the diagnosis of idiopathic subaortic stenosis co-existing with aortic valve disease. Circulation, 50: 752, 1974.

Popp, R., et al.: Echocardiographic findings in discrete subvalvular aortic stenosis. Circulation, 49: 226, 1974.

Roelandt, J., et al.: Long-segment (tunnel) subaortic stenosis. Chest, 72: 222, 1977.

Sung, C., et al.: Discrete subaortic stenosis in adults. Am. J. Cardiol., 42: 283, 1978.

TenCate, F., et al.: Fixed subaortic stenosis. Value of echocardiography for diagnosis and differentiation between various types. Br. Heart J., 41: 159, 1979.

Weyman, A., et al.: Cross-sectional echocardiography in evaluating patients with discrete subaortic stenosis. Am. J. Cardiol., 37: 358, 1976.

Weyman, A., et al.: Localization of left ventricular outflow obstruction by cross-sectional echocardiography. Am. J. Med., 60: 33, 1976.

Wilcox, W., et al.: Discrete subaortic stenosis: two-dimensional echocardiographic features with angiographic and surgical correlation. Mayo Clin. Proc., 55: 425, 1980.

Williams, E., et al.: Cross-sectional echocardiographic localization of sites of left ventricular outflow tract obstruction. Am. J. Cardiol., 37: 250, 1976.

Supravalvular

Bolen, J., et al.: Echocardiographic features of supravalvular aortic stenosis. Circulation, 52: 817, 1975.

Chang, S., et al.: Recent echocardiographic evaluation of the great vessels and their valves. In Progress in Medical Ultrasound. Vol. 1. Edited by A. Kurjak. Amsterdam, Excerpta Medica, 1980.

Mori, Y., et al.: Echocardiographic and angiocardiographic features of supravalvular aortic stenosis in children. Jpn. Circ. J., 43: 137, 1979.

Nasrallah, A., et al.: Supravalvular aortic stenosis: echocardiographic features. Br. Heart J., 37: 662, 1975.

Shaub, Michael, et al.: Echocardiographic diagnosis of supravalvular aortic stenosis: a case report. J. Clin. Ultrasound, 3: 2, 1975.

Usher, B., et al.: Echocardiographic detection of supravalvular aortic stenosis. Circulation, 49: 1257, 1974.

Weyman, A., et al.: Cross-sectional echocardiographic characterization of aortic obstruction. 1. Supravalvular aortic stenosis and aortic hypoplasia. Circulation, 57: 491, 1978.

Valvular

Bass, J., et al.: Echocardiographic screening to assess the severity of congenital aortic valve stenosis in children. Am. J. Cardiol., 44: 82, 1979.

Blackwood, R., et al.: Aortic stenosis in children. Experience with echocardiographic prediction of severity. Circulation, 57: 263, 1978.

Broderic, T., et al.: Critical aortic stenosis in neonates. Radiology, 129: 393, 1978.

Chang, S., et al.: Aortic stenosis; echocardiographic cusps separation and surgical description of aortic valve in 22 patients. Am. J. Cardiol., 39: 499, 1977.

Clinical conferences at the Johns Hopkins Hospital. Aortic stenosis in the elderly. Johns Hopkins Med. J., *146*: 33, 1980.

DeMaria, A., et al.: Value and limitations of cross-sectional echocardiography of the aortic valve in the diagnosis and quantification of valvular aortic stenosis. Circulation, *62*: 304, 1980.

Feizi, O., et al.: Echocardiography of the aortic valve. I: studies of normal aortic valve, aortic stenosis, aortic regurgitation and mixed aortic valve disease. Br. Heart J., *36*: 341, 1974.

Fowles, R., et al.: Two-dimensional echocardiographic features of bicuspid aortic valve. Chest, *75*: 434, 1979.

Gramiak, R., et al.: Echocardiography of the normal and diseased aortic valve. Radiology, *96*: 1, 1970.

Hernberg, J., et al.: The ultrasonic recording of aortic valve motion. Radiology, *94*: 361, 1970.

Morgan, D., et al.: Occult aortic stenosis as cause of intractable heart failure. Br. Med. J., *1*: 784, 1979.

Nanda, N., et al.: Echocardiographic recognition of the congenital bicuspid aortic valve. Circulation, *49*: 870, 1974.

Radford, D., et al.: Echocardiographic assessment of bicuspid aortic valves: angiographic and pathological correlates. Circulation, *53*: 80, 1976.

Shah, P., et al.: Diagnosis and treatment of aortic valve stenosis. Curr. Probl. Cardiol., *2*: 1, 1977.

Tremblay, G.: Echocardiography. III. Aortic stenosis. Union Med. Can., *106*: 746, 1977.

Vignola, P.: Echocardiographic evaluation of aortic valve and root disease. Med. Clin. North Am., *64*: 205, 1980.

Voelkel, A., et al.: Noninvasive tests to evaluate the severity of aortic stenosis. Limitations and reliability. Chest, *77*: 155, 1980.

Weyman, A., et al.: Cross-sectional echocardiography in assessing the severity of valvular aortic stenosis. Circulation, *52*: 828, 1975.

Weyman, A., et al.: Cross-sectional echocardiographic assessment of the severity of aortic stenosis in children. Circulation, *55*: 773, 1977.

Yeh, H., et al.: Echocardiographic aortic valve orifice dimension; its use in evaluating aortic stenosis and cardiac output. J. Clin. Ultrasound, *1*: 182, 1973.

CORONARY ARTERIES

Chandraratna, P., et al.: Left main coronary arterial patency assessed with cross-sectional echocardiography. Am. J. Cardiol., *46*: 91, 1980.

Chen, C., et al.: Detecting left main coronary artery disease by apical, cross-sectional echocardiography. Circulation, *62*: 288, 1980.

Karlsberg, R., et al.: Noninvasive visualization of right coronary artery aneurysms. Cardiology, *66*: 18, 1980.

Ogawa, S., et al.: A new approach to visualize the left main coronary artery using apical cross-sectional echocardiography. Am. J. Cardiol., *45*: 301, 1980.

Reeder, G., et al.: Visualization of coronary artery fistula by two-dimensional echocardiography. Mayo Clin. Proc., *55*: 185, 1980.

Rogers, E., et al.: Evaluation of left coronary artery anatomy in vitro by cross-sectional echocardiography. Circulation, *62*: 782, 1980.

ENDOCARDITIS

DeMaria, A., et al.: Echography and phonocardiography of acute aortic regurgitation in bacterial endocarditis. Ann. Intern. Med., *82*: 329, 1975.

Dillon, J., et al.: Echocardiographic manifestations of valvular vegetations. Am. Heart J., *86*: 698, 1973.

Fox, S., et al.: Echocardiographic diagnosis of acute aortic valve endocarditis and its complications. Arch. Intern. Med., *137*: 85, 1977.

Gottlieb, S., et al.: Echocardiographic diagnosis of aortic valve vegetations in candida endocarditis. Circulation, *50*: 826, 1974.

Hirschfeld, D., et al.: Localization of aortic valve vegetations by echocardiography. Circulation, *53*: 280, 1976.

Mardelli, T., et al.: Cross-sectional echocardiographic detection of aortic ring abscess in bacterial endocarditis. Chest, *74*: 576, 1978.

Martinez, E., et al.: Echocardiographic diagnosis of vegetative aortic bacterial endocarditis. Am. J. Cardiol., *34*: 845, 1974.

Moorthy, K., et al.: Echocardiographic appearance of aortic valve vegetations in bacterial endocarditis due to Actinobacillus actinomycetemcomitans. J. Clin. Ultrasound, 5: 49, 1977.

Orita, Y., et al.: Detection of flail aortic valve in bacterial endocarditis with real-time, two-dimensional echocardiography. A case report. Jpn. Heart J., *21*: 141, 1980.

Pease, H., et al.: Lethal obstruction by aortic valvular vegetation: echocardiographic studies of endocarditis without apparent aortic regurgitation. Chest, *73*: 658, 1978.

Petersen, J., et al.: Single and multiple beam echocardiography in aortic valve endocarditis. Report of three cases. Acta Med. Scand., *204*: 315, 1978.

Ramirez, J., et al.: Echocardiographic diagnosis of ruptured aortic valve leaflet in bacterial endocarditis. Circulation, *57*: 634, 1978.

Rinke, H., et al.: The echocardiogram in bacterial endocarditis of the aortic valve. *In* Noninvasive Cardiovascular Diagnosis. Edited by E. B. Dietrich. Baltimore, University Park Press, 1978.

Shimada, T., et al.: Acute aortic regurgitation with congestive heart failure due to bacterial endocarditis: diagnosed by echocardiogram and treated successfully by surgery (a case report). Jpn. Circ. J., *43*: 59, 1979.

Shiu, M., et al.: Echocardiographic findings in prolapsed aortic cusp with vegetation. Br. Heart J., *41*: 118, 1979.

Sternberg, L., et al.: Echocardiographic features of an unusual case of aortic valve endocarditis. Can. Med. Assoc. J., *115*: 1022, 1976.

Wray, T.: Echocardiographic manifestations of flail aortic valve leaflets in bacterial endocarditis. Circulation, *51*: 832, 1975.

Wray, T.: The variable echocardiographic features in aortic valve endocarditis. Circulation, *52*: 658, 1975.

Yoshikawa, J., et al.: Cord-like aortic valve vegetation in bacterial endocarditis: demonstration by cardiac ultrasonography. Report of a case. Circulation, *53*: 911, 1976.

9
Tricuspid Valve

The tricuspid valve is located between the right atrium and the right ventricle, medial and inferior in relation to the aortic root. Composed of three cusps, a large anterior leaflet and small septal and posterior leaflets, the tricuspid valve is separated from the pulmonary root by the conus arteriosus. Thus, the tricuspid valve does not have fibrous continuity with the pulmonary root.

Debilitating cardiac disease in the adult patient is primarily confined to the mitral and aortic valves, coronary vessels, myocardium, and pericardium. A patient is practically never referred to an echocardiographer for evaluation of isolated tricuspid valve disease.

Examination of the tricuspid valve should be undertaken when mitral stenosis or left heart myxoma has been identified, to exclude tricuspid stenosis or a prolapsing right atrial tumor. Patients with Marfan's syndrome and prolapse of the mitral valve have a higher incidence of associated tricuspid valve prolapse than do patients with a prolapsing mitral valve from another cause. Intravenous drug abuse is a common source of damage to the tricuspid leaflets secondary to infective endocarditis. An inability to record tricuspid leaflet motion from the right or left parasternum or subcostally suggests tricuspid atresia in the pediatric patient. An increased association between type-B Wolff-Parkinson-White syndrome and Ebstein's anomaly has been shown in the pediatric patient.

RECORDING TECHNIQUE

The examiner should turn the patient to a partial or steep left lateral decubitus position. One should place the transducer in a selected intercostal space along the left parasternum and direct the sound beam toward the aortic root. Then one should angle the sound beam from the aorta directly toward the sternum and inferiorly toward the patient's right flank. The echogram will show transition from anterior aortic wall motion to tricuspid valvular motion (Fig. 9–1).

Anterior and septal tricuspid leaflet motion can be recorded from some older children and adults by placing the transducer along the right parasternum (Fig. 9–2). One should place the patient in a supine or right lateral decubitus position to displace the heart and the lung rightward. After locating mitral

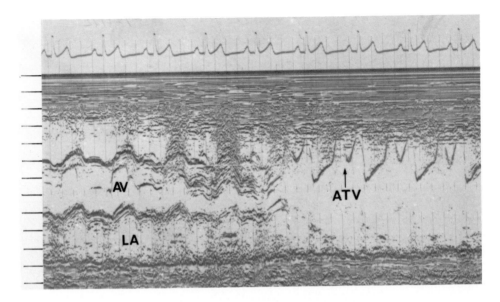

Fig. 9–1. A continuous scan from the aorta to the tricuspid valve. The transducer was at the left parasternum; the sound beam was directed medially and inferiorly from the position required to see the aortic root and leaflet movement. The tricuspid valve was in closer proximity to the transducer than was the anterior aortic wall. The empty space posterior to the tricuspid leaflet motion represented some portion of the right atrium. AV, aortic valve motion; LA, left atrium; ATV, anterior tricuspid leaflet motion.

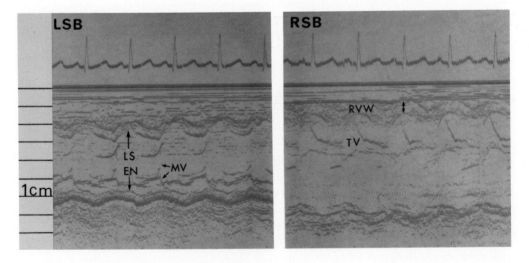

Fig. 9–2. A ten-year-old female patient with left-to-right shunt at the ventricular level, QpQs ratio, 1.2:1. The right ventricular wall (RVW) and the tricuspid leaflet motion (TV) could be recorded only at the right parasternum (RSB). LS, left septum-blood interface; EN, endocardium-blood interface of posterior left ventricular wall; MV, mitral leaflet motion; LSB, left sternal border.

valve motion along the left parasternum, one should relocate the transducer in the same right intercostal space along the right parasternum and direct the sound beam posteriorly and medially. If leaflet motion is incompletely recorded throughout a cardiac cycle, the transducer should be relocated to other right intercostal spaces. The probe's angulation should be manipulated superiorly or inferiorly, as necessary, to visualize leaflet motion. Tricuspid valve motion can be recorded through a supine infant's sternum or subcostally when studies are inadequate along the parasternum.

TRICUSPID VALVE MOTION

In the presence of sinus rhythm, tricuspid and mitral leaflet motion are similar (Fig. 9–3). Alphabetical labels, identical to those designating individual components of mitral valve motion, have been assigned to the opening and closing phases of tricuspid valve movement (Fig. 9–4). Shortly after the completion of systole, the tricuspid leaflets begin to separate and allow blood to flow rapidly from the right atrium into the right

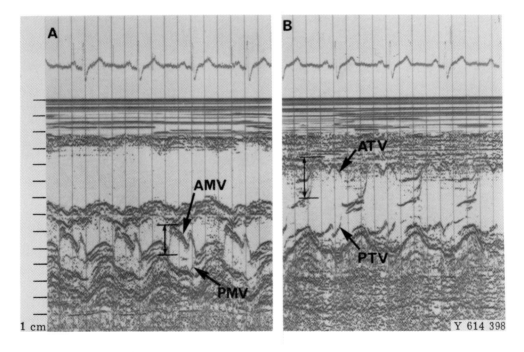

Fig. 9–3. A 48-year-old male patient with an atrial septal defect. Note the increased opening excursion of the anterior tricuspid leaflet (B), as compared to the opening excursion of the anterior mitral leaflet (A). Increased tricuspid leaflet separation is consistent with, but not diagnostic of, right atrial volume overload as from atrial septal defect, partial anomalous pulmonary venous return, or tricuspid regurgitation. AMV, anterior mitral leaflet motion; PMV, posterior mitral leaflet motion; ATV, anterior tricuspid leaflet motion; PTV, septal tricuspid leaflet motion.

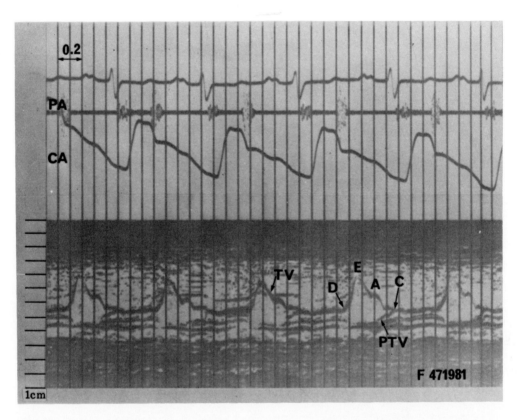

Fig. 9–4. A 47-year-old male patient with chronic renal failure, cardiomyopathy, and pulmonary hypertension. D, onset of tricuspid valve opening; E, maximum valve opening; A, valve opening in response to right atrial contraction; C, tricuspid valve closure; TV, anterior tricuspid leaflet motion; PTV, septal tricuspid leaflet motion; PA, phonocardiogram recorded at third left intercostal space; CA, right carotid pulse.

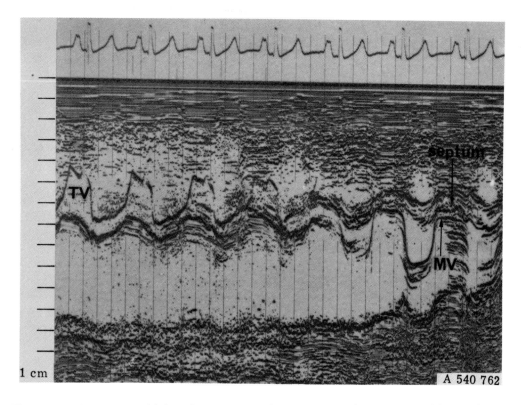

Fig. 9–5. A 21-year-old female patient with severe mitral stenosis, mild mitral and tricuspid regurgitation and pulmonary hypertension. The transducer was at the left parasternum; the sound beam was directed medially to record the tricuspid leaflet motion (TV). Paper recording was continuous while the transducer was redirected laterally toward the mitral valve (MV). When tricuspid and mitral leaflets cannot be recorded simultaneously, this maneuver is adequate to obtain tracings of both valves for the comparative measurement of valve opening or closing time intervals.

ventricle. The leaflets then float toward a semiclosed position. Following atrial depolarization, the valve opens in response to right atrial contraction. It returns to a fully closed position following ventricular depolarization. In the presence of bradycardia, a normal tricuspid valve may close prior to ventricular depolarization.

Whenever tricuspid valve motion is recorded, it should be related to the chest wall, the septum, and the mitral valve. Normally, the tricuspid valve is positioned nearer to the chest wall and is separated from the more posteriorly positioned mitral valve by the interventricular septum (Fig. 9–5). The tricuspid valve should open first and close within 30 msec after mitral valve closure. Delayed tricuspid valve closure occurs with right bundle branch block, type-A Wolff-Parkinson-White syndrome, and Ebstein's anomaly. Generally, the velocity of leaflet opening is comparable to that of the

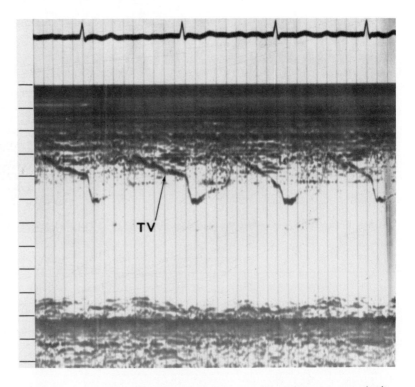

Fig. 9–6. A 53-year-old female patient with moderate, noncalcific mitral stenosis, minimal to mild aortic regurgitation and minimal tricuspid regurgitation, and mild pulmonary hypertension. At catheterization, there was no pressure gradient across the tricuspid valve (TV). The absence of a pressure gradient does not exclude leaflet obstruction when cardiac output is decreased. This patient's cardiac index was low, measuring 2.1 L/min/M².

mitral valve, as is the rate of early diastolic closure prior to atrial contraction.

TRICUSPID STENOSIS

The presence of hemodynamically significant tricuspid stenosis is difficult to establish with M-mode echocardiography. Because of the lower pressures in the right heart, the valve must be badly diseased before a pressure gradient is produced. Although a diminished velocity of early diastolic tricuspid valve closure is compatible with elevated right atrial pressure, a low cardiac output can produce an identical echocardiographic pattern of movement (Fig. 9–6). Unlike the mitral valve, the tricuspid leaflets rarely develop calcification. Hence, the leaflets seldom become excessively echoreflective. Tricuspid opening snaps could be attributed to the mitral valve unless movement of both valves is recorded simultaneously with a phonocardiogram (Fig. 9–7).

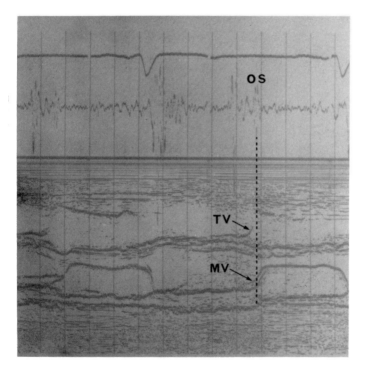

Fig. 9–7. A 41-year-old female patient with an atrial septal defect and an anomalous pulmonary vein. Opening snap (OS) was coincident with maximum opening of the tricuspid valve (TV). Although both atrioventricular valves exhibited an obstructed pattern of movement, no gradients were demonstrated at cardiac catheterization. Cardiac output was not measured.

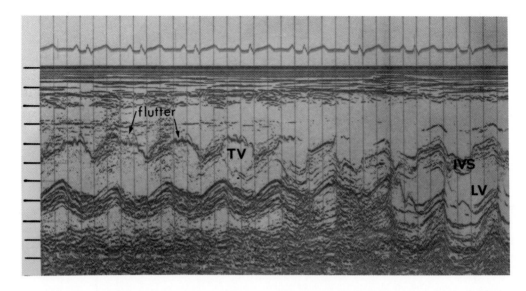

Fig. 9–8. A 24-year-old female patient with pulmonary regurgitation secondary to excision of the pulmonary valve, following two faulty fascia lata repairs for congenital pulmonary stenosis. The fluttering of the anterior tricuspid leaflet was consistent with the localized area of turbulence. TV, tricuspid valve; IVS, interventricular septum; LV, left ventricle.

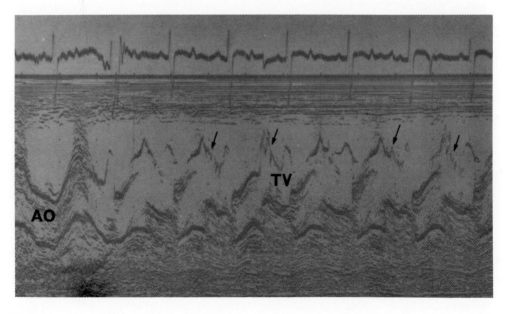

Fig. 9–9. An eight-year-old male patient with a fluttering tricuspid valve (TV), owing to turbulence secondary to high, atrial left-to-right shunt, QpQs ratio, 3:1. AO, aorta. (Tracing recorded by Barbara Keen, St. Vincent's Hospital, Toledo, Ohio.)

FLUTTERING TRICUSPID VALVE

Some coarse fluttering of the tricuspid leaflets may accompany normal blood flow during diastole. High-frequency vibration of the tricuspid leaflets occurs with turbulent blood flow, as from pulmonary regurgitation (Fig. 9–8). Similar high-frequency leaflet vibration has occurred in the presence of an atrial, left-to-right shunt (Fig. 9–9).

INFECTIVE ENDOCARDITIS

Figure 9–10 is an echocardiogram from a patient who had a surgically proven rupture of the right aortic sinus of Valsalva, secondary to infective endocarditis. A mass attached to the

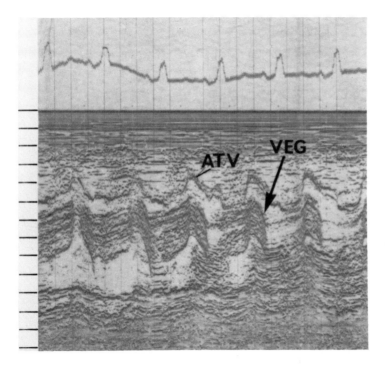

Fig. 9–10. A 24-year-old male patient with infective endocarditis, a ruptured sinus of Valsalva aneurysm, and massive aortic regurgitation. The vegetation (VEG) attached to the right aortic cusp prolapsed through the ruptured sinus into the right atrium and the tricuspid valve orifice. The following data were obtained from catheterization: right atrium, 29 mm Hg (mean); right ventricle, 57/26 mm Hg; pulmonary artery, 56/26 mm Hg; mean pulmonary wedge, 27 mm Hg. ATV, anterior tricuspid leaflet motion. (From Weyman, A., Dillon, D., Feigenbaum, H., and Chang, S.: Premature pulmonic valve opening following sinus of Valsalva aneurysm rupture into the right atrium. Circulation, *51*: 556, 1975. By permission of American Heart Association.)

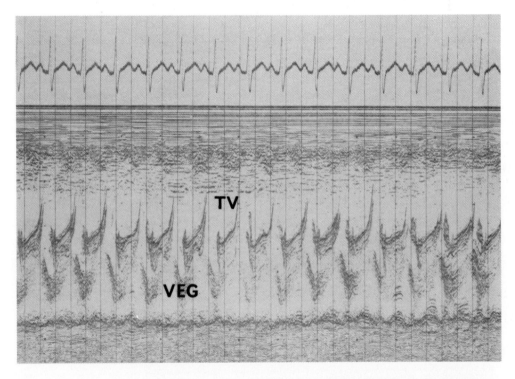

Fig. 9–11. An M-mode echocardiogram of a tricuspid valve vegetation (VEG) from the patient shown in Figure 9–12, *A* and *B*. While the movement of the mass could be appreciated, its size could not be accurately assessed. TV, tricuspid valve motion. (Tracing recorded by Julie Arthur, Medical College of Ohio, Toledo, Ohio.)

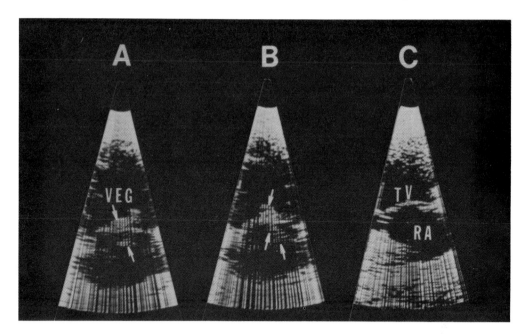

Fig. 9–12. *A* and *B,* A 30-year-old female patient with infective endocarditis secondary to illicit drug use. These single frames from a parasternal, two-dimensional echocardio-gram show the closed tricuspid valve with a large vegetation (VEG) attached to a leaflet. *C,* An 11-year-old female patient with Turner's syndrome. This single frame shows a normal, closed tricuspid valve. RA, right atrium; TV, tricuspid valve. (Tracings *A* and *B* recorded by Julie Arthur, Medical College of Ohio, Toledo, Ohio.)

right aortic leaflet prolapsed through the ruptured sinus into the right atrium and into the tricuspid valve's orifice. Without knowledge of the patient's clinical data, this movement of a vegetation would be indistinguishable from that produced by a right atrial tumor.

Large, mobile vegetations attached to the tricuspid valve frequently result from infective endocarditis, secondary to intravenous drug abuse. Whereas movement of the vegeta-tions is detectable on an M-mode echocardiogram (Fig. 9–11), their size is appreciated better with two-dimensional echocar-diography (Fig. 9–12).

BIBLIOGRAPHY

EBSTEIN'S ANOMALY

Anderson, K., et al.: Pathologic anatomy of Ebstein's anomaly of the heart revisited. Am. J. Cardiol., *41*: 739, 1978.

Barbero-Marcial, M., et al.: Surgical treatment of Ebstein's anomaly. Early and late results in twenty patients subjected to valve replacement. J. Thorac. Cardiovasc. Surg., *78*: 416, 1979.

Crews, T., et al.: Auscultatory and phonocardiographic findings in Ebstein's anomaly. Correlation of the first heart sound with ultrasonic records of tricuspid valve movement. Br. Heart J., *34*: 681, 1972.

Daniel, W., et al.: Value of M-mode echocardiography for noninvasive diagnosis of Ebstein's anomaly. Br. Heart J., 43: 38, 1980.

Farooki, Z., et al.: Echocardiographic spectrum of Ebstein's anomaly of the tricuspid valve. Circulation, 53: 63, 1976.

Giuliani, E., et al.: Ebstein's anomaly: the clinical features and natural history of Ebstein's anomaly of the tricuspid valve. Mayo Clin. Proc., 54: 163, 1979.

Gussenhoven, W., et al.: Echocardiographic criteria for Ebstein's anomaly of tricuspid valve. Br. Heart J., 43: 31, 1980.

Henry, J., et al.: Corrected transposition of great vessels and Ebstein's anomaly of tricuspid valve. Echocardiographic findings. Br. Heart J., 41: 249, 1979.

Hirschklau, M., et al.: Cross-sectional echocardiographic features of Ebstein's anomaly of the tricuspid valve. Am. J. Cardiol., 40: 400, 1977.

Kambe, T., et al.: Apex and subxiphoid approaches to Ebstein's anomaly using cross-sectional echocardiography. Am. Heart J., 100: 53, 1980.

Koiwaya, Y., et al.: Early closure of the tricuspid valve in a case of Ebstein's anomaly with type-B Wolff-Parkinson-White syndrome. Circulation, 60: 446, 1979.

Kotler, M.: Tricuspid valve in Ebstein's anomaly. Circulation, 49: 194, 1974.

Lo, K., et al.: Familial Ebstein's anomaly. Cardiology, 64: 246, 1979.

Lundström, N.: Echocardiography in the diagnosis of Ebstein's anomaly of the tricuspid valve. Circulation, 47: 597, 1973.

Marcelletti, C., et al.: Fontain's operation for Ebstein's anomaly. J. Thorac. Cardiovasc. Surg., 79: 63, 1980.

Matsumoto, M., et al.: Visualization of Ebstein's anomaly of the tricuspid valve by two-dimensional and standard echocardiography. Circulation, 53: 69, 1976.

Monibi, A., et al.: Left ventricular anomalies associated with Ebstein's malformation of the tricuspid valve. Circulation, 57: 303, 1978.

Ng, R., et al.: Ebstein's anomaly: late results of surgical correction. Eur. J. Cardiol., 9: 39, 1979.

Ports, T., et al.: Two-dimensional echocardiographic assessment of Ebstein's anomaly. Circulation, 58: 336, 1978.

Sealy, W.: The cause of the hemodynamic disturbances in Ebstein's anomaly based on observations at operation. Ann. Thorac. Surg., 27: 536, 1979.

Seward, J., et al.: Ebstein's anomaly in an 85-year-old man. Mayo Clin. Proc., 54: 193, 1979.

Tajik, A., et al.: Echocardiogram in Ebstein's anomaly with Wolff-Parkinson-White pre-excitation syndrome, type-B. Circulation, 47: 813, 1973.

Yuste, P., et al.: Ultrasonics in the study of Ebstein's anomaly. Rev. Esp. Cardiol., 26: 339, 1973.

TRICUSPID VALVE

Endocarditis

Berger, M., et al.: Two-dimensional echocardiographic findings in right-sided infective endocarditis. Circulation, 61: 855, 1980.

Chandraratna, P., et al.: Spectrum of echocardiographic findings in tricuspid valve endocarditis. Br. Heart J., 42: 528, 1979.

Crawford, F., et al.: Tricuspid endocarditis in a drug addict; detection of tricuspid vegetations by two-dimensional echocardiography. Chest, 74: 473, 1978.

Kisslo, J., et al.: Echocardiographic evaluation of tricuspid valve endocarditis; an M-mode and two-dimensional study. Am. J. Cardiol., 38: 502, 1976.

Lee, C., et al.: Detection of tricuspid valve vegetations by echocardiography. Chest, 66: 432, 1974.

Lundström, N., et al.: Mitral and tricuspid valve vegetations in infancy diagnosed by echocardiography. Acta Paediatr. Scand., 68: 345, 1979.

Mintz, G., et al.: Wide splitting of the first heart sound secondary to tricuspid valve endocarditis. A phonocardiographic-echocardiographic study. Am. J. Med., 66: 523, 1979.

Sheikh, M., et al.: Right-sided infective endocarditis: an echocardiographic study. Am. J. Med., 66: 283, 1979.

Ward, C., et al.: Tricuspid endocarditis complicating pacemaker implantation demonstrated by echocardiography. Br. J. Radiol., *52*: 501, 1979.

General

Alam, M., et al.: Tricuspid valve fluttering: echocardiographic features of ventricular septal defect. Chest, *77*: 517, 1980.

Edler, I.: The movements of the heart valves recorded by ultrasound. Nord. Med., *64*: 1178, 1960.

Fye, W., et al.: Right atrial angiosarcoma: echocardiographic diagnosis and surgical correlation. Johns Hopkins Med. J., *147*: 111, 1980.

Godman, M., et al.: Echocardiography in the evaluation of the cyanotic newborn infant. Br. Heart J., *36*: 154, 1974.

Hagan, A., et al.: Echocardiographic criteria for normal newborn infants. Circulation, *48*: 1221, 1973.

Kronik, G., et al.: Continuous systolic and diastolic tricuspid valve fluttering: occurrence in a patient with chest pain, dyspnea, and palpitations. Arch. Intern. Med., *138*: 1841, 1978.

Lundström, N.: Clinical applications of echocardiography in infants and children. I. Investigation of infants and children without heart disease. Acta Paediatr. Scand., *63*: 23, 1974.

Lundström, N., et al.: Ultrasoundcardiography in infants and children. Acta Paediatr. Scand., *60*: 117, 1971.

Matsumoto, M., et al.: Echocardiography for the evaluation of the tricuspid valve, right ventricle and atrium. Prog. Cardiovasc. Dis., *21*: 1, 1978.

Milner, S., et al.: Mitral and tricuspid valve closure in congenital heart disease. Circulation, *53*: 513, 1976.

Nanda, N., et al.: Echocardiography of the tricuspid valve in congenital left ventricular-right atrial communication. Circulation, *51*: 268, 1975.

Nimura, Y., et al.: The ultrasound cardiogram of the tricuspid valve in healthy subjects. Jpn. Heart J., *13*: 394, 1972.

Silver, M. et al.: Morphology of the human tricuspid valve. Circulation, *43*: 333, 1971.

Solinger, R., et al.: Echocardiography in the normal neonate. Circulation, *47*: 108, 1973.

Starling, M., et al.: Value of the tricuspid valve echogram for estimating right ventricular end-diastolic pressure during vasodilator therapy. Am. J. Cardiol., *45*: 966, 1980.

Tavel, M., et al.: Opening snap of the tricuspid valve in atrial septal defect: a phonocardiographic and reflected ultrasound study of sounds in relationship to movements of the tricuspid valve. Am. Heart J., *80*: 555, 1970.

Waider, W., et al.: First heart sound and ejection sounds: echocardiographic and phonocardiographic correlation with valvular events. Am. J. Cardiol., *35*: 346, 1975.

Obstruction

Anderson, R., et al.: Atresia of the right atrioventricular orifice. Br. Heart J., *39*: 414, 1977.

Beppu, S., et al.: Two-dimensional echocardiography in diagnosing tricuspid atresia: differentiation from other hypoplastic right heart syndromes and common atrioventricular canal. Br. Heart J., *40*: 1174, 1978.

Durairaj, M., et al.: Tricuspid atresia. Indian Heart J., *30*: 303, 1978.

Joyner, C., et al.: Reflected ultrasound in the diagnosis of tricuspid stenosis. Am. J. Cardiol., *19*: 66, 1967.

Mehl, S., et al.: Combined tricuspid and pulmonic stenosis. Clinical, echocardiographic, hemodynamic, surgical and pathological features. J. Thorac. Cardiovasc. Surg., *74*: 55, 1977.

Seward, J., et al.: Echocardiographic spectrum of tricuspid atresia. Mayo Clin. Proc., *53*: 100, 1978.

Sharratt, G., et al.: Persistence and effects of sinus rhythm after Fontan procedure for tricuspid atresia. Br. Heart J., *42*: 74, 1979.

Silverman, N., et al.: Simulated tricuspid valve echoes in tricuspid atresia. Am. Heart J., *95*: 761, 1978.

Takahashi, O., et al.: Tricuspid and pulmonic valve echoes in tricuspid and pulmonary atresia. Chest, *76*: 437, 1979.

Vaseenon, T., et al.: Tricuspid atresia with double-outlet left ventricle and bilateral conus. Chest, 74: 676, 1978.

Prolapse

Chandraratna, P., et al.: Echocardiographic detection of tricuspid valve prolapse. Circulation, 51: 823, 1975.

Chandraratna, P., et al.: The association between atrial septal defect and prolapse of the tricuspid valve. An echocardiographic study. Chest, 73: 839, 1978.

Karayannis, E., et al.: Use of echocardiography in the diagnosis of prolapsed tricuspid valve. J. Med. Assoc. Ga., 67: 205, 1978.

Sassé, L., et al.: Echocardiographic tricuspid prolapse and non-ejection systolic click. Chest, 73: 869, 1978.

Shah, K., et al.: Tricuspid valve prolapse. An echocardiographic diagnosis. Indian Heart J., 32: 55, 1980.

Werner, J., et al.: Occurrence and significance of echocardiographically demonstrated tricuspid valve prolapse. Am. Heart J., 96: 180, 1978.

Regurgitation

Bardy, G., et al.: Acquired cyanotic heart disease secondary to traumatic tricuspid regurgitation. Am. J. Cardiol., 44: 1401, 1979.

Lieppe, W., et al.: Detection of tricuspid regurgitation with two-dimensional echocardiography and peripheral vein injections. Circulation, 57: 128, 1978.

Meltzer, R., et al.: Diagnosis of tricuspid regurgitation by contrast echocardiography. Circulation, 63: 1093, 1981.

Seides, S., et al.: Echocardiographic findings in isolated, surgically created tricuspid insufficiency. Am. J. Cardiol., 35: 679, 1974.

Yoshikawa, J., et al.: Reappraisal of jugular phlebogram in the diagnosis of tricuspid regurgitation. Relationship between echocardiographic interventricular septal motion and jugular phlebogram. Jpn. Heart J., 18: 31, 1977.

10
Pulmonary Valve and Artery

The pulmonary valve and root are positioned superior to the mitral valve and anterior, lateral, and superior to the aortic root. Three pouched cusps occupy the pulmonary root. Unlike the aortic root, the normal pulmonary root does not contain coronary ostia.

In the older child and the adult patient, left pulmonary leaflet motion is most often recorded, since it is more perpendicular to the sound beam (Fig. 10–1). Absent or incomplete pulmonary leaflet motion results when the leaflets are parallel to the sound beam or when the great vessels are positioned side by side with an unusual rightward displacement. The inability to record leaflet motion does not confirm a diagnosis of hypoplasia or atresia of the pulmonary leaflets and root, but this possibility should be considered in the "blue" infant with appropriate clinical findings. I have recorded normal pulmo-

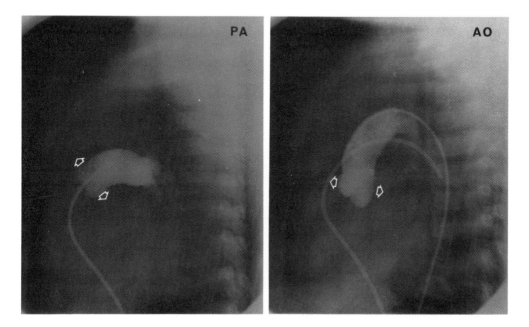

Fig. 10–1. An eight-month-old male patient with endocardial fibroelastosis. Lateral cineangiograms of the pulmonary root (PA) and the aortic root (AO) show the orientation of these vessels and their valves in relation to the anterior chest wall. Arrows indicate the direction of valvular movement during systole.

nary valve motion from the right parasternum when it was unavailable through the neonatal sternum or from any site over the left precordium.

RECORDING TECHNIQUE

The patient may be either supine or positioned in a shallow left lateral decubitus position to displace the lung leftward. The transducer should be placed over the precordial pulmonary artery pulsation and should be carefully angled in any direction necessary to record left pulmonary leaflet motion.

Using the mitral valve as an initial landmark, pulmonary valve motion can be recorded from lower intercostal spaces. One should angle the transducer cephalad from the mitral valve toward the left ear. Many echoes will be reflected from the conus arteriosus (Figs. 10–2 and 10–3). More cephalad and medial transducer angulation causes the sound beam to pass through the posterior aspect of the pulmonary root and the left pulmonary leaflet. The relation of the pulmonary valve to the aortic valve may be established by angling the transducer medially and inferiorly toward the right shoulder. The pulmo-

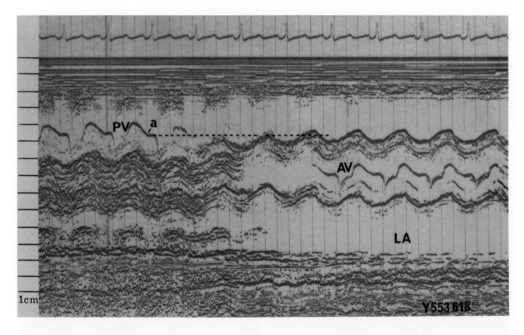

Fig. 10–2. A 30-year-old female patient with renal failure. In this scan from the pulmonary valve (PV) to the aortic valve (AV), the conus arteriosus is located posterior to the pulmonary leaflet movement and is an excellent landmark when searching for pulmonary leaflet motion. The pulmonary valve lies in closer proximity to the chest wall than does the aortic valve, which is confined by the aortic walls. a, "a-wave" or movement of pulmonary leaflet secondary to pressure changes initiated by right atrial contraction; LA, left atrium.

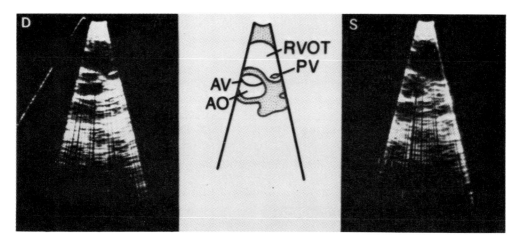

Fig. 10–3. A normal ten-year-old male patient. The anatomic orientation of the aortic root, the right ventricular outflow tract, and the pulmonary valve are shown in selected frames from a parasternal short-axis, two-dimensional echocardiogram. The left pulmonary leaflet is visible during diastole (D), but disappears during systole (S) as it opens away from the transducer. AO, aorta; AV, aortic valve; RVOT, right ventricular outflow tract; PV, pulmonary valve.

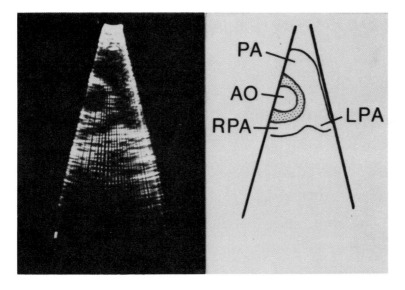

Fig. 10–4. A still frame and its diagram from a two-dimensional echocardiogram from the patient in Figure 10–3. The orientation of the transducer was long axis to the pulmonary artery trunk (PA) and short axis to the proximal ascending aorta (AO). This view was obtained by a slight superior transducer angulation from the view shown in Figure 10–3. Minimal clockwise or counterclockwise transducer rotation may be required to visualize the pulmonary artery bifurcation. This view is useful to evaluate the presence of the right (RPA) and left (LPA) pulmonary arteries and the diameter of the pulmonary artery trunk.

nary root and leaflets are positioned near the transducer. The aortic valve is positioned more posteriorly and is confined by well-defined aortic walls (Figs. 10–2 and 10–3).

Short-axis, two-dimensional echocardiography shows the relationship between the right ventricular outflow tract and the aorta. Normally, the distal right ventricular infundibulum is positioned anteriorly to the aortic root, curving around this structure toward the right (Fig. 10–3). During diastole, aortic and pulmonary leaflets are visible. During systole, the pulmonary leaflet disappears as it opens away from the transducer. With minimum superior angulation, the main pulmonary artery and its bifurcation become visible (Fig. 10–4). This is a good view by which to obtain the diameter of the pulmonary artery and to detect areas of dilatation (idiopathic, poststenotic) or narrowing (subpulmonic stenosis, pulmonary banding, supravalvular stenosis, congenital hypoplasia).

M-mode echographic records are more easily analyzed if they are recorded at 50 to 75 mm/sec on ultraviolet recorders and at 100 mm/sec on black-white recorders. Time line intervals of 40 msec may be superimposed over the tracing if desired. A simultaneous phonocardiogram assists in the identification of pulmonary valve closure (Fig. 10–5).

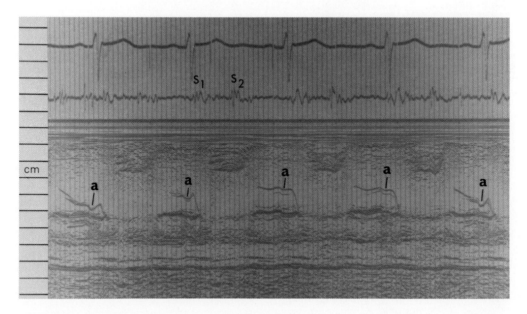

Fig. 10–5. A normal 23-year-old female patient. The normal pulmonary valve demonstrated an "a-wave" response during quiet expiration. The "a-wave" depth increased during inspiration. Valve closure was not seen on this tracing, but the P_2 component of the second heart sound (S_2) could be used to identify the right heart end-systole. S_1, first heart sound.

NORMAL PULMONARY VALVE MOTION

Alphabetical labels assist in the discussion of the individual components of left pulmonary leaflet motion (Fig. 10–6). Appropriately, the valve's opening response to right atrial contraction has been designated "a-wave" or "a-dip," followed by rapid posterior movement away from the transducer as the valve opens into the pulmonary artery (b to c). The pulmonary valve remains open throughout systole (c to d) with rapid closure following the onset of isovolumic relaxation (d to e). The c–d component is often not recorded in the normal person. The open leaflet is parallel to the interrogating sound beam, and echoes are not reflected back to the transducer.

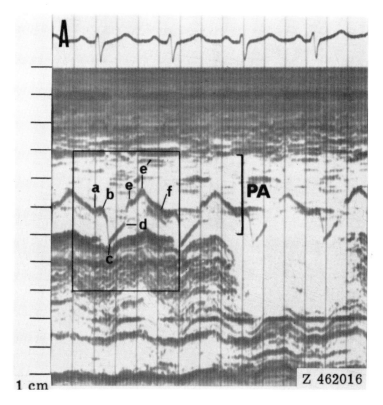

Fig. 10–6. A female patient with renal failure and clinical pulmonary hypertension. The motion of the left pulmonary leaflet throughout diastole and systole was: a, "a-wave" response to right atrial contraction; b to c, rapid opening of the leaflet during diastole; c to d, leaflet fully open throughout systole; d to e, rapid leaflet closure; e', termination of pulmonary valve closure. e' to f, diastolic displacement of the pulmonary root and leaflet; PA, pulmonary artery. (From Weyman, A., Dillon, J., Feigenbaum, H., and Chang, S.: Echocardiographic patterns of pulmonary valve motion in valvular pulmonary stenosis. Am. J. Cardiol., 34: 644, 1974.)

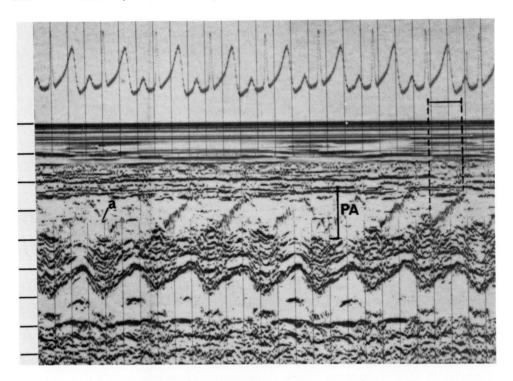

Fig. 10–7. This marked systolic and early diastolic pulmonary leaflet fluttering was consistent with infundibular pulmonary stenosis. However, this finding is not pathognomonic for this anatomic abnormality. The "a-wave" (a) is absent in most cases of significant subpulmonary valve obstruction. PA, pulmonary artery. (From Weyman, A., Dillon, J., Feigenbaum, H., and Chang, S.: Echocardiographic differentiation of infundibular from valvular pulmonary stenosis. Am. J. Cardiol., 36: 21, 1975.)

Early pulmonary valve closure may be followed by some anterior displacement of the valve throughout the remainder of systole (e to e'). The valve moves rapidly posteriorly during atrial emptying and ventricular filling (e' to f). Mild systolic fluttering of the c–d component has no known clinical significance. Accentuated leaflet fluttering, persisting throughout systole and into early diastole, has been compatible with subpulmonary valve obstruction (Fig. 10–7).

"a-wave"

Examination of the normal pulmonary valve from several different precordial locations should reveal "a-wave" movement during quiet expiration. Within 120 msec of the onset of atrial depolarization, the left pulmonary leaflet is displaced 3 to 7 mm posteriorly (Fig. 10–8). Since "a-wave" displacement is increased during inspiration, the quantity of displacement should be evaluated only during quiet expiration. "A-wave" depth increases in the presence of bradycardia and severe

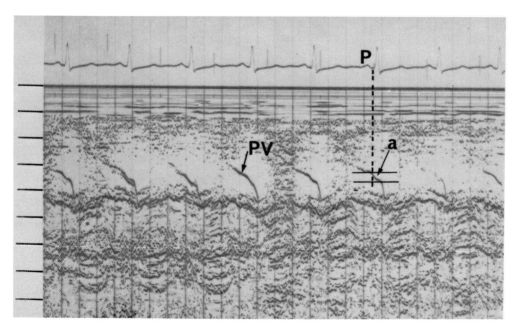

Fig. 10–8. Normal left pulmonary leaflet motion (PV). The late diastolic and early systolic movement of the valve was most commonly recorded in older children and adults. The late systolic valve movement was poorly recorded, since the sound beam and the leaflet motion are nearly parallel. a, "a-wave" response to pressure changes secondary to atrial contraction; P, atrial depolarization.

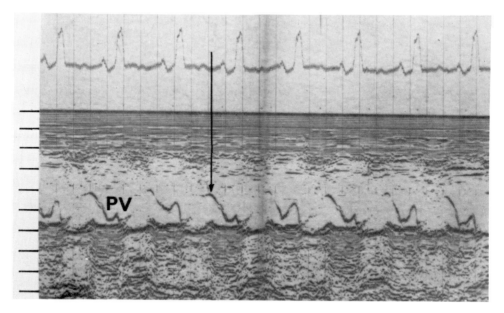

Fig. 10–9. A 24-year-old male patient with a ruptured sinus of Valsalva aneurysm with massive aortic regurgitation shunted into the right atrium. Pulmonary valve opening began before atrial contraction (arrow). Presystolic pulmonary valve opening was consistent with an acute rise in ventricular diastolic pressure. The following pressures were obtained at cardiac catheterization: right atrium, 29 mm Hg (mean); right ventricle, 57/26 mm Hg; pulmonary artery, 56/26 mm Hg; mean pulmonary wedge, 27 mm Hg; descending aorta, 140/39 mm Hg. PV, pulmonary leaflet motion.

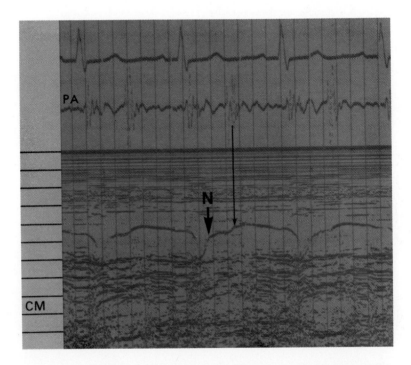

Fig. 10–10. A 30-year-old female patient with a postoperative atrial septal defect repair and severe pulmonary hypertension. Immediately following the maximum systolic leaflet opening, the pulmonary leaflet moved rapidly toward closure. Its movement was abruptly diminished at midsystole (N). This pattern of movement is a sensitive sign of elevated pulmonary pressure and resistance to flow, but it is not specific for pulmonary hypertension. PA, phonocardiogram recorded at third left intercostal space.

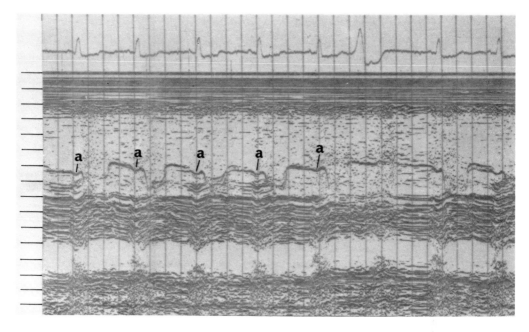

Fig. 10–11. A 72-year-old coal miner with restrictive lung disease, tricuspid regurgitation, and congestive heart failure. Although this patient had severe pulmonary hypertension, the pulmonary valve exhibited an "a-wave" (a) secondary to elevated right atrial pressure. The following pressures were obtained at catheterization: right atrium, 14 mm Hg (mean); a wave, 21 mm Hg; v wave, 17 mm Hg; right ventricle, 73/16 mm Hg; pulmonary artery, 73/30 mm Hg; pulmonary wedge, 15 mm Hg (mean); cardiac output, 2.7 L/min; cardiac index, 1.5 L/min/m². Pulmonary vascular resistance, 12 units. There was no evidence of constrictive pericardial disease.

pulmonary stenosis. Severe constrictive pericarditis or a ruptured sinus of Valsalva aneurysm may cause the valve to open before ventricular depolarization, if the right ventricular diastolic pressure exceeds pulmonary diastolic pressure (Fig. 10–9). The "a-wave" disappears in the presence of atrial fibrillation and is diminished or absent in the presence of pulmonary hypertension (Fig. 10–10). Extreme elevation of the right atrial pressure causes the "a-wave" to reappear, even though significant pulmonary hypertension is present (Fig. 10–11).

RIGHT HEART SYSTOLIC TIME INTERVALS

Calculation of right heart systolic time intervals provides a noninvasive method by which to evaluate diastolic pulmonary artery pressure and right ventricular function. These time intervals are particularly useful to follow a patient with progressive pulmonary hypertension or to monitor the effect of medical or surgical treatment altering right heart hemodynamics. The data are influenced by many variables, and their clinical compatibility must be constantly evaluated.

Right Ventricular Pre-ejection Period (RPEP)

Some time is required for the right ventricle to raise its diastolic pressure enough to exceed the diastolic pulmonary artery pressure and to open the pulmonary valve. This time is known as the pre-ejection period, measured from the onset of ventricular depolarization to the onset of rapid pulmonary valve opening. Often the valve appears to open in two phases, *b to b'* and *b' to c*. For consistency, I prefer to measure from the onset of ventricular depolarization to the *b'* component, where valve opening accelerates (Fig. 10–12). At comparable heart rates, the right heart pre-ejection period is shorter than the left heart pre-ejection period. It increases in the presence of a right bundle branch block.

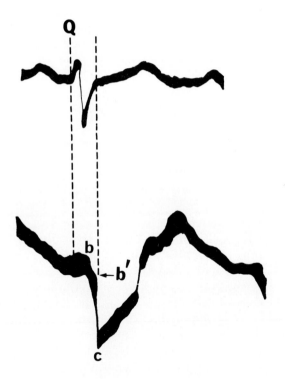

Fig. 10–12. A diagram of the left pulmonary leaflet motion from Figure 10–6. PEP, the time interval required to raise the right ventricular diastolic pressure to exceed the pulmonary diastolic pressure and the open valve. This time interval was measured from the electrocardiographic "Q" or onset of ventricular depolarization to b'. c, the maximum opening of the left pulmonary leaflet.

Right Ventricular Ejection Time (RVET)

The ejection time interval is the duration of time the pulmonary valve remains open (Fig. 10–13). End-systolic coaptation of the anterior and left pulmonary leaflets is most easily recorded in the infant or young child. Whenever possible, one should record a simultaneous phonocardiogram to identify valve closure coincident with the P_2 component of the second heart sound (see Figs. 10–5 and 10–10). At comparable heart rates, the right heart ejection time is longer than the left heart ejection time. The length of this time interval decreases with tachycardia and with low stroke volume.

Systolic Time Intervals Ratio

To derive a ratio between pre-ejection and ejection time intervals, one should divide the former by the latter, RPEP/RVET. This ratio is insignificantly influenced by age or by

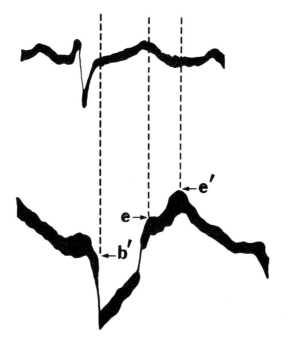

RVET

Fig. 10–13. A diagram of the left pulmonary leaflet motion from Figure 10–6. RVET, right ventricular ejection time; that is, the duration of the blood flow into the pulmonary artery from the right ventricle. The addition of a phonocardiogram is essential to identify the absolute end of systole, e or e'.

heart rate. For practical purposes, a ratio under 0.30 is consistent with normal diastolic pulmonary artery pressure unless both pre-ejection and ejection time intervals are unusually shortened or prolonged. Ratios exceeding 0.40 suggest an elevation of diastolic pulmonary pressure exceeding 25 mm Hg. Ratios exceeding 0.50 may reflect faulty right ventricular myocardial contraction rather than pure elevation of pulmonary pressure or resistance. Clinical correlation is always essential.

BIBLIOGRAPHY

PULMONARY ARTERY AND VALVE

Acquatella, H., et al.: Lack of correlation between echocardiographic pulmonary valve morphology and simultaneous pulmonary arterial pressure. Am. J. Cardiol., 43: 946, 1979.

Asayama, J., et al.: Echocardiographic findings of idiopathic dilatation of the pulmonary artery. Chest, 71: 671, 1977.

Atsuchi, Y., et al.: Echocardiographic detection of pulmonic valve vegetation. Jpn. Heart J., 18: 138, 1977.

Bauman, W., et al.: Mid-systolic notching of the pulmonary valve in the absence of pulmonary hypertension. Am. J. Cardiol., 43: 1049, 1979.

Bracchi, G., et al.: Relation between echocardiography of the pulmonary valve and the hemodynamics of chronic cor pulmonale. Bronchopneumologie, 27: 131, 1977.

Chandraratna, P., et al.: Echocardiographic observations on the mechanism of the second heart sound. Circulation, 51: 292, 1975.

Ebina, T., et al.: The ultrasono-tomography for the heart and great vessels in living human subjects by means of the ultrasonic reflection technique. Jpn. Heart J., 8: 331, 1967.

Edler, I., et al.: Ultrasound-cardiography. Acta Med. Scand. (Suppl.), 170: 37, 1961.

Fenichel, N., et al.: The effect of respiratory motion on the echocardiogram. Chest, 69: 655, 1976.

French, J., et al.: Echocardiographic findings in Uhl's anomaly: demonstration of diastolic pulmonary valve opening. Am. J. Cardiol., 36: 349, 1975.

Glasser, S., et al.: Pulmonary valve fluttering in subpulmonic ventricular septal defect. Am. Heart J., 94: 3, 1977.

Goodman, D., et al.: Echocardiographic features of primary pulmonary hypertension. Am. J. Cardiol., 33: 438, 1974.

Gramiak, R., et al.: Echocardiographic detection of the pulmonary valve. Radiology, 102: 153, 1972.

Green, E., et al.: Right-sided Austin Flint murmur: documentation of intracardiac phonocardiography, echocardiography and postmortem findings. Am. J. Cardiol., 32: 370, 1973.

Hada, Y., et al.: Echocardiogram of the pulmonary valve. Variability of the pattern and the related technical problems. Jpn. Heart J., 18: 298, 1977.

Hada, Y., et al.: Echocardiographic patterns of normal pulmonary valve motion. Jpn. Heart J., 18: 421, 1977.

Heger, J., et al.: A review of M-mode and cross-sectional echocardiographic findings of the pulmonary valve. J. Clin. Ultrasound, 7: 98, 1979.

Karmarkar, S.: Pulmonary valve echocardiography. J. Postgrad. Med., 25: 219, 1979.

Kasper, W., et al.: Echocardiography in assessing acute pulmonary hypertension due to pulmonary embolism. Am. J. Cardiol., 45: 567, 1980.

Kerber, R., et al.: Effects of acute hemodynamic alterations on pulmonic valve motion. Circulation, 60: 1074, 1979.

Kramer, N., et al.: Pulmonary valve vegetations detected with echocardiography. Am. J. Cardiol., 39: 1064, 1977.

Lew, W., et al.: Assessment of pulmonary valve echogram in normal subjects and in patients with pulmonary arterial hypertension. Br. Heart J., 42: 147, 1979.

McAlpine, W.: Heart and Coronary Arteries. New York, Springer-Verlag, 1975.

Millard, D., et al.: Dissecting aortic aneurysm diagnosed by echocardiography in a patient with rupture of the aneurysm into the right atrium. Am. J. Cardiol., 30: 427, 1972.

Mills, P., et al.: Noninvasive assessment of pulmonary hypertension from right ventricular isovolumic contraction time. Am. J. Cardiol., 46: 272, 1980.

Nanda, N., et al.: Evaluation of pulmonary hypertension by echocardiography. J. Clin. Ultrasound, 1: 255, 1973.

Nanda, N.: Echocardiography of tricuspid and pulmonary valves. Cardiovasc. Clin., 9: 97, 1978.

Nussbaum, E., et al.: Echocardiographic changes in children with pulmonary hypertension secondary to upper airway obstruction. J. Pediatr., 93: 931, 1978.

Pocoski, D., et al.: Physiologic correlates of echocardiographic pulmonary valve motion in diastole. Circulation, 58: 1064, 1978.

Rothbaum, D., et al.: Echocardiographic manifestation of right sinus of Valsalva aneurysm. Circulation, 49: 768, 1974.

Sakamoto, T., et al.: Echocardiogram of the pulmonary valve. Jpn. Heart J., 15: 360, 1974.

Sakamoto, T., et al.: Echocardiogram and phonocardiogram related to the movement of the pulmonary valve. Jpn. Heart J., 16: 107, 1975.

Sakamoto, T., et al.: Echocardiography of the semilunar valves. Jpn. Circ. J., 43: 313, 1979.

Shah, P.: Echocardiography of the aortic and pulmonary valves. Prog. Cardiovasc. Dis., 10: 451, 1978.

Silverman, N., et al.: Evaluation of pulmonary hypertension by M-mode echocardiography in children with ventricular septal defect. Circulation, 61: 1125, 1980.

Wann, L., et al.: Premature pulmonary valve opening. Circulation, 55: 128, 1977.

Weyman, A.: Pulmonary valve echo motion in clinical practice. Am. J. Med., 62: 843, 1977.

Weyman, A., et al.: Echocardiographic patterns of pulmonary valve motion with pulmonary hypertension. Circulation, 50: 905, 1974.

Yoshida, Y., et al.: Echocardiographic evaluation of pulmonary hypertension by oxygen inhalation method. Tohoku J. Exp. Med., 127: 199, 1979.

Yoshikawa, J., et al.: Echocardiographic features of congenital pulmonary regurgitation. Jpn. Heart J., 19: 58, 1978.

PULMONARY OBSTRUCTION

Assad-Morell, J., et al.: Echo-phonocardiographic and contrast studies in conditions associated with systemic arterial trunk over-riding the ventricular septum: truncus arteriosus, tetralogy of Fallot, and pulmonary atresia with ventricular septal defect. Circulation, 53: 663, 1976.

Caldwell, R., et al.: Right ventricular outflow tract assessment by cross-sectional echocardiography in tetralogy of Fallot. Circulation, 59: 395, 1979.

Eslam, B., et al.: Paradoxical septal motion in a patient with pulmonic stenosis. Chest, 67: 244, 1975.

Flanagan, W., et al.: Echocardiographic correlate of pre-systolic pulmonary ejection sound in congenital valvular pulmonic stenosis. Am. Heart J., 94: 633, 1977.

Garcia, E., et al.: Echocardiographic assessment of the adequacy of pulmonary arterial banding. Am. J. Cardiol., 44: 487, 1979.

Kasper, W., et al.: Echocardiography in assessing acute pulmonary hypertension due to pulmonary embolism. Am. J. Cardiol., 45: 567, 1980.

Lewis, B., et al.: Echocardiographic diagnosis of pulmonary atresia with intact ventricular septum. Am. Heart J., 97: 92, 1979.

Lutz, J., et al.: "Pseudo-tumor" of the right ventricular outflow tract and congenital pulmonary valve regurgitation: a case report. Am. Heart J., 100: 349, 1980.

Mahoney, L., et al.: Cardiac rhabdomyoma simulating pulmonic stenosis. Cathet. Cardiovasc. Diagn., 5: 385, 1979.

Mehl, S., et al.: Combined tricuspid and pulmonic stenosis. Clinical, echocardiographic, hemodynamic, surgical and pathological features. J. Thorac. Cardiovasc. Surg., 74: 55, 1977.

Nagai, Y., et al.: Echocardiographic findings of congenital absence of the pulmonary valve with tetralogy of Fallot. Chest, 75: 481, 1979.

Takahashi, O., et al.: Tricuspid and pulmonic echoes in tricuspid and pulmonary atresia. Chest, 76: 437, 1979.

Weyman, A., et al.: Echocardiographic pattern of pulmonary valve motion in valvular pulmonary stenosis. Am. J. Cardiol., 34: 644, 1974.

Weyman, A., et al.: Echocardiographic differentiation of infundibular from valvular pulmonary stenosis. Am. J. Cardiol., 36: 21, 1975.

Weyman, A., et al.: Cross-sectional echocardiographic visualization of the stenotic pulmonary valve. Circulation, 56: 769, 1977.

RUPTURED SINUS OF VALSALVA ANEURYSM

Cooperberg, P., et al.: Rupture of a sinus of Valsalva aneurysm. Report of a case diagnosed pre-operatively by echocardiography. Radiology, 113: 171, 1974.

DeSa'Neto, A., et al.: Right sinus of Valsalva-right atrial fistula secondary to nonpenetrating chest trauma: a case report with description of noninvasive diagnostic features. Circulation, 60: 205, 1979.

Matsumoto, M., et al.: Echocardiographic diagnosis of ruptured aneurysm of sinus of Valsalva: report of two cases. Circulation, 53: 382, 1976.

Millward, D., et al.: Dissecting aortic aneurysm diagnosed by echocardiography in a patient with rupture of the aneurysm into the right atrium. Am. J. Cardiol., 30: 427, 1972.

Oberhänsli, I., et al.: Aneurysm of the left sinus of Valsalva draining into the right atrium. Chest, 76: 322, 1979.

Rothbaum, D., et al.: Echocardiographic manifestation of right sinus of Valsalva aneurysm. Circulation, 49: 768, 1974.

Sher, R., et al.: Aneurysm of the sinus of Valsalva: its natural history. Postgrad. Med., 65: 191, 1979.

Weyman, A., et al.: Premature pulmonic valve opening following sinus of Valsalva aneurysm rupture into the right atrium. Circulation, 51: 556, 1975.

Wong, B., et al.: Echocardiographic features of an aneurysm of the left sinus of Valsalva. Chest, 73: 105, 1978.

Yoshida, S., et al.: Ruptured sinus of Valsalva aneurysm into the left ventricle. Jpn. Heart J., 19: 954, 1978.

SYSTOLIC TIME INTERVALS

Gutgesell, H.: Echocardiographic estimation of pulmonary artery pressure in transposition of the great arteries. Circulation, 57: 1151, 1978.

Halliday, H., et al.: Echographic ventricular systolic time intervals in normal term and preterm neonates. Pediatrics, 62: 317, 1978.

Hedvall, G.: Systolic time intervals in newborn infants. Acta Paediatr. Scand., 64: 839, 1975.

Hirschfeld, S., et al.: Measurement of right and left ventricular systolic time intervals by echocardiography. Circulation, 51: 304, 1975.

Hirschfeld, S., et al.: The echocardiographic assessment of pulmonary artery pressure and pulmonary vascular resistance. Circulation, 52: 642, 1975.

Johnson, G., et al.: Echocardiographic assessment of pulmonary arterial pressure in children with complete right bundle branch block. Am. J. Cardiol., 41: 1264, 1978.

Kerber, R., et al.: Effects of acute hemodynamic alterations on pulmonic valve motion. Circulation, 60: 1074, 1979.

Leighton, R., et al.: Right and left ventricular systolic time intervals. Effects of heart rate, respiration and atrial pacing. Am. J. Cardiol., 27: 66, 1971.

Riggs, T., et al.: Neonatal circulatory changes: an echocardiographic study. Pediatrics, 59: 338, 1977.

Riggs, T., et al.: Assessment of the pulmonary vascular bed by echocardiographic right ventricular systolic time intervals. Circulation, 57: 939, 1978.

Spooner, E., et al.: Estimation of pulmonary/systemic resistance ratios from echocardiographic systolic time intervals in young patients with congenital or acquired heart disease. Am. J. Cardiol., *42*: 810, 1978.

Tsuda, S.: Studies on right ventricular performance by noninvasive measurement of systolic and diastolic time intervals in patients with chronic right ventricular overloading. Jpn. Circ. J., *42*: 1319, 1978.

11

Prosthetic Valves

Patients with prosthetic valves are referred to echocardiography for evaluation of poppet movement, thrombotic obstruction, and intracardiac chamber size and ventricular function. Single examinations contribute little information concerning a valve's function, particularly progressive dysfunction. Serial studies are more useful when compared to early postoperative tracings. Changes in echo intensity, with clinical findings of embolic episodes, fever, fainting, or the onset of new murmurs, assist in the identification of causes of valvular dysfunction. However, even serial evaluations have not heralded a catastrophic systemic embolism or dehiscence of the prosthesis.

RECORDING TECHNIQUE

Starr-Edwards Prosthesis—Aortic Position

The echocardiographer should place the transducer in the supraclavicular fossa (Fig. 11–1) or at the second intercostal space along the right parasternal border. The sound beam should be aligned perpendicularly to the poppet as it moves *toward* the transducer at the onset of systole (Fig. 11–2A, arrow). The poppet should remain open throughout systole and should move away from the transducer to a closed position at the end of systole.

When the motion of the poppet cannot be recorded from the supraclavicular position, the transducer should be moved to the cardiac apex. The sound beam should be directed through the long axis of the left ventricle (Fig. 11–1). Poppet motion will be *away* from the transducer at the onset of systole and will return toward the transducer at the completion of systole (Figs. 11–2B and 11–3).

Long-axis, two-dimensional echocardiography (see Fig. 8–1) is useful to detect significant changes in the quantity of echoes reflected from prosthetic aortic valves when infective endocarditis is a tenable diagnosis. Large abscesses become apparent as unusually echo-reflective areas near the suture lines. Dilatation of a sinus of Valsalva or of the whole aortic root can be detected with M-mode and two-dimensional echocardiography, even though a prosthetic valve is in place (Figs. 11–4 and 11–5).

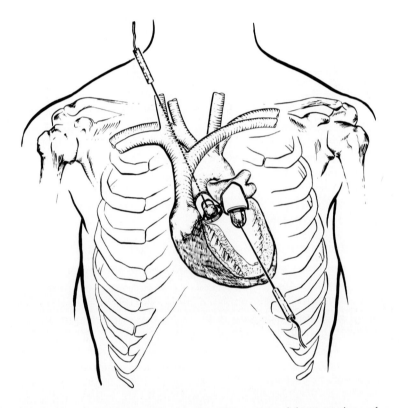

Fig. 11–1.   A diagram showing the placement of the transducer for examination of prosthetic ball-and-cage mitral and aortic valves. (From Schuchman, H., Feigenbaum, H., Dillon, J., and Chang, S.: Intracavitary echoes in patients with mitral prosthetic valves. J. Clin. Ultrasound, 3: 107, 1975.)

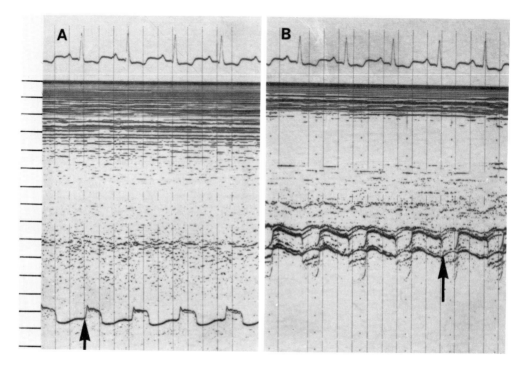

Fig. 11–2. A 63-year-old female patient. *A,* The normal poppet motion of a Starr-Edwards aortic prosthesis, recorded from the right supraclavicular fossa. At the onset of systole, the poppet opened rapidly toward the transducer (arrow) with a slight rebound movement following full opening. The poppet remained open throughout systole, followed by rapid closure at the end of systole. *B,* The motion of the same valve, recorded from the left ventricular apex. The opening systolic movement is away from the transducer (arrow).

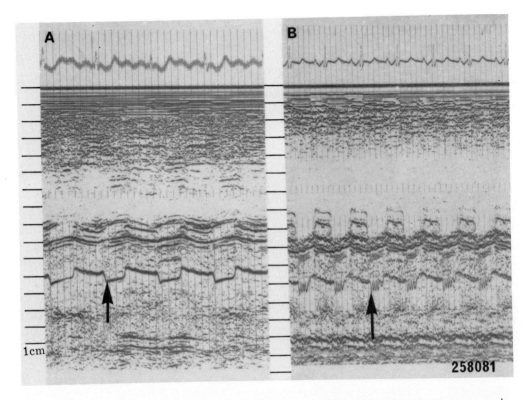

Fig. 11–3. A 50-year-old female patient who had a mitral valve commissurotomy and a Starr-Edwards aortic valve replacement in 1968. *A,* The aortic prosthetic poppet's motion was recorded from the cardiac apex in April, 1973. *B,* The poppet's motion was recorded in August, 1973, following embolic episodes in July. A murmur of aortic regurgitation was heard for the first time. The cause of the poppet's systolic fluttering was unclear. Arrows, maximum systolic poppet displacement.

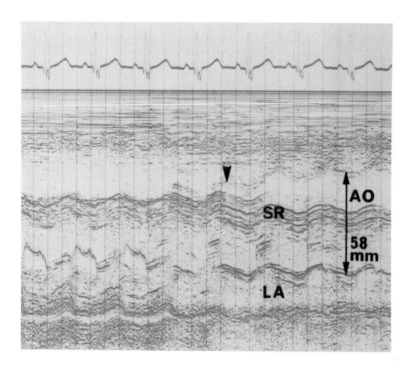

Fig. 11–4. A 32-year-old female patient with Candida parapsilosis infection, Marfan's syndrome, and a history of illicit drug use. The patient had a Starr-Edwards aortic valve replacement in 1975 for aortic stenosis and insufficiency secondary to rheumatic heart disease. This scan from the mitral valve to the aorta shows the anterior aortic wall diverging from the prosthetic suture ring (arrowhead). (See Fig. 11–5.) Computerized tomography showed a marked dilatation of the ascending aorta without evidence of dissection or rupture. The patient refused further surgical procedures and is being medically managed. SR, suture ring; LA, left atrium; AO, aorta.

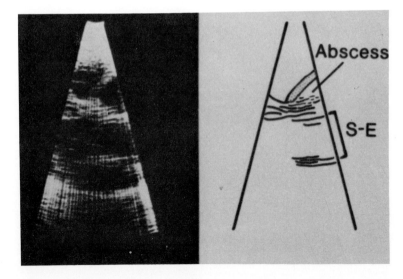

Fig. 11–5. A long-axis, two-dimensional echocardiogram (systolic frame) from the patient in Figure 11–4. The movement of the prosthesis was synchronous with the aortic root's motion, excluding significant dehiscence. The aortic root began to dilate at the suture ring and extended into the proximal ascending aorta. During real-time monitoring, low-intensity echoes were reflected from the junction of the anterior aortic root and the suture ring (abscess). The cause of these echoes was thought to be sepsis. S-E, Starr-Edwards prosthesis, aortic position.

Starr-Edwards and Cutter-Smeloff Prosthesis—Mitral Position

One should place the transducer at the cardiac apex and direct the sound beam perpendicularly to the poppet's movement. The poppet should open *toward* the transducer at the onset of diastole, remain open throughout diastole, and then move rapidly away from the transducer at the end of systole (Fig. 11–6). Paper recording speed should exceed 75 mm/sec, with superimposed time line intervals of 40 msec if available. A simultaneous phonocardiogram assists in the measurement of the time interval between aortic valve closure (A_2) and the poppet's opening click (OC) (Fig. 11–6). At rest, the A_2–OC interval ranges from 70 to 110 msec. With normal sinus rhythm, beat-to-beat variation should not exceed 20 msec. Beat-to-beat variation of 30 msec can occur with atrial fibrillation. If desired, the A_2–OC time interval may be corrected for the heart rate by using the following formula:

$$\frac{A_2\text{–OC}}{\sqrt{\text{preceding R–R interval}}}$$

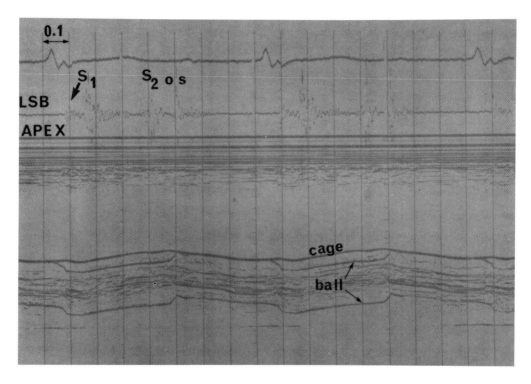

Fig. 11–6. A 44-year-old male patient five years after a Starr-Edwards mitral and aortic valve replacement. The patient was referred for an echocardiogram following an embolic episode. The mitral poppet's movement was recorded from the left ventricular apex at 100 mm/sec with a simultaneous phonocardiogram obtained from the left sternal border (LSB). The time interval between the aortic valve's closure (S_2) and the mitral poppet's opening snap (os) was approximately 100 msec (normal = 70 to 110 msec). The poppet opened with good excursion and approximated the prosthetic cage throughout diastole.

A short A_2–OC time interval is consistent with an elevation of left atrial pressure and probable prosthetic valve obstruction. Regular or intermittent prolongation of the A_2–OC time interval is consistent with a sticking poppet.

A normally functioning prosthesis shows simultaneous anterior movement of the cage and the poppet at the onset of diastole (Fig. 11–7). In one case, the movement of the prosthetic cage was used to identify the initial onset of diastole. Asynchronous poppet opening and cage movement suggested an impaction of the poppet; this diagnosis was confirmed by cardiac catheterization and surgical procedures (Figs. 11–8 to 11–10).

A significant number of patients have exhibited extraneous, high-velocity echoes moving anteriorly to the mitral prosthesis (Fig. 11–11). In these patients, the transducer was positioned at the left ventricular apex with a low reject setting

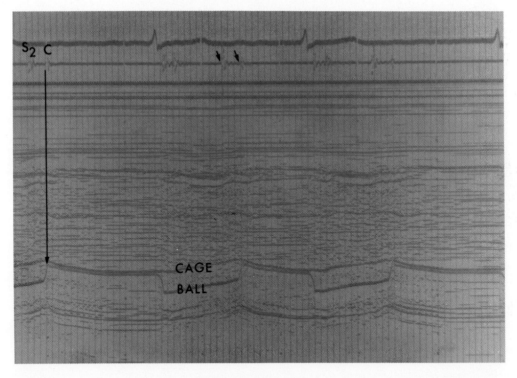

Fig. 11–7. A 68-year-old female patient, who had aortic and mitral Starr-Edwards prosthetic valve replacements in 1970, with atrial fibrillation and coronary artery disease. The mitral poppet's motion was recorded from the left ventricular apex with a simultaneous phonocardiogram eight years after valve replacement. The time interval between the onset of the second heart sound (S_2) and the poppet's opening click (C) was approximately 133 msec, averaging 120 msec when more complexes were compared. Catheterization showed normally functioning mitral and aortic prostheses. There was a significant left ventricular dysfunction secondary to coronary artery disease. Cardiac output, 3.4 L/min; cardiac index, 1.9 L/min/m²; ejection fraction, 47%.

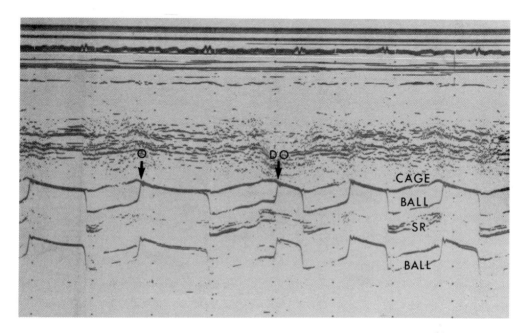

Fig. 11–8. A 53-year-old male patient with a Cutter-Smeloff mitral valve prosthesis, chronic obstructive lung disease, and atrial fibrillation. The mitral valve cage and poppet motion were recorded from the left ventricular apex. An intermittent delay of the poppet's opening (DO) suggested that the poppet was sticking (see Fig. 11–9). O, normal diastolic movement of cage followed by full opening of the poppet; SR, suture ring. (From Behi, F., Chang, S., and Welch, T.: Malfunction of Cutter-Smeloff mitral prosthesis: an echocardiographic diagnosis. J. Thorac. Cardiovasc. Surg., 75: 313, 1978.)

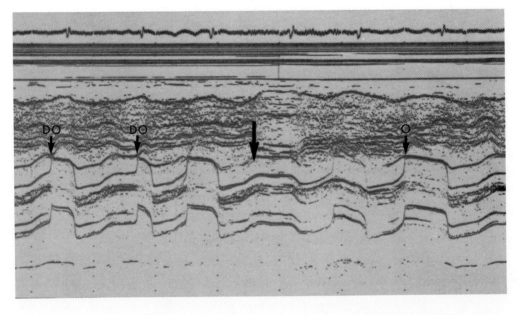

Fig. 11–9. A tracing from the patient in Figure 11–8 recorded three months later. The intermittent delay in the poppet's opening persisted with occasional failure to open at all (large arrow). Catheterization revealed elevated right heart pressures: right ventricle, 74/0 mm Hg; pulmonary artery, 74/38 mm Hg; pulmonary wedge, 38 mm Hg (mean). The cardiac output was depressed at 3.5 L/min. The patient was referred for operation (see Fig. 11–10). (From Behi, F., Chang, S., and Welch, T.: Malfunction of Cutter-Smeloff mitral prosthesis: an echocardiographic diagnosis. J. Thorac. Cardiovasc. Surg., 75: 313, 1978.)

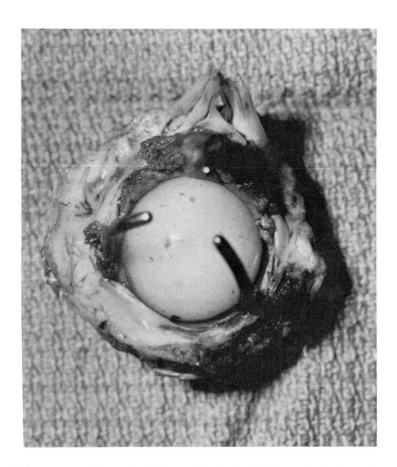

Fig. 11-10. The excised Cutter-Smeloff mitral prosthesis from the patient in Figures 11-8 and 11-9. At operation, the annulus and struts were completely thrombosed. Most of the thrombotic tissue fell off during removal of the valve. The poppet barely moved inside the cage, stuck midway between a systolic and diastolic position. There was fibrinous growth involving one strut on the ventricular side of the prosthesis. The suture ring was epithelialized. The appearance of the silastic poppet was unremarkable. (From Behi, F., Chang, S., and Welch, T.: Malfunction of Cutter-Smeloff mitral prosthesis: an echocardiographic diagnosis. J. Thorac. Cardiovasc. Surg., 75: 313, 1978.)

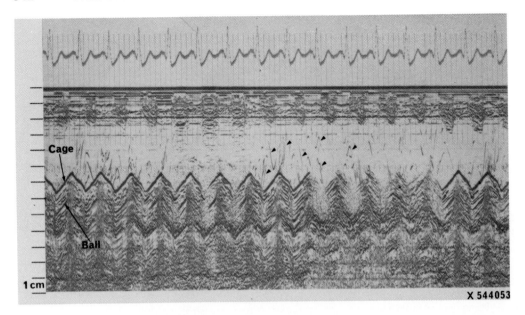

Fig. 11–11. The second of three Starr-Edwards mitral prostheses placed in a 20-year-old female patient between February and September, 1973. The prosthetic valve motion was recorded from the left ventricular apex. Extraneous, high-velocity echoes (arrowheads) were present following all three valve replacements. The patient was anemic throughout her hospitalization. At operation, this prosthesis showed partial dehiscence and extensive clotting on the valve. Six months after placement of the third prosthesis, the patient died of liver failure. (From Schuchman, H., Feigenbaum, H., Dillon, J., and Chang, S.: Intracavitary echoes in patients with mitral prosthetic valves. J. Clin. Ultrasound, 3: 107, 1975.)

on the echograph. These low-intensity echoes moved from the mitral valve toward the apex, then swirled away from the transducer toward the left ventricular outflow tract. The echoes occurred in preoperative patients, before the excision of dysfunctioning cloth-covered mitral prostheses, and in early postoperative patients. These echoes could have been due to early postoperative fibrinous infiltration of the prosthetic valve or to the breaking away of debris from deteriorating cloth-covered struts. Hemolysis of red blood cells traumatized by the poppet-to-cage movement was another possibility. Filtration of left ventricular blood samples from patients referred for cardiac catheterization was negative for particulate matter. More sensitive tests were never performed. The most significant finding was a predictable development of clinical symptoms in patients exhibiting this peculiar phenomenon.

BIBLIOGRAPHY

BEALL

Kawai, N., et al.: Delayed opening of Beall mitral prosthetic valve detected by echocardiography. Chest, 67: 239, 1975.

Oliva, P., et al.: Dysfunction of the Beall mitral prosthesis and its detection by cinefluoroscopy and echocardiography. Am. J. Cardiol., *31*: 393, 1973.

Smith, R., et al.: Noninvasive diagnostic evaluation of the normal Beall mitral prosthesis. Cathet. Cardiovasc. Diagn., *2*: 289, 1976.

BJÖRK-SHILEY

Bernal-Ramirez, J., et al.: Echocardiographic study of malfunction of the Björk-Shiley prosthetic heart valve in the mitral position. Am. J. Cardiol., *40*: 449, 1977.

Carliner, N., et al.: Misleading noninvasive signs of Björk-Shiley mitral valve dysfunction. Johns Hopkins Med. J., *143*: 160, 1978.

Chun, P., et al.: Björk-Shiley mitral valvular dehiscence. Documented by radiography, echocardiography, fluoroscopy, and cineangiography. Am. Heart J., *99*: 230, 1980.

Clements, S., et al.: Malfunction of a Björk-Shiley prosthetic heart valve in the mitral position producing an abnormal echocardiographic pattern. J. Clin. Ultrasound, *6*: 334, 1978.

Copans, H., et al.: Thrombosed Björk-Shiley mitral prostheses. Circulation, *61*: 169, 1980.

Douglas, J., et al.: Echocardiographic evaluation of the Björk-Shiley prosthetic valve. Circulation, *50*: 52, 1974.

Escarous, A.: The Björk-Shiley tilting disc valve prosthesis. Echocardiographic findings. Scand. J. Thorac. Cardiovasc. Surg., *9*: 192, 1975.

Holen, J., et al.: Obstructive characteristics of Björk-Shiley, Hancock and Lillehei-Kaster prosthetic mitral valves in the immediate postoperative period. Acta Med. Scand., *204*: 5, 1978.

Johnson, M., et al.: Echocardiographic determination of mitral disc valve excursion. Circulation, *47*: 1274, 1973.

Kato, I., et al.: Successful replacement of a thrombosed Björk-Shiley mitral valve prosthesis. Jpn. Heart J., *17*: 791, 1976.

McLeod, A., et al.: Near fatal puerperal thrombosis on Björk-Shiley mitral valve prosthesis. Br. Heart J., *40*: 934, 1978.

Orzan, F., et al.: Ultrasonic evaluation of thrombosis of Björk-Shiley aortic valve prosthesis. J. Thorac. Cardiovasc. Surg., *74*: 11, 1977.

Srivastava, T., et al.: Echocardiographic diagnosis of a stuck Björk-Shiley aortic valve prosthesis. Chest, *70*: 94, 1976.

Yoganathan, A., et al.: In vitro velocity measurements in the near vicinity of the Björk-Shiley aortic prosthesis using a laser-Doppler anemometer. Med. Biol. Eng., *17*: 453, 1979.

CUTTER-SMELOFF

Behi, F., et al.: Malfunction of Cutter-Smeloff mitral prosthesis. J. Thorac. Cardiovasc. Surg., *75*: 313, 1978.

Belenkie, I., et al.: Malfunction of a Cutter-Smeloff mitral ball valve prosthesis: diagnosis by phonocardiography and echocardiography. Am. Heart J., *86*: 339, 1973.

GENERAL

Alderman, E., et al.: Normal and prosthetic atrioventricular valve motion in atrial flutter. Circulation, *45*: 1206, 1972.

Anderson, E., Jr., et al.: Failure of auscultation and echocardiography to detect prosthetic mitral valve thrombosis. J. Tenn. Med. Assoc., *73*: 11, 1980.

Assad-Morell, J., et al.: Malfunctioning tricuspid valve prosthesis. Clinical, phonocardiographic, echocardiographic and surgical findings. Mayo Clin. Proc., *42*: 443, 1974.

Brodie, B., et al.: Diagnosis of prosthetic mitral valve malfunction with combined echo-phonocardiography. Circulation, *53*: 93, 1976.

Cunha, C., et al.: Echo-phonocardiographic findings in patients with prosthetic heart valve malfunction. Mayo Clin. Proc., *55*: 231, 1980.

Denbow, C., et al.: The role of echocardiography in the selection of mitral valve prosthesis. Am. Heart J., *99*: 586, 1980.

Fowler, N., et al.: Indications for surgical replacement of the mitral valve. With particular reference to common and uncommon causes of mitral regurgitation. Am. J. Cardiol., *44*: 148, 1979.

Henry, W., et al.: Evaluation of aortic valve replacement in patients with valvular aortic stenosis. Circulation, 61: 814, 1980.

Hoie, J., et al.: Paravalvular fistula in mitral valve implant. Intimation of malfunction of implant and quantification of regurgitant flow from effective area measurements. Scand. J. Thorac. Cardiovasc. Surg., 13: 103, 1979.

Holen, J., et al.: Evaluation of obstructive characteristics of mitral valve disc valve implants with ultrasound Doppler techniques. Acta Med. Scand., 201: 429, 1977.

Horowitz, M., et al.: Echocardiographic evaluation of the stent-mounted aortic bioprosthetic valve in the mitral position. In vitro and in vivo studies. Circulation, 54: 91, 1976.

Ikäheimo, M., et al.: Echocardiography after mitral valve replacement and criteria of paraprosthetic regurgitation. Ann. Clin. Res., 9: 25, 1977.

Jacovella, G., et al.: Phonocardiographic and echocardiographic diagnosis of prosthetic valve malfunction. In Noninvasive Cardiovascular Diagnosis. Edited by E. Diethrich. Baltimore, University Park Press, 1978.

Kesler, K., et al.: Pseudo-mitral-valve echogram following prosthetic mitral valve replacement. J. Clin. Ultrasound, 8: 35, 1980.

Kloster, F.: Diagnosis and management of complications of prosthetic heart valves. Am. J. Cardiol., 35: 872, 1975.

Kotler, M., et al.: Echocardiographic and phonocardiographic evaluation of prosthetic heart valves. Cardiovasc. Clin., 9: 187, 1978.

Lewis, B., et al.: Echocardiography and valve replacement in the critically ill patient with acute rheumatic carditis. Ann. Thorac. Surg., 27: 529, 1979.

Mahringer, W., et al.: Ultrasound cardiogram in patients with mitral valve disc prostheses. Angiology, 21: 336, 1970.

Nanda, N., et al.: Echocardiographic assessment of left ventricular outflow width in the selection of mitral valve prosthesis. Circulation, 48: 1208, 1973.

Popp, R.: Echocardiographic assessment of prosthetic mitral valves. In The Mitral Valve. Edited by D. Kalmanson. Acton, Mass., Publishing Sciences Group, 1976.

Raj, M., et al.: Thrombotic jamming of a tricuspid prosthesis. Br. Heart J., 38: 1355, 1976.

Roelandt, J.: Echocardiographic evaluation of patients with prosthetic heart valves. In Noninvasive Cardiovascular Diagnosis. Edited by E. Diethrich. Baltimore, University Park Press, 1978.

Salem, B., et al.: Major dehiscence of a prosthetic aortic valve: detection by echocardiography. Chest, 75: 513, 1979.

Schapira, J., et al.: Two-dimensional echocardiographic assessment of patients with bioprosthetic valves. Am. J. Cardiol., 43: 510, 1979.

Schuchman, H., et al.: Intracavitary echoes in patients with mitral prosthetic valves. J. Clin. Ultrasound, 3: 107, 1975.

Skorton, D., et al.: Noninvasive diagnosis of prosthetic mitral valve dysfunction. Radiology, 131: 185, 1979.

Stefadouros, M., et al.: First-degree atrioventricular block: a cause of false malfunction of a mitral disc-valve prosthesis. Case report. J. Thorac. Cardiovasc. Surg., 69: 776, 1975.

Strunk, B., et al.: The assessment of mitral stenosis and prosthetic mitral valve obstruction, using the posterior aortic wall echocardiogram. Circulation, 55: 885, 1977.

Veenendaal, M., et al.: Noninvasive diagnosis of mitral prosthesis malfunction. Am. J. Med., 69: 458, 1980.

Wann, L., et al.: Ball variance in the Harken mitral prosthesis. Echocardiographic and phonocardiographic features. Chest, 72: 785, 1977.

Watts, E., et al.: Echocardiography in evaluation of mitral valve prostheses. J. Clin. Ultrasound, 3: 2, 1975.

HANCOCK (PORCINE)

Alam, M., et al.: M-mode and two-dimensional echocardiographic features of porcine valve dysfunction. Am. J. Cardiol., 43: 502, 1979.

Alam, M., et al.: Echocardiographic features of a stenotic porcine aortic valve. Am. Heart J., 100: 517, 1980.

Bloch, W., et al.: Echocardiogram of the porcine aortic bioprosthesis in the mitral position. Am. J. Cardiol., 38: 293, 1976.

Bloch, W., et al.: The echocardiogram of the porcine aortic bioprosthesis in the aortic position. Chest, 72: 640, 1977.

Brown, J., et al.: Late spontaneous disruption of a porcine xenograft mitral valve. Clinical, hemodynamic, echocardiographic and pathological findings. J. Thorac. Cardiovasc. Surg., 75: 606, 1978.

Chandraratna, P., et al.: Echocardiographic features of the normal and malfunctioning porcine xenograft valve. Am. Heart J., 95: 548, 1978.

Crupi, G., et al.: Severe late failure of a porcine xenograft mitral valve: clinical, echocardiographic, and pathological findings. Thorax, 35: 210, 1980.

Harston, W., et al.: Echocardiographic evaluation of porcine heterograft valves in the mitral and aortic positions. Am. Heart J., 96: 448, 1978.

Holen, J., et al.: Obstructive characteristics of Björk-Shiley, Hancock and Lillehei-Kaster prosthetic mitral valves in the immediate postoperative period. Acta Med. Scand., 204: 5, 1978.

Horowitz, M., et al.: Echocardiographic evaluation of the stent-mounted aortic bioprosthetic valve in the mitral position. Circulation, 54: 91, 1976.

Magilligan, D., et al.: Hemolytic anemia with porcine xenograft aortic and mitral valves. J. Thorac. Cardiovasc. Surg., 79: 628, 1980.

Nagara, H., et al.: Mitral valve replacement using a porcine xenograft for treatment of IHSS—a case report. Jpn. J. Surg., 8: 326, 1978.

LILLEHEI-KASTER

Bomba, M., et al.: Morphology of the echoes of the Lillehei-Kaster prosthesis in aortic and mitral sites. Boll. Soc. Ital. Cardiol., 20: 1775, 1975.

Estevez, R., et al.: Phonocardiographic and echocardiographic features of Lillehei-Kaster mitral prosthesis. J. Clin. Ultrasound, 5: 153, 1977.

Gibson, T., et al.: Echocardiographic and phonocardiographic characteristics of the Lillehei-Kaster mitral valve prosthesis. Circulation, 49: 434, 1974.

Holen, J., et al.: Obstructive characteristics of Björk-Shiley, Hancock and Lillehei-Kaster prosthetic mitral valves in the immediate postoperative period. Acta Med. Scand., 204: 5, 1978.

Vardan, S., et al.: Echo- and phonocardiographic studies in patients with Lillehei-Kaster aortic valve prostheses. Jpn. Heart J., 20: 277, 1979.

STARR-EDWARDS

Gimenez, J., et al.: Dynamics of Starr-Edwards ball valve prosthesis: a cinefluorographic and ultrasonic study in humans. Am. J. Med. Sci., 250: 652, 1965.

Hultgren, H., et al.: A phonocardiographic study of patients with the Starr-Edwards mitral valve prosthesis. Am. Heart J., 69: 306, 1965.

Johnson, M., et al.: Ultrasonic evaluation of prosthetic valve motion. Circulation, 4: 3, 1970.

Miller, H., et al.: Echocardiographic features of mitral Starr-Edwards paraprosthetic regurgitation. Br. Heart J., 35: 560, 1973.

Miller, H., et al.: Role of echocardiography and phonocardiography in diagnosis of mitral paraprosthetic regurgitation with Starr-Edwards prosthesis. Br. Heart J., 35: 1217, 1973.

Pfeifer, J., et al.: Malfunction of mitral ball valve prosthesis due to thrombus. Am. J. Cardiol., 29: 95, 1972.

Schelbert, H., et al.: Detection of fungal vegetations involving a Starr-Edwards mitral prosthesis by means of ultrasound. Vasc. Surg., 6: 20, 1972.

Schuchman, H., et al.: Intracavitary echoes in patients with mitral prosthetic valves. J. Clin. Ultrasound, 3: 2, 1975.

Siggers, D., et al.: Analysis of dynamics of mitral Starr-Edwards valve prosthesis using reflected ultrasound. Br. Heart J., 32: 552, 1970.

Siggers, D., et al.: Analysis of dynamics of mitral Starr-Edwards valve prosthesis using reflected ultrasound. Br. Heart J., 33: 401, 1971.

Suwansirikul, S., et al.: Late thrombosis of Starr-Edwards tricuspid ball valve prosthesis. Am. J. Cardiol., 34: 737, 1974.

Winters, W., et al.: Clinical applications of ultrasound in the analysis of prosthetic ball valve function. Am. J. Cardiol., 19: 97, 1967.

Appendix

BODY SURFACE NOMOGRAM
(Adults)

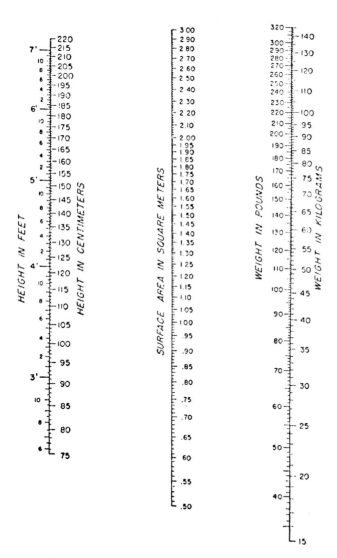

Fig. Appendix–1. Place ruler on the patient's height (left column) and weight (right column). Read the body surface area in square meters from the center column. (Reprinted with permission from Boothby, W., and Sandiford, R.: Boston Med. Surg. J., *185*: 337, 1921. Courtesy of the New England Journal of Medicine.)

POLAROID PHOTOGRAPHS

Many problems concerning the graphic appearance of an echocardiographic tracing taken on Polaroid film have nothing to do with the technical skill in obtaining the tracing. Basic adjustments must be made on the echograph that will optimize the focusing, intensity, and clipping. The interplay of these three controls affect the quality of the tracing on the film. Usually, these adjustments are made and then remain stable, but if many persons use the echograph for different types of examination, then these control settings should be checked frequently.

One should follow the recommendation in the echograph service manuals, but also proceed as follows:

1. Panel C in Figure Appendix–2 is out of focus. One should focus the instrument with fine focus while the M-mode is sweeping or set on B-mode, and focus on the calibration dots until they are pinpoint. It is not necessary to do this often unless a malfunction of the instrument causes the focusing to become unstable.

2. Panel A in Figure Appendix–2 shows that the intensity is set too high. One should place the damping (attenuation) on level 5 or turn the coarse gain all the way down. One should adjust the intensity control until there is a faint band of light sweeping across the oscilloscope. If this adjustment is set too high, the whole photograph, including the background, will be too light and poorly defined.

3. Panel D in Figure Appendix–2 demonstrates an effect called "bloom." The clip control is set too high. One should apply jelly to the transducer and press against the palm of the hand. Then one should place the damping on settings 1, 2, or 3, depending on the instrument and set the near gain and coarse gain at moderate levels and the reject on 3, 4, or 5. One should turn the clip completely clockwise, then counterclockwise until every individual echo being received from the transducer can be distinguished.

   If the clip adjustment is too high, as seen in panel D, echoes close to each other bleed into large, fuzzy images with poor resolution.

4. One should take a picture of the oscilloscope with echoes being displayed. If the picture is too dark as in panel B in Figure Appendix–2, one should turn the clip up and take another picture. If the oscilloscope display looks good, but the picture is still too dark, one should increase the size of the camera aperture to admit more light. A setting of $f5.6$ is usual, but settings between $f8$ and $f16$ have been used by different examiners. If the picture seems

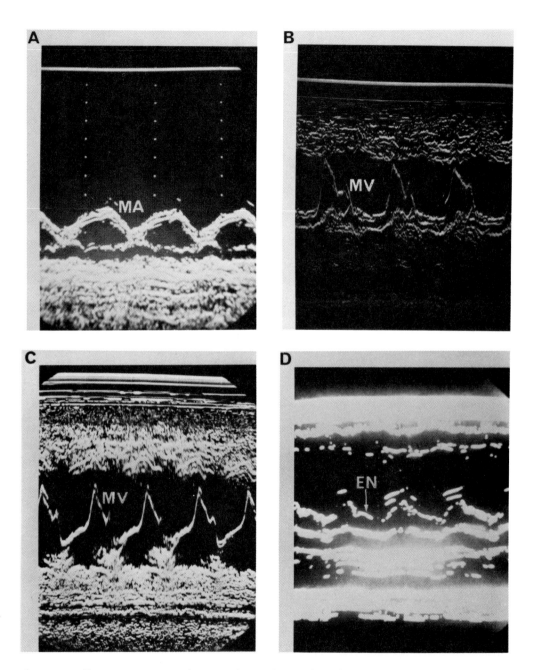

Fig. Appendix–2.   Features of poor echocardiographic photography on Polaroid film. *A*, The intensity is too high. *B*, The clipping is too low, or the camera aperture is too small, or the intensity is too low. *C*, This tracing is out of focus. *D*, "Blooming" or a blending of close-lying movement patterns occurs when the clipping is set too high. MA, mitral annulus; MV, mitral valve motion; EN, endocardial surface of the posterior left ventricular wall.

overexposed, the size of the camera aperture should be decreased to admit less light.

5. One should not be concerned if calibration markers are not seen on the photographs. Quality tracings of the echocardiogram are desired first. Calibrations may be taken at the end of the examination on a separate photograph without any tracing.

WORKSHEETS AND CONSULTATION FORMS

At Riverside Hospital, Toledo, Ohio, a consultation request form is sent to the echocardiography laboratory with the patient's vital statistics, the name of the referring physician, and the clinical diagnosis or reason for the examination. In addition, the laboratory's personnel indicate findings from other sources (i.e., electrocardiography, x-ray examination,

M-MODE
ECHOCARDIOGRAPHIC WORKSHEET

PATIENT'S NAME _____ DATE: _____ BSA _____ M²

INTRACARDIAC DIMENSIONS (cm): (Normal)

Right ventricular wall	(0.3–0.7)	_____
Right ventricular dimension	(< 1.7 cm/m²)	_____
Left ventricular dimension (D)	(< 3.2 cm/m²)	_____
Left ventricular dimension (S)		_____
Left atrial dimension	(< 2.2 cm/m²)	_____
Posterior LV wall thickness	(0.8–1.2)	_____
Septal wall thickness	(0.7–1.2)	_____
Aortic root dimension (sinuses)	(2.5–3.7)	_____
Aortic annulus dimension	(> 2.0)	_____

LEFT VENTRICULAR FUNCTION:

Heart rate (beats per min)		_____
Minor axis shortening	(24–42%)	_____
Relative velocity of contraction	(> 0.85 dia/sec)	_____

SYSTOLIC TIME INTERVALS: (left heart)

PEP/LVET	(< 0.42)	_____
PEP, corrected for heart rate	(120–140 msec)	_____
LVET, corrected for heart rate	(400–429 msec)	_____

SYSTOLIC TIME INTERVALS: (right heart)

RPEP/RVET (children)	(0.16–0.30)	_____
RPEP/RVET (newborn) (>5 days)	(0.28 ± 0.04)	_____
RPEP/RVET (pre-term) (>5 days)	(0.28 ± 0.04)	_____

Additional measurements, calculations, references, and comments:

Fig. Appendix–3. M-Mode Echocardiographic Worksheet. Preliminary measurements, calculations, and data evaluations, with appropriate references, are compiled during detailed analysis of the paper tracing.

stress testing, surgical procedures). Medications and emotional status (e.g., anxiety, anger, depression) are included, since their presence may significantly alter the echocardiographic data. I have found that the diagnostic quality of the examination and its interpretation improves in direct relation to the amount of information known about the patient.

Following completion of the M-mode echocardiogram (and two-dimensional echocardiogram, if necessary), preliminary measurements, calculations, and diagrams are compiled on a worksheet. I describe the appearance of specific echocardiographic patterns and offer possible causes for changes that deviate from the normal values. For example, the distinction between calcification and fibrosis and vegetations, and the recognition of abnormal movement of valves, walls, or vessels secondary to changes in the anatomic structure, pressure, or

---

TWO-DIMENSIONAL ECHOCARDIOGRAPHIC WORKSHEET

PATIENT'S NAME _____ DATE: _____
Tape Number _____ From _____ To _____
Clinical diagnosis or reason for examination _____
_____

PARASTERNAL LONG AXIS:

    Right heart:

    Left heart:

    Apical:

SHORT AXIS:

    Great vessels:

    Ventricular base:

    Papillary muscles:

APICAL:

    Four-chamber:

    Two-chamber:

ADDITIONAL COMMENTS:

Fig. Appendix–4. Two-dimensional Echocardiographic Worksheet. Systematic evaluation of a patient's two-dimensional echocardiogram.

RIVERSIDE HOSPITAL
Toledo, Ohio 43604
Form 507001-6 Rev. 2/80

ECHOCARDIOGRAPHIC
CONSULTATION REQUEST

Imprint

Date of Request _____ Blood Pressure _____
Age _____ Height _____ Weight _____ BSA _____ m²
Inpatient _____ Outpatient _____ Referring Physician _____
Clinical diagnosis and reason for examination _____
_____
_____
_____

INTRACARDIAC DIMENSIONS: (in centimeters) (Normal values)
    Right ventricular wall thicknesses   (0.3–0.7) _____
    Right ventricular dimension   (< 1.7 cm/m²) _____
    Left ventricular dimension   (< 3.2 cm/m²) _____
    Left atrial dimension   (< 2.2 cm/m²) _____
    Posterior wall thickness   (0.8–1.2) _____
    Septal wall thickness   (0.7–1.2) _____
    Aortic root dimension (sinuses)   (2.5–3.7) _____
    Aortic root dimension (annulus)   (> 2.0) _____
LEFT VENTRICULAR FUNCTION:
    Heart rate   _____ (beats per min)
    Minor axis shortening   (24–42) _____ %
    Contraction velocity   (> 0.85) _____ (dia/sec)
SYSTOLIC TIME INTERVALS:
    PEP/LVET   (Less than 0.42) _____
    PEP, corrected for heart rate   (120–140 msec) _____ msec
    LVET, corrected for heart rate   (400–429 msec) _____ msec

Additional measurements, references, and comments:

Director, Echocardiographic
Laboratory

M.D.

Fig. Appendix–5. Echocardiographic Consultation Request. Pertinent M-mode and two-dimensional echocardiographic data are integrated and reported on this form, which becomes a permanent addition to the patient's hospital record.

cardiac rhythm, require descriptive analysis rather than measurement techniques. Occasionally, a reference is offered for
elucidation of the data's validity and clinical value. All these
data are reviewed by the hospital's consulting cardiologist.

Examples of my worksheets and Riverside Hospital's echocardiographic consultation request form are provided in this
appendix as Figures Appendix–3, 4, and 5.

Normal echocardiographic values used in Riverside Hospital, Toledo, Ohio, are shown in Tables Appendix–1 and 2. The
data were derived from 60 adults without cardiovascular
disease and were combined with the original measurements
for adult normal values in the appendix of the first edition of
this book. Prior to the echocardiogram, each person was

Table Appendix–1.   Adult Normal Values

	Mean (cm)	Range (cm)	Number
AGE (years)	33.8	13–65	194
BODY SURFACE AREA (m²)	1.81	1.45–2.35	190
RIGHT VENTRICULAR WALL THICKNESS			
Supine	0.48	0.3–0.9	56
Left Lateral	0.53	0.3–1.0	58
Subcostal	0.67	0.3–0.9	56
RIGHT VENTRICULAR DIMENSION			
Supine	1.6	0.6–2.9	139
Left Lateral	2.8	0.9–3.7	93
Subcostal	1.2	0.3–2.7	55
LEFT VENTRICULAR DIMENSION			
Supine	4.6	3.7–5.6	126
Left Lateral	4.6	3.5–5.8	139
Subcostal	4.5	3.8–5.1	49
Morbidly Obese	4.7	4.2–5.8	26
LEFT ATRIAL DIMENSION			
Normal Body Size	3.0	1.9–4.1	183
Morbidly Obese	3.4	2.3–4.2	30
AORTIC ROOT DIMENSION	2.8	2.0–3.9	183
SEPTAL WALL THICKNESS			
Supine	0.94	0.5–1.2	45
Left Lateral	0.91	0.7–1.2	194
Subcostal	0.97	0.7–1.1	52
POSTERIOR LV WALL THICKNESS			
Supine	0.99	0.7–1.2	46
Left Lateral	0.93	0.6–1.2	196
Subcostal	0.97	0.7–1.2	50
SEPTAL AMPLITUDE			
Supine	0.69	0.3–1.1	45
Left Lateral	0.68	0.4–1.3	60
Subcostal	0.61	0.3–1.1	54
POSTERIOR LV WALL AMPLITUDE			
Supine	0.80	0.8–1.3	55
Left Lateral	0.98	0.7–1.7	60
Subcostal	1.03	0.8–1.7	53

Table Appendix–2.   Adult Normal Values, Corrected for Body Surface Area

	Mean (cm/m²)	Range (cm/m²)	Number
RIGHT VENTRICULAR DIMENSION			
Supine	0.99	0.4–2.0	141
Left Lateral	0.87	0.3–1.5	132
Subcostal	0.66	0.2–1.4	55
LEFT VENTRICULAR DIMENSION			
Supine	2.5	1.9–3.2	119
Left Lateral	2.5	1.9–3.2	137
Subcostal	2.5	2.0–3.2	49
Morbidly Obese	2.1	1.8–2.7	26
LEFT ATRIAL DIMENSION			
Normal Body Size	1.7	1.2–2.2	177
Morbidly Obese	1.5	1.1–2.0	30
AORTIC ROOT DIMENSION	1.5	1.1–2.2	175

evaluated with a chest roentgenogram, an electrocardiogram, and a physical examination. The echocardiograms were obtained with a 2.25-MHz, medium-focused transducer and were recorded on an 1856 Honeywell or an Ekoline E21 ultraviolet visicorder. The obese patients were examined with echocardiography following a thorough evaluation for an ileobypass operation. Although many of the obese patients were hypertensive, all were without clinical evidence of cardiovascular disease.

Index

Page numbers followed by *b* indicate bibliographic listings; page numbers followed by *t* indicate tables.